AF710834

Therapy Dogs in Cancer Care

Dawn A. Marcus, MD

Therapy Dogs in Cancer Care

A Valuable Complementary Treatment

Springer

Dawn A. Marcus, MD
Department of Anesthesiology
University of Pittsburgh
PA, USA

ISBN 978-1-4614-3377-4 ISBN 978-1-4614-3378-1 (eBook)
DOI 10.1007/978-1-4614-3378-1
Springer NewYork Heidelberg Dordrecht London

Library of Congress Control Number: 2012935101

© Springer Science+Business Media New York 2012
This work is subject to copyright. All rights are reserved by the Publisher, whether the whole or part of the material is concerned, specifically the rights of translation, reprinting, reuse of illustrations, recitation, broadcasting, reproduction on microfilms or in any other physical way, and transmission or information storage and retrieval, electronic adaptation, computer software, or by similar or dissimilar methodology now known or hereafter developed. Exempted from this legal reservation are brief excerpts in connection with reviews or scholarly analysis or material supplied specifically for the purpose of being entered and executed on a computer system, for exclusive use by the purchaser of the work. Duplication of this publication or parts thereof is permitted only under the provisions of the Copyright Law of the Publisher's location, in its current version, and permission for use must always be obtained from Springer. Permissions for use may be obtained through RightsLink at the Copyright Clearance Center. Violations are liable to prosecution under the respective Copyright Law.
The use of general descriptive names, registered names, trademarks, service marks, etc. in this publication does not imply, even in the absence of a specific statement, that such names are exempt from the relevant protective laws and regulations and therefore free for general use.
While the advice and information in this book are believed to be true and accurate at the date of publication, neither the authors nor the editors nor the publisher can accept any legal responsibility for any errors or omissions that may be made. The publisher makes no warranty, express or implied, with respect to the material contained herein.

Printed on acid-free paper

Springer is part of Springer Science+Business Media (www.springer.com)

Foreword

I must admit a certain lack of objectivity in any discussion of dogs. For the past 25+ years, our family has been blessed as we shared our home and our lives with a series of dogs (including several at any one time), specifically Golden Retrievers. These remarkable creatures have added incredible joy to our lives. Thus, when asked if I would be willing to review and write the foreword for this unique book, written by Dr. Dawn Marcus, I leaped at the chance. And I was not disappointed.

Therapy Dogs in Cancer Care: A Valuable Complementary Treatment is a wonderful effort which includes a comprehensive summary of truly impressive research demonstrating the ability of dogs to serve an important therapeutic role within the cancer arena and in other serious medical conditions. Further, the text provides highly practical advice and very helpful "tips" to insure those who desire to employ these magnificent animals to assist the cancer patient have the necessary knowledge and "tools" to optimize outcomes.

Therapy Dogs in Cancer Care is a well-organized, appropriately researched, and highly readable book that will inform and delight both the casual reader and anyone desiring a "how-to" text. In summary, Dawn Marcus has created a book that is a thoroughly enjoyable and spectacularly educational read. And the product once again confirms that *dogs are truly man's (and woman's) best friend.*

Cancer Treatment Centers of America
Maurie Markman, MD

Preface

According to the American Cancer Society, over 11 million people in the USA have cancer. Cancer treatment usually involves a holistic approach addressing medical management, emotional needs, and lifestyle changes. About half of cancer patients add complementary therapies to their treatment regimens, citing benefits for symptomatic improvement and an increased sense of control over the treatment process when complementary treatments are incorporated into traditional cancer programs.

I have spent my medical career in academic medicine, focused primarily on pain management. Decades of caring for patients have taught me that reducing symptoms and easing suffering usually involve more than just a pill. Although I have found nontraditional, alternative, and complementary treatments to be beneficial in clinical practice and research studies, I was skeptical when my veterinarian suggested I have my Wheaten Terrier trained as a therapy dog to visit hospital patients. My terrier and I began our hospital therapy experience working with a palliative care team, and before long, I was convinced that the research was true—therapy dog visits are therapeutic. My experiences inspired me to write *The Power of Wagging Tails: A Doctor's Guide to Dog Therapy and Healing* to showcase both medical research and first-person anecdotal stories about the impact of the human-canine encounter.

Therapy dog visits will not cure cancer; however, these visits have been convincingly shown to reduce stress, loneliness, and mood disturbance that may complicate cancer care. Furthermore, dogs may provide important motivation for patients to maintain rehabilitation programs that have been shown to reduce cancer risk and improve cancer survival. *Therapy Dogs in Cancer Care: A Valuable Complementary Treatment* is a resource to provide detailed descriptions of possible roles for therapy dogs as a useful complementary treatment for cancer patients, including details of available evidence of expected benefits from therapy dog visits. Medical studies consistently show benefits from therapy dog visits. Brief therapy dog visits lower blood pressures and heart rates, raise endorphin levels, decrease stress hormones, and boost the immune system. Improvements in physical and emotional health have been linked to measurable changes in human physiology which occur after spending a few minutes petting and connecting with a therapy dog. Studies have also shown that therapy dogs can play an important role for cancer patients. Dogs have been used as cancer detectors and as companions to patients undergoing cancer treatment. Therapy dogs have been used during chemotherapy treatments to reduce patient distress and discomfort.

Today, both of my Wheaten Terrier therapy dogs make regular rounds at hospital cancer centers, bringing joy and smiles to patients, their family members, and the staff.

Understanding the potential benefits from brief therapy dog visits can motivate cancer caregivers to include helpful therapy dog visits as part of a complementary management strategy for cancer patients. *Therapy Dogs in Cancer Care: A Valuable Complementary Treatment* provides practical suggestions to effectively incorporate dogs into cancer care, with detailed instructions about requirements for therapy dogs to ensure visits are safe and limit unwanted spread of infection.

Dawn A. Marcus, MD
www.FitAsFido.com

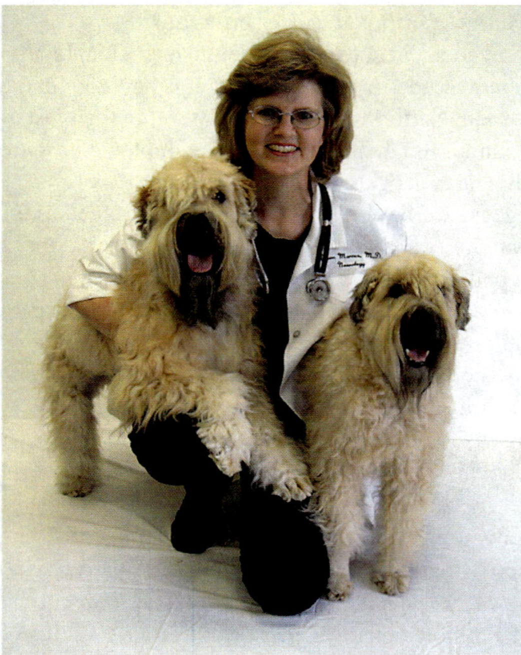

Dr. Marcus with Wheaten Terrier therapy dogs Toby and Wheatie (photo courtesy of Natalie Larocco)

Acknowledgments

This book was substantially assisted by the many individuals who contributed to my research. Paula Breuer was instrumental in developing a dog-themed exercise program for cancer patients. Her extensive work in clinical physical therapy treatment and personal experiences as a cancer survivor were invaluable for providing a practical program that can be used by patients with a broad range of abilities. Expert advice and program information were appreciated from individuals incorporating therapy dogs in programs designed for cancer patients, including Bernie Siegel, MD; Kristy Everette from Pets at Duke; Stephanie Samolovitch and Rebecca Whitlinger from the University of Pittsburgh's Cancer Caring program; and Deborah Erickson from the Angel Foundation. The data they provided about the effects of their unique programs may inspire others to similarly add therapy dog programs to their facilities. I would also like to thank Raymond Hanlon, MS who provided valuable insights into the psychological aspects of dog interactions. A special thanks is needed for oncologist Maurie Markman, MD from Cancer Treatment Centers of America who thoughtfully reviewed this project and provided support throughout the writing process.

I would also like to thank those cancer survivors, therapy dog handlers, and health-care workers who kindly shared their personal experiences and poignant stories of therapy dogs connecting with cancer patients, including Jay Brady, Beth Brown and the Dachshund pack, Amy Coglio and George, Sandy Golomb and Ike, DJ Goodell and Polly, Charmaine Hammond and Toby, Diana Hare and Sonia, Roberta Hoffman with Gráinne and Diarmuid, Lynn Huber Jablonski with Shen Li and Boy, Judith Kelly and Apple, Beth Kraimer and Petey, Patricia Larrabee and Magic, Becky Magnelli, Nancy Missildine and Gracie, Ellen Morrow and Charley, Lynn Ready and Max, Seadon Renfrow and Pearl, Patti Shanaberg and Sami, Priscilla Sharpe and Joy, Patricia Tirrell and Charlie, and Dori Weisbrod and Buster. Their stories confirm and expand upon the findings of scientific studies evaluating the impact of therapy dogs in cancer care. Another thank you is needed for the professional photographers who graciously shared their images that captured the impact of therapy dogs: Nick Barberio (www.nickbarberio.com/hospital-corners), Ann Cadman from Animal Friends, Leah Charbonneau from Charbonneau Photography (www.leahcphotography.com), Jasmine Goldband from the Pittsburgh *Tribune-Review*, Patricia A. M. Ingram from Ingram

Portrait Design (www.ingramportraitdesign.com), and Natalie Larocco. And finally, I need to recognize my personal instructors on the impact of therapy dog visits, my Wheaten Terrier therapy dogs, who have inspired me with their gentle touch and the joy they share when visiting patients, their family members, and staff in the hospital and chemotherapy suite.

Contents

1 Cancer Overview

Key Chapter Points

- According to the National Cancer Institute, two in every five people will be diagnosed with cancer at some point during their lives.
- Psychological distress, fear of rejection, and isolation can result in loneliness that may worsen cancer progression.
- Complementary treatments may address unmet patient needs and give patients a sense of empowerment and control over their cancer treatment.
- Therapy dogs can provide a cost-free complementary treatment to reduce stress and loneliness in cancer patients.

Keywords
Exercise • Isolation • Loneliness • Pain • Progression • Stress

"You've got cancer" are probably the three words that doctors dread telling patients and patients fear hearing the most. This seemingly simple diagnosis is charged with a wide range of physical and psychosocial issues. While health-care providers anticipate patient fear and anxiety about cancer-related symptoms, pain, and death, patients may also worry about isolation from family and friends when they share their diagnosis, experience hair loss with chemotherapy, or undergo disfiguring surgery. Consequently, medical treatments designed to target symptoms deemed most important by health-care providers may fail to attend to additional significant concerns for some cancer patients.

Addressing the complex concerns that develop throughout the course of a patient's cancer diagnosis, treatment, and recovery usually requires including practitioners from a wide range of disciplines, incorporating both drug and nondrug therapies [1]. For example, a recent review concluded that including nondrug complementary therapies with cancer management improves patient quality of life [2]. Incorporating complementary options within a comprehensive cancer management program may help address unmet patient needs and fears. Among various complementary options, hospitals, hospices, etc. may include visits from certified therapy dogs to benefit cancer patients. Therapy dogs have been trained to be calm and

D.A. Marcus, *Therapy Dogs in Cancer Care: A Valuable Complementary Treatment*,
DOI 10.1007/978-1-4614-3378-1_1, © Springer Science+Business Media New York 2012

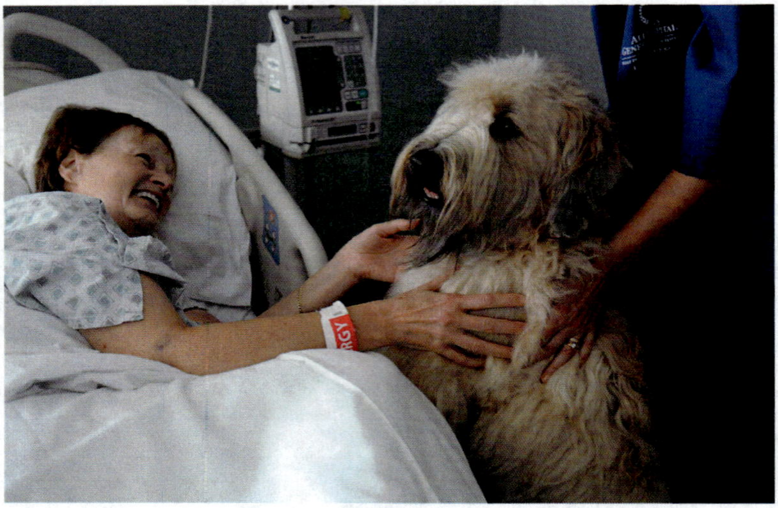

Fig. 1.1 Therapy dog visits can be incorporated as a complementary therapy to provide pleasure, comfort, stress relief, and distraction from worry to a broad range of patients. (Photo courtesy of Jasmine Goldband, Pittsburgh Tribune-Review)

provide comfort and pleasure to strangers (Fig. 1.1). The care of the therapy dog is the responsibility of the dog's handler who provides therapy dog services as a volunteer complementary intervention. As will be described throughout this book, numerous studies have documented consistent benefits from therapy dog visits for reducing symptoms that commonly occur in patients with cancer. Benefits include both emotional and physical changes that can provide immediate and long-term improvements.

In *The Power of Wagging Tails: A Doctor's Guide to Dog Therapy and Healing*, a patient with metastatic prostate cancer shared his story about how isolated cancer patients can feel:

> *Cancer is an island....We speak a different language there—where simple words like "mets" and "nodes" can strike terror, and time is measured in checkups and treatment cycles. It is a strange place where things that can kill you, like radiation and poisons, are used as cures* [3].

Although this patient had a strong support network of caregivers and family, working with therapy dogs helped keep him from dwelling on his "cancer island" and helped him focus on the positives in his present and pleasures he could still enjoy in his daily life. For this patient and others with cancer, therapy dog visits may address important psychosocial factors that may not be adequately addressed through traditional therapies.

Health-care providers may fail to recognize the importance of certain concerns and issues for some patients. In an interesting study surveying 80 breast cancer patients, researchers compared concerns reported by patients with issues their health-care providers believed patients would have [4]. Health-care providers surveyed included 41 oncology nurses and 49 physicians (including oncologists, hematologists, and internists). While there was very high concordance for responses between oncology nurses and doctors (0.90), concordance between health-care providers and patients was only moderate (0.62–0.66). Both health-care providers and patients ranked fear of metastases and fatigue among the top three concerns for patients with cancer. Hair loss, however, was ranked number four by patients, dropping to ninth for nurses, and not included among the top ten factors by doctors. This study highlights the potential discord that can occur between patient and health-care provider expectations. Identifying the broad range of cancer-related concerns for patients may also suggest symptoms that might be effectively targeted through complementary therapy dog visits.

Case 1

In 1963, Adsett wrote an article describing emotional reactions cancer patients might have to disfiguring surgery, concluding that the "fear of isolation and rejection by others may be more terrifying than fear of death" [5]. How therapy dogs can help address this isolation is highlighted by the case of SR, a 67-year-old woman with aggressive head and neck cancer who had undergone extensive treatments. SR was hospitalized on a palliative care unit after radical surgery had removed most of her left mandible, which resulted in significant facial deformity and speech that was often incomprehensible. Her supervising physician noted that the staff tended to avoid SR's room, stating that they found the gaping opening on the left side of her face disconcerting and that communication was tedious. The palliative care team requested a pet therapy visit as part of her complementary treatment.

An initial pet therapy visit was made by a soft-coated Wheaten Terrier therapy dog (Wheatie) who greeted SR with enthusiasm. SR's disfigurement and inability to speak clearly were erased as she connected with her four-legged therapist with the ease of close physical contact and petting. Wheatie and SR formed a fast bond and spent the next 15 min nose to snout, with SR chatting happily to Wheatie while he gazed into her eyes and wagged his tail. SR was able to share secrets, fears, and tears, which the dog absorbed without judgment, comment, or unnecessary feedback. Wheatie never questioned SR's disease or treatment, commented on her difficult speech, or showed signs of sorrow over SR's plight. These moments connected with the therapy dog took SR away from her cancer, her fears, and her suffering. For those moments, she was no longer "the lady with terminal cancer" but became "Wheatie's new friend."

Cancer Statistics

According to data from the World Health Organization, cancer is a leading cause of mortality worldwide, accounting for about 13% of all deaths [6]. The National Cancer Institute estimates that over 1.5 million people were diagnosed with cancer in 2010 and that 41% of people would be diagnosed with cancer at some point during their lives [7].

The most common cancer in men is lung cancer, accounting for 17% of new cancer cases and 23% of cancer deaths [8]. Breast cancer is the most common cancer in women, resulting in 23% of total cancer cases and 14% of cancer deaths [8]. According to data available at the National Cancer Institute web site, national costs for cancer care in the United States in 2010 nearly reached $125 billion and costs for 2020 are projected to reach at least $158 billion in 2010 dollars [9].

Modifiable Cancer Risk Factors

Health-care providers can help reduce individual patient risk and potentially improve survival by reinforcing reduction of modifiable cancer risk factors. The National Cancer Institute notes that 50–75% of cancer deaths in the United States can be attributed to potentially modifiable risk factors, including smoking, poor diet, and physical inactivity [10]. Furthermore, obesity is estimated to cause 14% of cancer deaths in men and 20% of cancer deaths in women. According to a recent report on global cancer statistics, promoting healthy lifestyle habits is an important component of cancer reduction [8]. This report describes decreases in breast cancer death in developing countries, due to earlier detection and treatment; however, incidence and mortality of breast cancer are rising in Africa and Asia. This increase is at least partially attributed to lifestyle changes with reduced physical activity and increased obesity.

Table 1.1 Impact of physical activity on cancer

Reference	Data source	Cancer type	Effect of physical activity
Cancer prevention			
[12]	Literature review	Breast	25% average risk reduction among physically active women versus least active
[13]	Literature review	Colon	Physical activity reduces risk by 25%
[14]	Literature review	Lung	Physical activity reduces risk by 20–30% in women and 20–50% in men
[15]	Meta-analysis	Ovarian	20% risk reduction for most versus least active women
[15]	Literature review	Endometrial	Sedentary behavior linked to increased risk
[16]	Literature review	Prostate and renal	< 10% average risk reduction among those with high versus low activity
Cancer survival			
[17]	Literature review	Breast and colon/colorectal	Cancer-related mortality was reduced with higher levels of physical activity

Table 1.2 Different levels of exercise intensity

	Light intensity exercise	Moderate intensity exercise	Vigorous exercise
Examples of common exercises	• Walking slowly (≤2 miles per hour) • Golfing with a power cart • Bowling	• Brisk walking (≥3 miles per hour) • Climbing stairs • Leisurely swimming or bicycling • Golfing, carrying clubs • Dancing	• Jogging • Hiking • Bicycling > 10 miles per hour • Swimming laps • Skating • Skiing
Respiratory stress during exercise	Able to sing while exercising	Able to have a conversation but not sing	Unable to carry on a conversation

Physical Activity

Higher levels of physical activity have been linked to reduced risk for the development of breast, colon, lung, prostate, and endometrial cancers [11]. Clinical trials have consistently shown prevention benefits from a more physically active lifestyle across a range of cancers (Table 1.1) [12–18]. Limited data suggest a possible protective effect from physical activity for hematologic cancer prevention [19].

The American Cancer Society recommends at least 30 min of moderate-to-vigorous physical exercise at least 5 days per week for cancer prevention (Table 1.2) [20]. Dog walking has been shown to be an effective tool for achieving exercise targets among individuals who own dogs and non-dog owners able to walk a therapy dog. Dog ownership has been linked to improved overall health, with studies supporting improvements in physical exercise, autonomic activity, and psychosocial factors [21]. Living with a companion dog can serve as motivation to encourage people to adhere to a healthy exercise program. Data from 5,902 participants in the 2005 Michigan Behavioral Risk Factor Survey revealed that dog owners were 69% more likely to participate in leisure-time physical activity and 34% more likely to walk at least 150 min per week compared with individuals not owning dogs [22]. Another study showed that non-dog owners became motivated to maintain walking programs when they were assigned a therapy dog to walk, reporting that participants developed a sense of responsibility for the well-being of the dog that resulted in a 72% mean walking program adherence rate and an average weight loss of 14.4 pounds (6.5 kg) over the 50-week study ($P=0.013$).

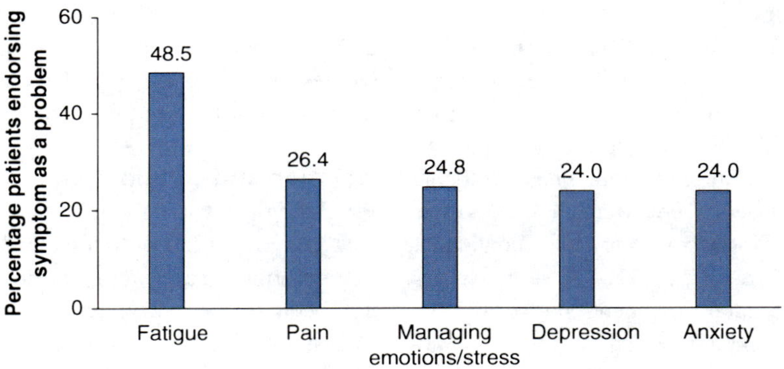

Fig. 1.2 Somatic symptoms in adults with cancer (Based on [23])

Practical Pointer: The American Cancer Society recommends a total of ≥150 min of at least moderate intensity exercise weekly for cancer prevention. This can be successfully achieved with brisk dog walking.

Cancer-Related Symptoms

A variety of somatic complaints occur commonly in patients with cancer. Adult patients ($N=2{,}776$) seen at a tertiary cancer center for any reason (diagnosis, new consultation, follow-up, or treatment) were screened to identify problems they were currently having or expected to have, using a problem checklist [23]. The average number of symptoms endorsed was three, with those most commonly identified as problems including psychological distress, fatigue, and pain (Fig. 1.2).

Practical Pointer: Symptoms commonly occurring in patients with cancer can be problematic during and after completing cancer treatment, with both physical and psychosocial symptoms continuing to be a problem in long-term cancer survivors.

Psychological Distress

Psychological distress is common among patients with cancer. Relevant distress was identified in nearly half (48%) of patients with newly diagnosed brain tumors in one survey [24]. A systematic review reported anxiety as an important concern in women undergoing a wide range of breast cancer treatments, with anxiety particularly problematic among women undergoing chemotherapy [25]. The high prevalence and significant impact of distress in cancer patients has resulted in the development of screening measures of distress for cancer [26, 27] and recommendations to add distress as the sixth vital sign in cancer patients [28–30].

The Distress Thermometer is a single-item question asking cancer patients to rate distress on a 0 (no distress) to 10 (extreme distress) severity scale. This tool is a practical and valid measure of distress [27, 28].

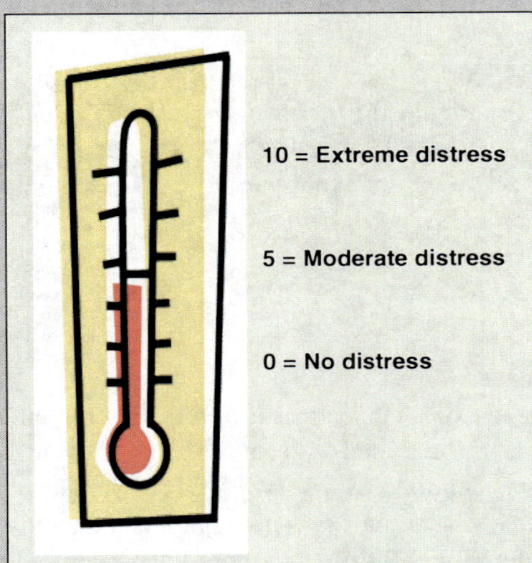

Mood Disorders

Anxiety and depression are the most common emotional disorders seen in cancer patients. A study comparing the prevalence of mood disorders in a sample of 150 adult cancer patients (median illness duration = 6 months) and 268 controls reported cancer patients were 2.83 times more likely to have a mood disorder (95% confidence interval [CI] 1.89–4.25) [31]. A large survey screening 8,265 adult outpatients presenting to a tertiary cancer center reported depressive symptoms in 18% of patients and anxiety in 24% [32]. In another sample, intense levels of anxiety and depression, respectively, were reported in 27% and 20% of adult outpatients prior to initiating chemotherapy [33]. Not unexpectedly, mood disorders were negatively related to quality of life. Other surveys screening patients at different points during their cancer management have reported depression in 17–22% and anxiety in 19–39% [34–36].

Mood disorders can continue to be a problem throughout cancer care, with depression and anxiety affecting patients who have been recently diagnosed, undergoing treatment, and long-term survivors. For example, a survey of 214 patients admitted to the hospital for treatment 2 weeks after receiving their diagnosis of gynecological cancer identified a mood disorder in 55% of patients [37]. Another study evaluating 45 gynecological cancer survivors who had completed primary cancer treatment (mean time since diagnosis = 4 ± 2.8 years) reported anxiety and depression, respectively, in 29% and 20% of patients [38].

> **Practical Pointer:** Mood disorders occur in about half of cancer patients undergoing treatment and continue to be a substantial problem in one in three to five cancer survivors.

Stress

Not unexpectedly, stress is a frequent problem in patients diagnosed with cancer. High stress levels were identified in a survey of 100 women with breast cancer, half of whom had been diagnosed within 3 months of study enrollment and half of whom had completed treatment at least 6 months before enrollment [39]. Seventy percent of women surveyed described having a stress level rated ≥ 5 on a 1–7 severity scale.

Isolation and Loneliness

Psychological distress can continue after patients have completed cancer treatment, and both physical and emotional scars can contribute to what has been termed survivor loneliness [40, 41]. This sense of aloneness has been described as the consequence of several factors, including perceiving a more acute sense of mortality, changes in self-identify and connections, and alterations in life priorities and threshold for distress.

A survey of 633 men with prostate cancer diagnosed 1.5–2 years before the survey revealed that 23% reported having no one in whom they could confide [42]. Among those men living with a partner, 70% reported being able to confide in their partner with only 10% confiding in someone other than the partner. Among those men without a partner, 70% reported not sharing emotional feelings with anyone. Furthermore, men without someone in whom they could confide were more likely to feel tired (relative risk [RR] 1.5, 95% CI 1.1–2.0) and not happy (RR 1.7, 95% CI 1.3–2.2).

Health-care providers are becoming increasingly aware of the emotional needs of family members caring for cancer patients [43]. Loneliness has also been described in the parents of children completing cancer treatment [44] and in family members of men with advanced prostate cancer [45]. These data highlight that both patients and their families can experience isolation and rejection, which should be addressed during cancer treatment visits.

Significance of Stress and Isolation on Cancer Progression

Basic science and clinical studies have linked depression, stress, and lack of social support with increased risk for cancer growth and metastasis [46, 47]. Stress results in a range of neurochemical changes. Moreno-Smith and colleagues cataloged negative influences on cancer metastasis from stress-related increases in norepinephrine, epinephrine, and cortisol (Fig. 1.3) [48]. While acute stress increases dopamine, chronic stress has been

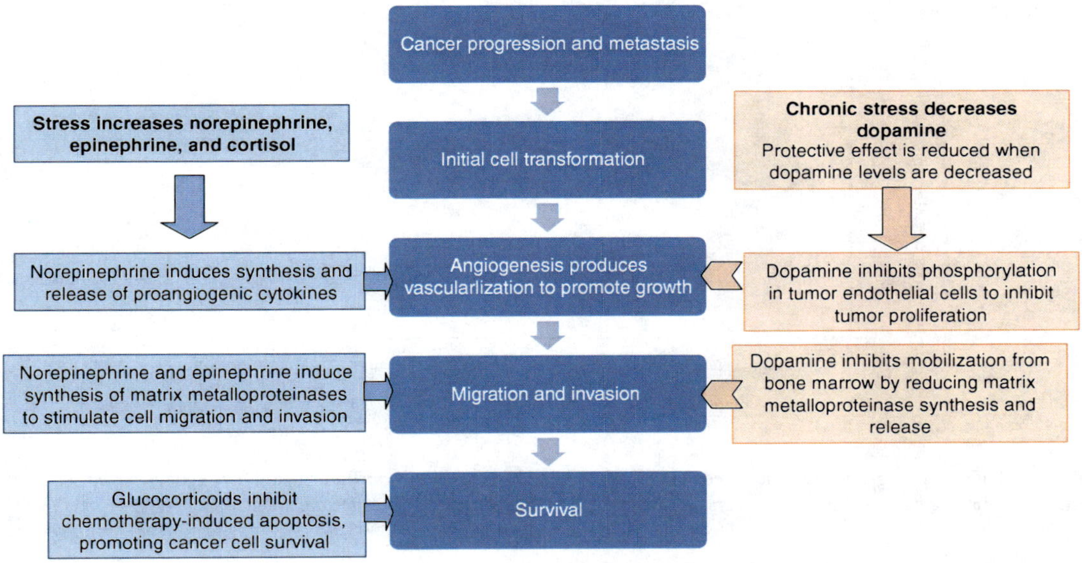

Fig. 1.3 Steps in cancer metastasis and effects of stress hormones (Based on [48])

linked to reduce dopamine release [48, 49]. Dopamine is expected to inhibit phosphorylation of tumor endothelial cells to reduce tumor proliferation. Dopamine also inhibits mobilization from the bone marrow by reducing matrix metalloproteinase-9 synthesis and release. Reductions in dopamine's inhibitory influence on cancer growth and metastasis may be another important negative consequence of untreated chronic stress.

Social isolation has also been linked to cancer progression. Lutgendorf and colleagues at the University of Iowa linked social isolation and ovarian cancer [50]. Higher norepinephrine levels were identified in advanced stage and higher grade tumors. After adjusting for stage, grade, and perisurgical beta-blockers, patients lacking social support had significantly higher tumor norepinephrine ($P = 0.012$). Because beta-adrenergic signaling is important for tumor growth, researchers postulated that social isolation may increase patients' risk for cancer progression.

Practical Pointer: Emotional factors, including psychological distress and social isolation, can have important physical consequences that can worsen cancer outcome.

Fatigue

Cancer-related fatigue is defined as a persistent and disabling tiredness related to cancer or cancer treatment that is not relieved by rest or sleep [51, 52]. Incidence of cancer-related fatigue across treatment studies varies between 15% and 90%, with variability between and within cancer diagnoses [51]. In recent reviews of available literature, fatigue was reported to be a common symptom across the full spectrum of cancer management (Fig. 1.4) [51, 53].

Practical Pointer: Terms most commonly used by patients to describe cancer-related fatigue include [54]:
- Easy fatigue
- Weakness
- Lack of energy

Cancer-related fatigue substantially reduces patient functioning and has been linked to psychological distress [51]. One study asked 379 cancer patients (79% female) who had received chemotherapy (most commonly for breast cancer [62%] or genitourinary cancer [12%]), about fatigue and its impact [55]. A total of 76%

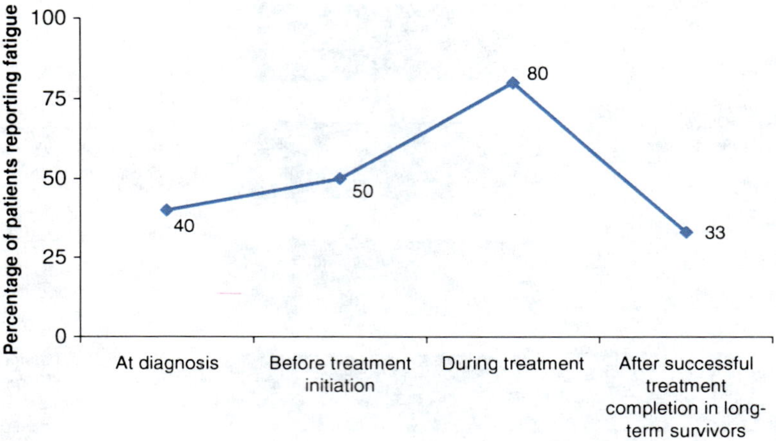

Fig. 1.4 Fatigue during the course of cancer care. Cancer-related fatigue is a common symptom throughout cancer management, with fatigue persisting in many patients for months to years after completing cancer treatment (Based on [51] and [53])

reported fatigue during or after their most recent chemotherapy, with fatigue lasting >4 days for 62% and >2 weeks for 33%. In addition, 60% reported that fatigue was the symptom that most affected their daily life. Negative effects from fatigue were reported for a wide range of daily activities, including household chores, exercise, and social activities. Fatigue was also linked with decreased motivation or interest in usual activities, cognitive problems, and depression. Among patients employed at the start of chemotherapy, 75% had to change their work status due to fatigue. Another survey of 969 cancer patients (median age = 65 years; 55% male) with a variety of diagnoses (most commonly lung [24%], breast, [9%], colorectal [8%], and prostate [7%] cancers) linked cancer-related fatigue with significantly shorter duration survival [54].

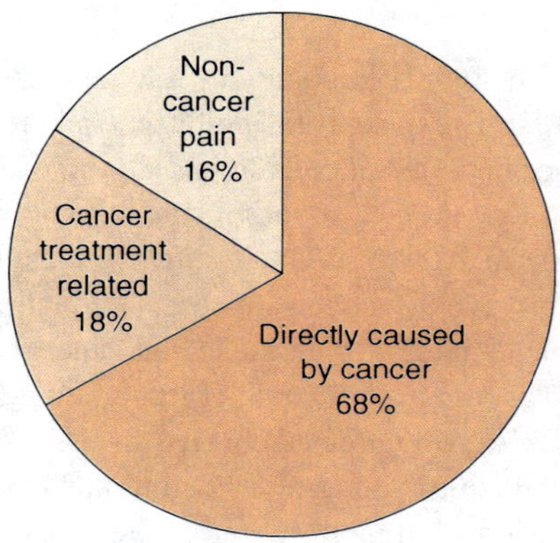

Fig. 1.5 Cause of pain in cancer patients (Based on [57])

Pain

Pain is a presenting symptom in 20–50% of patients with cancer [56]. Cancer pain is most commonly caused by the cancer itself (Fig. 1.5) [57]. A meta-analysis of 52 studies calculated pooled prevalence rates of cancer pain, with over half of cancer patients experiencing pain (Fig. 1.6) [58]. Cancer pain was prevalent throughout the course of cancer care, including in cancer survivors who had completed curative treatment. Pain prevalence was highest among patients with head/neck cancer, although pain was reported by over half of patients with a broad range of cancer types (Fig. 1.7).

Pain is reported by at least half of patients actively involved in cancer treatment. A survey of 179 cancer patients seen at the Cleveland Clinic identified cancer pain in 65% of patients [59]. Interestingly, patients <65 years old were significantly more likely to experience pain compared with older patients. A longitudinal study likewise showed more pain flares in younger patients with cancer pain [60]. The Indiana

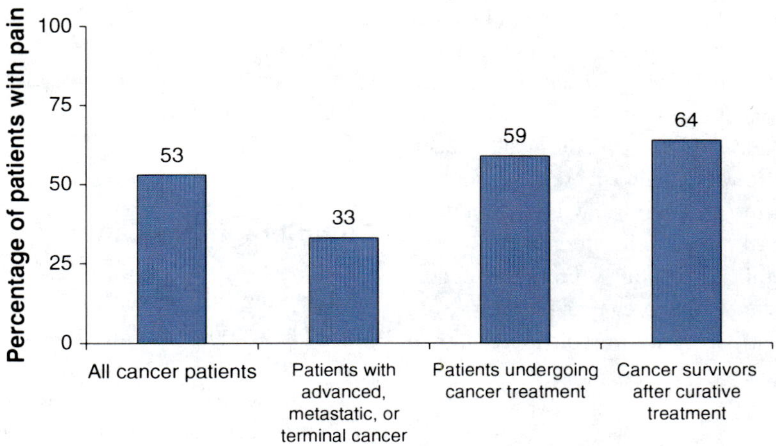

Fig. 1.6 Prevalence of cancer pain (Based on meta-analysis data from [58])

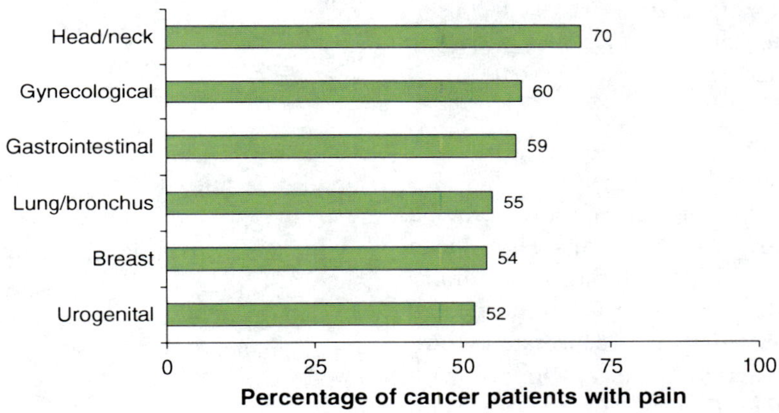

Fig. 1.7 Pooled cancer pain prevalence by cancer type (Based on meta-analysis data from [58])

Cancer Pain and Depression study identified pain as a symptom in two of three (68%) community-based oncology patients [61]. Pain was considered to be cancer related for 67% of patients reporting pain. Among patients with cancer-related pain, the most common pain locations were the back (32%), abdomen (16%), shoulders (13%), and hips (11%). Most patients (56%) rated their average pain severity as moderate (4–6 on a 0–10-point pain severity scale); however, worst pain was rated ≥ 6 for 77% of patients. Not unexpectedly, pain was significantly associated with worse quality of life and overall disability. A survey of 312 Chinese-American oncology patients likewise identified frequent or persistent pain in 52% of patients [62].

Pain is also a frequent chronic sequela in long-term cancer survivors. For example, chronic pain may occur in up to half of patients after having cancer surgery [63]. A recent literature review reported the following statistics for pain in cancer survivors [64]:

- Pain and functional limitations related to breast cancer treatment were reported for 26–47% during the first 6 months after treatment. Pain or functional limitations occurred in 20–23% at 6–12 months after treatment, 21–41% at 1–2 years after treatment, and 19–41% at 2–5 years after treatment.
- Pain/functional limitations were reported by 54% of prostate cancer survivors up to 5 years after treatment.

- Pain was present in 27% of colorectal cancer survivors more than 5 years after their diagnosis. Pain was attributed to cancer by 12% of colorectal cancer survivors.
- Among patients with gynecological cancer, one study showed pain decreased slightly 6 months after treatment and then remained stable up to 24 months after treatment.

These data highlight the fairly common occurrence of persistent pain in cancer patients, even among those patients who are considered cured from their cancer.

Practical Pointer: Pain is a common symptom reported by about two in five patients at the time of cancer diagnosis, at least half of patients undergoing cancer treatment, and about one in three long-term survivors.

Impact of Cancer Pain

Cancer pain has been linked to increased emotional distress, with this distress reduced with pain treatment [65]. Longer pain duration and greater pain severity are correlated with increased risk for depression [66]. Furthermore, among cancer patients with pain in the Indiana Cancer Pain and Depression study reported above, patients with pain were disabled an average of 12–20 days over the preceding 4 weeks, with 28–55% reporting being unable to work due to health-related reasons [61].

Pain in long-term survivors may be particularly difficult for patients who many not have anticipated needing to deal with chronic pain after they were no longer actively involved with cancer care [67]. For some patients experiencing long-term pain, coping with pain without the support that was provided by health-care providers during cancer treatment leads to worsened quality of life. Pain may also result in concerns about disease recurrence, as well as impairments in sleep and mood. Pain has also been shown to contribute to long-term disability in cancer survivors.

Practical Pointer: Cancer-related pain has been linked to psychological distress and functional disability.

Complementary Cancer Treatment

Recognizing and screening for common symptoms that accompany cancer care need to be coupled with effective strategies for reducing symptom severity. For example, a recent review evaluating screening for distress and depression in cancer patients concluded that screening needs to be linked with treatment, follow-up, and engaging the patient in their care [68]. Complementary therapies can provide useful options for addressing both symptoms and unmet needs that frequently accompany cancer.

Practical Pointer: Complementary treatments typically target problematic symptoms that may be inadequately addressed through traditional medicine, including psychosocial distress, pain, and a sense of loss of autonomy.

Nontraditional therapies are collectively referred to as *complementary and alternative medicine*. *Complementary* treatments are defined as therapies that support, enhance, or facilitate conventional disease management. *Alternative* therapies are used instead of conventional treatments. In most cases where cancer patients are using nonconventional therapies, these treatments are enhancing or supplementing standard treatment regimens as complementary therapy. Complementary treatments can fill important treatment gaps for patients. A survey of cancer patients identified a wide range of important needs that are often unmet during traditional treatment [69]. Several of these important needs might be effectively addressed through complementary therapy, including therapy dog visits (Fig. 1.8).

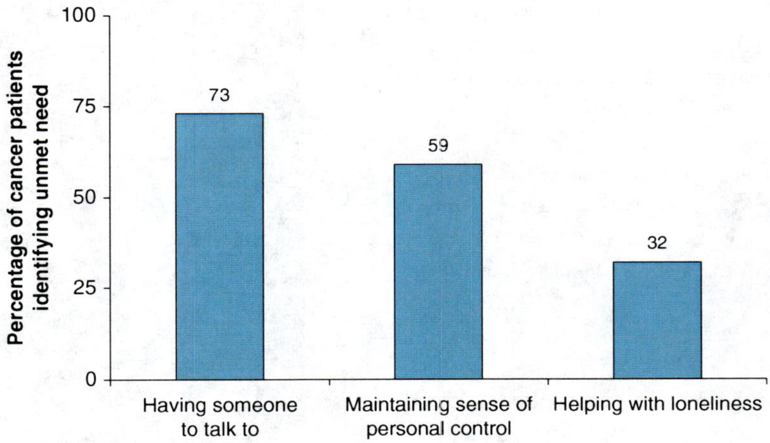

Fig. 1.8 Important needs identified by patients with cancer that might be addressed using complementary therapies (Based on [69])

> **Practical Pointer:** The term *complementary and alternative therapy* is often used to refer to nontraditional treatments.
>
> - *Complementary* treatments are used to supplement and enhance traditional medicine.
> - *Alternative* treatments are used instead of traditional care.
>
> Therapy dog visits are used as complementary treatment to augment patient benefits from other interventions.

Cancer patients are often interested in incorporating complementary treatments into their cancer care program. A survey of 172 patients undergoing radiation therapy showed that 24% used complementary care, with an additional 31% interested in using complementary treatments [70]. Patients using complementary treatments were neither experiencing higher distress nor were they poorly compliant with their conventional therapy. Rather these patients showed active coping behaviors, utilizing complementary techniques to avoid feeling passive and hopeless. Likewise, a survey of 621 neuro-oncology patients with glioma found that 40% use complementary therapies [71]. In this study, patients were motivated to use complementary therapy as a means to supplement standard care; complementary treatments were not used because patients were dissatisfied with conventional therapy. Complementary options can empower cancer patients to take an active and positive role in their care. Furthermore, a survey of chemotherapy nurses showed that those nurses familiar with the use of complementary treatment in a chemotherapy setting (such as relaxation therapy, music, and reflexology) found those treatments to be very useful for patients [72].

Acute cancer treatments and rehabilitative care in cancer survivors may be limited by economic and logistical issues. For example, a survey of Canadian breast cancer survivors identified lack of service availability, cost, and lack of support as important barriers to cancer rehabilitation [73]. In an interesting report, 56 studies describing economic evaluation of complementary and alternative medicine for a broad range of medical conditions were reviewed, including complementary stress management for cancer patients undergoing chemotherapy [74]. Self-administered stress management techniques were effective and lowered total cost in cancer patients. These data support recommendations to include complementary treatment routinely in cancer therapy as effective and cost-saving additions to enhance symptomatic reduction [75]. Dog therapy has specifically been recommended as a cost-saving intervention that also delivers effective therapy [76].

> "With the current intense focus on health care reform, increased use of animals as therapy may serve as a cost-effective strategy for improving and maintaining health ...." [76], page 19

Complementary treatments are often selected by patients because of perceived safety, a belief in potential benefit despite lack of rigorous evidence, and a need to assume a sense of control over treatment [77, 78]. An interesting study surveyed cancer patients, long-term survivors, and health-care provides to determine reasons why complementary treatments were not included as part of cancer management [79]. The most commonly cited reasons included cost or time constraints, fear or distrust of complementary treatments, lack of evidence proving benefits from complementary treatments, and satisfaction with conventional therapy. This study suggests a need for health-care providers to be familiar with available and effective complementary treatments so that patients may benefit from increased information about complementary treatments that might improve their cancer care experience. In some cases, health-care providers raise concerns that patients will opt to abandon life-saving conventional treatments in favor of less effective alternative therapies [80]. This further highlights the need to understand the additive benefits that may occur from complementary treatments so patients can be best informed about both traditional and complementary treatment options.

Therapy Dogs in Cancer Care

Animal therapy, including therapy dog visits, may be included as complementary therapy for a range of medical conditions [81]. The American Cancer Society's *Complete Guide to Complementary & Alternative Cancer Therapies* [82] describes a wide range of complementary treatments, including acupuncture, aromatherapy, imagery, massage, meditation, music therapy, nutritional supplements, Reiki, therapeutic touch, yoga, water therapy, and more. While therapy dogs are not included in this list, visits from trained, certified dogs can provide a valuable and economically accessible component to cancer care that can positively impact many cancer patients (Fig. 1.9). Numerous studies have demonstrated reduction in problematic symptoms, like stress, loneliness, and pain, from therapy dog visits (see Chap. 4).

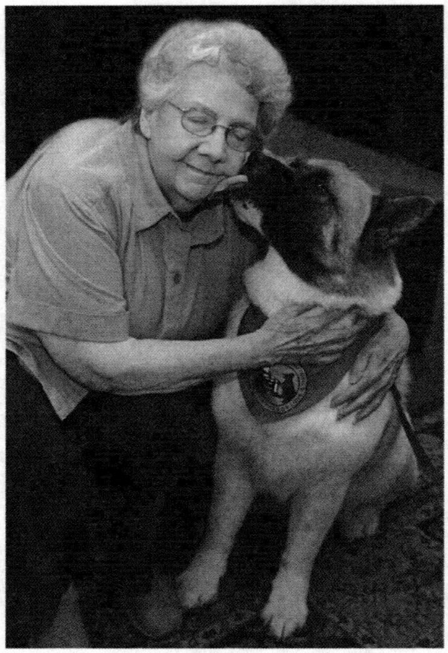

Fig. 1.9 Akita therapy dog Apple provided a welcome complementary intervention to 73-year-old breast cancer survivor Rose, while Rose was undergoing cancer treatment

Therapy dog visits are becoming more widely recognized, accepted, and incorporated into medical therapy, including cancer management [83]. For example, the National Home and Hospice Care Survey conducted in the United States in 2007

> **Practical Pointer:** Therapy dog interactions can effectively address a variety of psychosocial and physical needs for cancer patients that can result in improved quality of life and potentially improved cancer outcome.

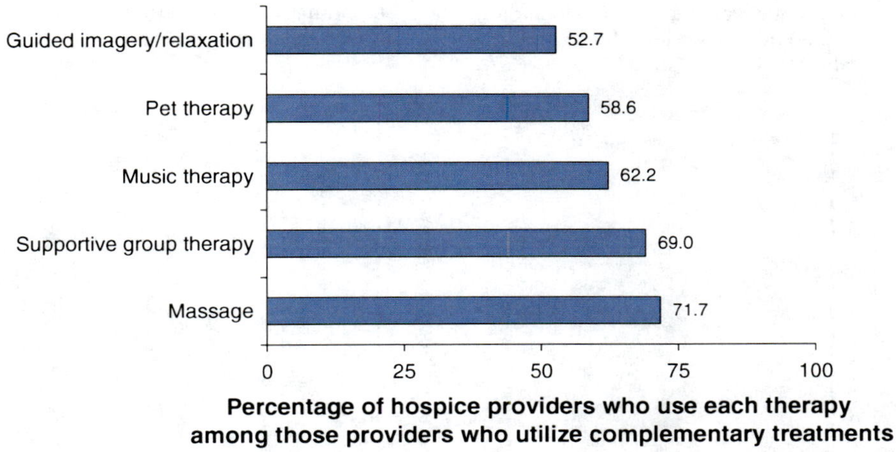

Fig. 1.10 Complementary treatments commonly included in hospice care (Based on [84])

reported that 42% of hospice care providers offered complementary therapies [84]. Among those therapies most commonly utilized, pet therapy ranked fourth and was offered by over half of those providers who utilized any complementary treatments in their practices (Fig. 1.10).

> **Practical Pointer:** Therapy dog visits are the fourth most common complementary treatment used in hospice.

Therapeutic dog interactions do not depend on individuals having a previous positive relationship with a dog or having a dog companion. Therapeutic interactions can occur when patients interact with dogs with whom they are not familiar, like therapy dogs. For example, a small study evaluating stress responses in seniors ($N=13$) found profound improvements when walking and daily household activities were performed with a therapy dog with whom participants were not familiar before the study [85]. In this study, electrocardiogram (ECG) monitors were used to assess heart variability to calculate high-frequency power as an index of parasympathetic activity. An increase in parasympathetic activity is generally associated with reduced stress effects. In this study, parasympathetic activity was determined when seniors were walking and conducting typical daily chores in the home. Each walk lasted 30 min, followed by a 20-min rest, and then a second 30-min walk. Continuous ECG recordings were obtained for 6 h while performing routine activities, which included two 30-min intervals during which the dog was present to interact with the person. Responses were compared when the senior walked or was in the home with a friendly 2-year-old Cavalier King Charles Spaniel or without the dog. The same dog was used to interact with each participant. Parasympathetic activity increased by 47% when participants walked with the dog (Fig. 1.11). When walking on three consecutive days, there was no change over time in parasympathetic activity when walks occurred without the dog, with a significant increase when walking with the dog. Interacting with the dog at home resulted in a nearly two times increase in desirable high-frequency power values.

Therapy dog visits can provide cancer patients with needed companionship, distraction from cancer and cancer treatment, and sensory stimulation and increased physical activity through petting, grooming, or walking with the dog (Fig. 1.12). Therapy dog visits have also been shown to reduce symptoms of psychosocial distress and improve well-being in cancer patients [86]. Social worker Irene Muschel conducted an interesting survey of cancer patients at a hospice

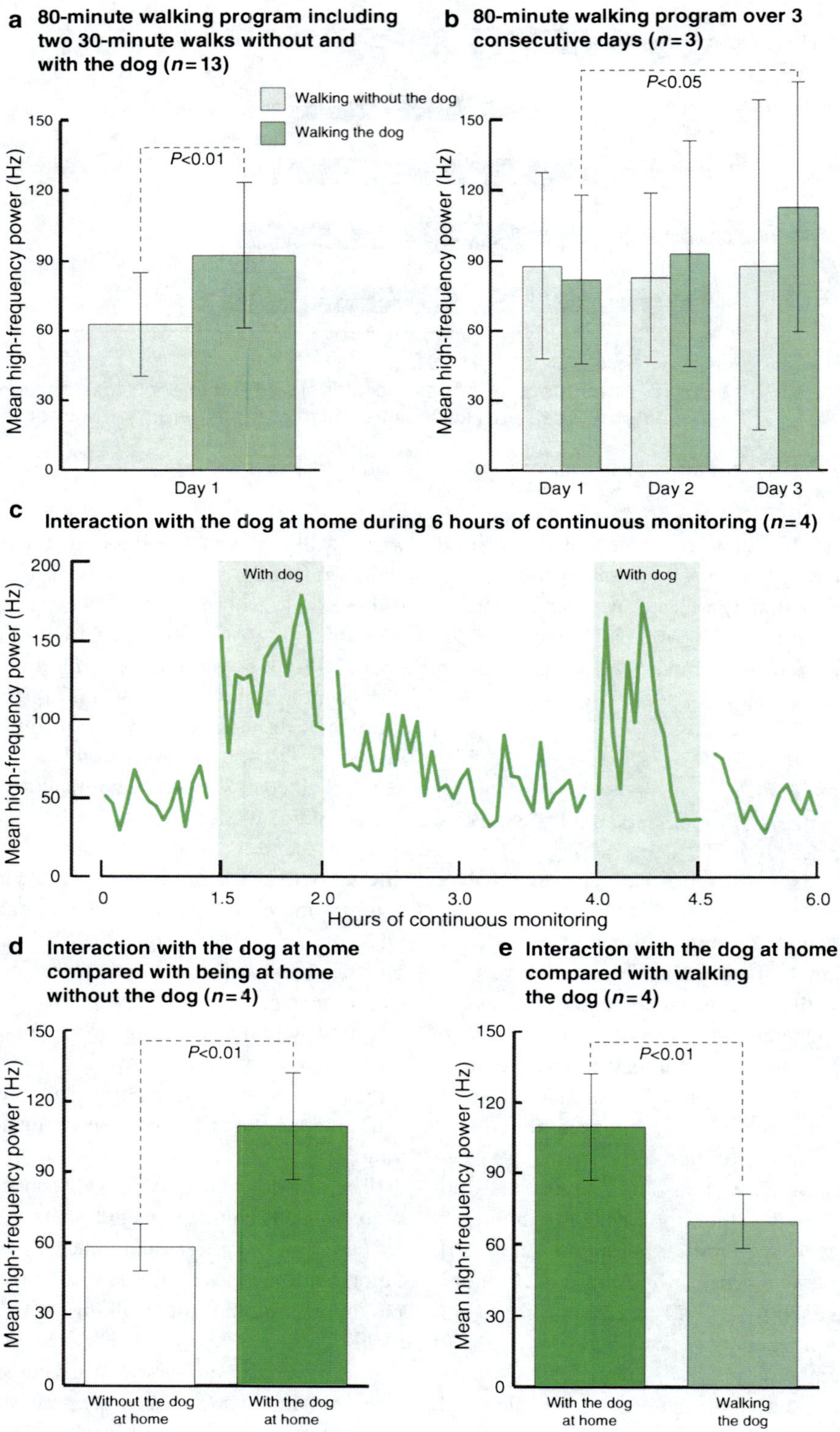

Fig. 1.11 Parasympathetic activity with walking and daily home activities when performed with or without being accompanied by an unfamiliar dog (Reproduced with permission [85])

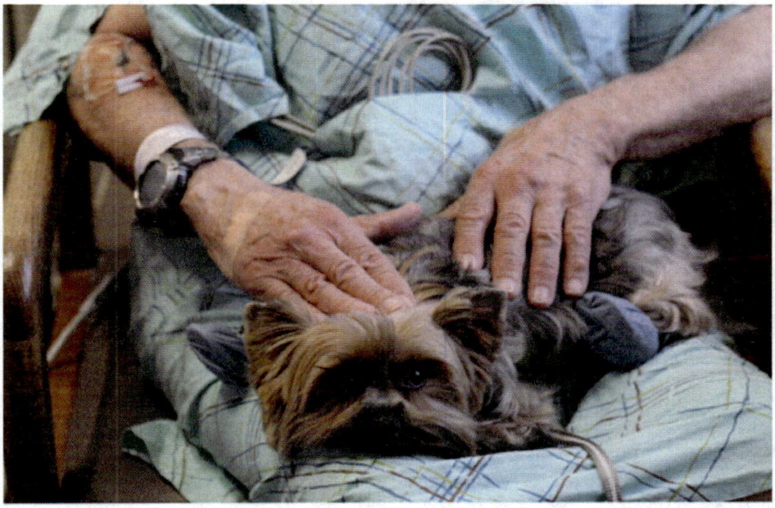

Fig. 1.12 During her friend's final weeks with cancer, Beth Kraimer's Yorkshire Terrier Petey provided comfort to both the friend and Beth. Trained and certified as a therapy dog, Petey has happily volunteered at Beth Israel Medical Center in New York City since 2006 (Photo courtesy of Nick Barberio)

center receiving visits from a pet therapy program including dogs and cats [86]:

- Physical and emotional isolation were common problems in these patients.
- Pet therapy visits reduced patient fears, isolation, loneliness, helplessness, anxiety, and despair.
- Relating to the animals facilitated patients externalizing and trying to reduce their concerns. For example, patients might tell the pet not to be scared, providing assurance that things would be all right.
- Caring for the pet gave patients a sense of control and reduced passivity and helplessness.
- Watching pets brought laughter and aroused a sense of playfulness in patients who often engaged in play activities with the pets.
- Pet visits facilitated positive reminiscing that improved mood and enhanced a sense of connectedness.

Muschel concluded, "The study suggests that animals may help individuals in ways people are not always able to. People who live and work with dying patients often bring to them their own concerns and fears about death. Animals, on the other hand, never avoid the dying patient. They do not intrude, moreover, upon the patient's attempts to come to terms with mortality. The animal's quiet, accepting, and nurturing presence strengthens and frees the patient to resolve his or her final experience successfully" (page 457) [86].

> One cancer patient in Muschel's hospice study described visits with a therapy dog:
>
> "He gives me comfort without a voice. I never feel alone with an animal. I can be open with my feelings with an animal." ([86], page 455)

Summary

- According to the World Health Organization, cancer is a leading cause of death worldwide.
- Fatigue and psychosocial distress are common throughout cancer care and can worsen the course of cancer.
- Comorbid pain occurs in over half of cancer patients and can lead to disability.
- Traditional medicine often fails to identify and address major concerns in patients with cancer.
- Patients with cancer are often interested in including complementary therapies with traditional cancer treatment to reduce symptom severity and empower patients with a sense of control.
- Therapy dog visits can provide a cost-free, effective complementary intervention that can address a variety of unmet patient needs.

References

1. Dy SM, Apostol CC. Evidence-based approaches to other symptoms in advanced cancer. Cancer J. 2010;16:507–13.
2. Blaes AH, Kreitzer MJ, Torkelson C, Haddad T. Nonpharmacologic complementary therapies in symptom management for breast cancer survivors. Semin Oncol. 2011;38:394–402.
3. Marcus DA. I have cancer: how can a dog help me? The power of wagging tails: a doctor's guide to dog therapy and healing. New York: Demos Health; 2011. p. 185.
4. Mulders M, Vingerhoets A, Breed W. The impact of cancer and chemotherapy: perceptual similarities and differences between cancer patients, nurses and physicians. Eur J Oncol Nurs. 2008;12:97–102.
5. Adsett CA. Emotional reactions to disfigurement from cancer therapy. Can Med Assoc J. 1963;89:385–91.
6. World Health Organization website. Available at http://www.who.int/cancer/en/. Accessed April 2011
7. National Cancer Institute website. Available at http://seer.cancer.gov/statfacts/html/all.html. Accessed September 2011
8. Jemal A, Bray F, Center M, et al. Global cancer statistics. CA Cancer J Clin. 2011;61:69–90.
9. National Cancer Institute at the National Institutes of Health website. Available at http://www.cancer.gov/aboutnci/servingpeople/cancer-statistics/costofcancer. Accessed June 2011
10. National Cancer Institute. Cancer trends progress report – 2009/2010 update. Available at http://progressreport.cancer.gov/. Accessed May 2011
11. Wiggins MS, Simonavice EM. Cancer prevention, aerobic capacity, and physical functioning in survivors related to physical activity: a recent review. Canc Manag Res. 2010;2:157–64.
12. Lynch BM, Neilson HK, Friedenreich CM. Physical activity and breast cancer prevention. Recent Results Cancer Res. 2011;186:13–42.
13. Wolin KY, Tuchman H. Physical activity and gastrointestinal cancer prevention. Recent Results Cancer Res. 2011;186:73–100.
14. Emaus A, Thune I. Physical activity and lung cancer prevention. Recent Results Cancer Res. 2011;186:101–33.
15. Cust AE. Physical activity and gynecologic cancer prevention. Recent Results Cancer Res. 2011;186: 159–85.
16. Leitzmann MF. Physical activity and genitourinary cancer prevention. Recent Results Cancer Res. 2011;186:43–71.
17. Barbaric M, Brooks E, Moore L, Cheifetz O. Effects of physical activity on cancer survival: a systematic review. Physiother Can. 2010;62:25–34.
18. Wolin KY, Yan Y, Colditz GA. Physical activity and risk of colon adenoma: a meta-analysis. Br J Cancer. 2011;104:822–5.
19. Pan SY, Morrison H. Physical activity and hematologic cancer prevention. Recent Results Cancer Res. 2011;186:135–58.
20. Doyle C, Kushi LH, Byers T, et al. Nutrition and physical activity during and after cancer treatment: an American Cancer Society guide for informed choices. CA Cancer J Clin. 2006;56:323–53.
21. Arhant-Sudhir K, Arhant-Sudhir R, Sudhir K. Pet ownership and cardiovascular risk reduction: supporting evidence, conflicting data, and underlying mechanisms. Clin Exp Pharmacol Physiol. 2011;38:734–8.
22. Reeves MJ, Rafferty AP, Miller CE, Lyon-Callo SK. The impact of dog walking on leisure-time physical activity: results from a population-based survey of Michigan adults. J Phys Act Health. 2011;8:436–44.
23. Carlson LE, Angen M, Cullum J, et al. High levels of untreated distress and fatigue in cancer patients. Br J Canc. 2004;90:2297–304.
24. Goebel S, Stark AM, Kaup L, von Harscher M, Mehdorn HM. Distress in patients with newly diagnosed brain tumors. Psychooncology. 2011;20:623–30.
25. Lim CC, Devi MK, Ang E. Anxiety in women with breast cancer undergoing treatment: a systematic review. Int J Evid Based Healthc. 2011;9:215–35.
26. Carlson LE, Bultz BD. Cancer distress screening. Needs, models, and methods. J Psychosom Res. 2003;55:403–9.
27. Mitchell AJ. Short screening tools for cancer-related distress: a review and diagnostic validity meta-analysis. J Natl Compr Canc Netw. 2010;8:487–94.
28. Bultz BD, Carlson LE. Emotional distress: the sixth vital sign in cancer care. J Clin Oncol. 2005;23: 6440–1.
29. Holland JC, Bultz BD. The NCCN guideline for distress management: a case for making distress the sixth vital sign. J Natl Compr Canc Netw. 2007;5:3–7.
30. Bultz BD, Groff SL, Fitch M, et al. Implementing screening for distress, the 6th vital sign: a Canadian strategy for changing practice. Psychooncology. 2011;20:463–9.
31. Jadoon NA, Munir W, Shahzah MA, Choudhry ZS. Assessment of depression and anxiety in adult cancer outpatients: a cross-sectional study. BMC Cancer. 2010;10:594.
32. Brintzenhofe-Szoc KM, Levin TT, Li Y, Kissane DW, Zabora JR. Mixed anxiety/depression symptoms in a large cancer cohort: prevalence by cancer type. Psychosomatics. 2009;50:383–91.
33. Iconomou G, Iconomou AV, Argyriou AA, et al. Emotional distress in cancer patients at the beginning of chemotherapy and its relation to quality of life. J BUON. 2008;13:217–22.
34. Ernstmann N, Neumann M, Ommen O, et al. Determinants and implications of cancer patients' psychosocial needs. Support Care Cancer. 2009;17: 1417–23.
35. Lueboonthavatchai P. Prevalence and psychosocial factors of anxiety and depression in breast cancer patients. J Med Assoc Thai. 2007;90:2164–74.
36. Vahdaninia M, Omidvari S, Montazeri A. What do predict anxiety and depression in breast cancer patients? A follow-up study. Soc Psychiatry Psychiatr Epidemiol. 2010;45:355–61.

37. Suzuki N, Ninomiya M, Maruta S, et al. Psychological characteristics of Japanese gynecologic cancer patients after learning the diagnosis according to the hospital anxiety and depression scale. J Obstet Gynaecol Res. 2011;37:800–8.
38. Urbaniec OA, Collins K, Denson LA, Whitford HS. Gynecological cancer survivors: assessment of psychological distress and unmet supportive care needs. J Psychosoc Oncol. 2011;29:534–51.
39. Koopman C, Angell K, Turner-Cobb JM, et al. Distress, coping, and social support among rural women recently diagnosed with primary breast cancer. Breast J. 2001;7:25–33.
40. Rosedale M. Survivor loneliness of women following breast cancer. Oncol Nurs Forum. 2009;36:175–83.
41. Jefferies H, Clifford C. Aloneness: the lived experience of women with cancer of the vulva. Eur J Cancer Care. 2011;20:738–46.
42. Helgason AR, Dickman PW, Adolfsson J, Steineck G. Emotional isolation: prevalence and the effect on well-being among 50-80-year-old prostate cancer patients. Scand J Urol Nephrol. 2011;35:97–101.
43. Harding R, Epiphaniou E, Hamilton D, et al. What are the perceived needs and challenges of informal caregivers in home cancer palliative care? Qualitative data to construct a feasible psycho-educational intervention. Support Care Cancer, in press.
44. Wakefield CE, McLoone JK, Butow P, Lenthen K, Cohn RJ. Parental adjustment to the completion of their child's cancer treatment. Pediatr Blood Cancer. 2011;56:524–31.
45. Carter N, Bryant-Lukosius D, DiCenso A, Blythe J, Neville AJ. The supportive care needs of family members of men with advanced prostate cancer. Can Oncol Nurs J. 2010;20:166–76.
46. Lutgendorf SK, Sood AK, Antoni MH. Lost factors and cancer progression: biobehavioral signaling pathways and interventions. J Clin Oncol. 2010;28:4094–9.
47. Armaiz-Pena GN, Lutgendorf SK, Cole SW, Sood AK. Neuroendocrine modulation of cancer progression. Brain Behav Immun. 2009;23:10–5.
48. Moreno-Smith M, Lutgendorf SK, Sood AK. Impact of stress on cancer metastasis. Future Oncol. 2010;6: 1863–81.
49. Moreno-Smith M, Lu C, Shahzad MM, et al. Dopamine blocks stress-mediated ovarian carcinoma growth. Clin Cancer Res. 2011;17:3649–59.
50. Lutgendorf SK, DeGeest K, Dahmoush L, et al. Social isolation is associated with elevated tumor norepinephrine in ovarian carcinoma patients. Brain Behav Immun. 2011;25:250–5.
51. Hofman M, Ryan JL, Figueroa-Moseley CD, Jean-Pierre P, Morrow GR. Cancer-related fatigue: the scale of the problem. Oncologist. 2007;12 suppl 1:4–10.
52. Campos MP, Hassan BJ, Riechelmann R, Del Giglio A. Cancer-related fatigue: a practical review. Ann Oncol. 2011;22:1273–9.
53. de Vries U, Reif K, Petermann F. Cancer-related fatigue and its psychosocial burden. Internist (Berl). 2011;52:1317–24.
54. Hauser K, Rybicki L, Walsh D. What's in a name? Word descriptors of cancer-related fatigue. Palliat Med. 2010;24:724–30.
55. Curt GA, Breitbart W, Cella D, et al. Impact of cancer-related fatigue on the lives of patients: new findings from the fatigue coalition. Oncologist. 2000;5: 353–60.
56. Fischer DJ, Villines D, Kim YO, Epstein JB, Wilkie DJ. Anxiety, depression, and pain: differences by primary cancer. Support Care Cancer. 2010;18:801–10.
57. Gutgsell T, Walsh D, Zhukovsky DS, Gonzales F, Lagman R. A prospective study of the pathophysiology and clinical characteristics of pain in a palliative medicine population. Am J Hosp Palliat Care. 2003;20:140–8.
58. van den Beuken-van Everdingen MH, de Rijke JM, Kessels AG, et al. Prevalence of pain in patients with cancer: a systematic review of the past 40 years. Ann Oncol. 2007;18:1437–49.
59. Shaheen PE, Legrand SB, Walsh D, et al. Errors in opioid prescribing: a prospective survey in cancer pain. J Pain Symptom Manage. 2010;39:702–11.
60. Green CR, Hart-Johnson T. Cancer pain: an age-based analysis. Pain Med. 2010;11:1525–36.
61. Kroenke K, Theobald D, Wu J, et al. The association of depression and pain with health-related quality of life, disability, and health care use in cancer patients. J Pain Symptom Manage. 2010;40:327–41.
62. Dhingra L, Lam K, Homel P, et al. Pain in underserved community-dwelling Chinese American cancer patients: demographic and medical correlates. Oncologist. 2011;16:523–33.
63. Raphael J, Hester J, Ahmedzai S, et al. Cancer pain: part 2: physical, interventional and complimentary therapies; management in the community; acute, treatment-related and complex cancer pain: a perspective from the British Pain Society endorsed by the UK Association of Palliative Medicine and the Royal College of General Practitioners. Pain Med. 2010;11: 872–96.
64. Harrington CB, Hansen JA, Moskowitz M, Todd BL, Feuerstein M. It's not over when it's over: long-term symptoms in cancer survivors – a systematic review. Int J Psychiatry Med. 2010;40:163–81.
65. O'Mahony S, Goulet JL, Payne R. Psychosocial distress in patients treated for cancer pain: a prospective observational study. J Opioid Manag. 2010;6:211–22.
66. Laird BJ, Boyd AC, Colvin LA, Fallon MT. Are cancer pain and depression interdependent? A systematic review. Psychooncology. 2009;18:459–64.
67. Chapman S. Chronic pain syndromes in cancer survivors. Nurs Stand. 2010;25:35–41.
68. Mitchell AJ, Vahabzadeh A, Magruder K. Screening for distress and depression in cancer settings: 10 lessons from 40 years of primary-care research. Psychooncology. 2011;20:572–84.
69. Soothill K, Morris SM, Thomas C, et al. The universal, situational, and personal needs of cancer patients and their main carers. Eur J Oncol Nurs. 2003; 7:5–16.

70. Söllner W, Maislinger S, DeVries A, et al. Use of complementary and alternative medicine by cancer patients is not associated with perceived distress or poor compliance with standard treatment but with active coping behavior. A survey. Cancer. 2000;89:873–80.
71. Heese O, Schmidt M, Nickel S, et al. Complementary therapy use in patients with glioma: an observational study. Neurology. 2010;75:2229–35.
72. Saltmarsh K, De Vries K. The paradoxical image of chemotherapy: a phenomenological description of nurses' experiences of administering chemotherapy. Eur J Cancer Care. 2008;17:500–8.
73. Miedema B, Easley J. Barriers to rehabilitative care for young breast cancer survivors: a qualitative understanding. Support Care Cancer, in press.
74. Herman PM, Craig BM, Caspi O. Is complementary and alternative medicine (CAM) cost-effective? A systematic review. BMC Complement Altern Med. 2005;5:11.
75. Block KI. Cost savings with clinical solutions: the impact of reforming health and health care economics with integrative therapies. Integr Cancer Ther. 2010;9:129–35.
76. Cangelosi PR, Sorrell JM. Walking for therapy with man's best friend. J Psychosoc Nurs Ment Health Serv. 2010;48:19–22.
77. Singh H, Maskarinec G, Shumay DM. Understanding the motivation for conventional and complementary/alternative medicine use among men with prostate cancer. Integr Cancer Ther. 2005;4:187–94.
78. Evans M, Shaw A, Thompson EA, et al. Decisions to use complementary and alternative medicine (CAM) by male cancer patients: information-seeking roles and types of evidence used. BMC Complement Altern Med. 2007;7:25.
79. Beatty L, Koczawara B, Knott V, Wade T. Why people choose to not use complementary therapies during cancer treatment: a focus group study. Eur J Cancer Care. 2012;21:98–106.
80. Trinidade A, Shakeel M, Hurman D, Hussain A. Traditional and complementary and alternative medicines make for unwilling bedfellows in the management of cancer: a case report with a tragic outcome. J Laryngol Otol. 2011;125:1193–5.
81. Snyder M, Lindquist R. Complementary & alternative therapies in nursing. 6th ed. New York: Springer; 2010.
82. American Cancer Society. Complete guide to complementary & alternative cancer therapies. 2nd ed. American Cancer Society Health Promotions Publishing: Atlanta; 2009.
83. Matuszek S. Animal-facilitated therapy in various patient populations: systematic literature review. Holist Nurs Pract. 2010;24:187–203.
84. Bercovitz A, Sengupta M, Jones A, Harris-Kojetin LD. Complementary and alternative therapies in hospice: the National Home and Hospice Care Survey: United States, 2007. National Health Statistics Report. 2011;33:1–20.
85. Motooka M, Koike H, Yokoyuki T, Kennedy NL. Effect of dog-walking on autonomic nervous activity in senior citizens. Med J Aust. 2006;184:60–3.
86. Muschel IJ. Pet therapy with terminal cancer patients. Soc Casework. 1984;65:451–8.

Introduction to Therapy Dogs

2

Key Chapter Points

- Complementary treatments may include goal-directed dog visits to specific populations, called *animal-assisted therapy*, or more casual encounters designed to provide socialization and increase comfort, called *animal-assisted activities*.
- Therapy dogs may be permitted into areas that may typically restrict animals (e.g., schools, hospitals, and hospices) during the time when the dogs are providing therapeutic services.
- Therapy dog visits have been shown to provide both subjective and objective improvements in pediatric, adult, and geriatric populations with a broad range of medical conditions.
- Studies have shown significant physiological changes in humans after experiencing therapy dog visits.
- Ethical issues surrounding therapy dog visits have been addressed.

Keywords

Animal-assisted • Assistance dog • Chromogranin A • Cortisol • Ethics • IgA • Service dog

Working dogs have been helping people with medical disabilities by serving as service or assistance dogs for centuries. The concept of deriving comfort and cheer from trained dogs as a therapeutic intervention is a newer model of the working dog. Nurse Elaine Smith began formal therapy dog work after noticing improvements in patients visited by a chaplain who was accompanied by his Golden Retriever. In 1976, nurse Smith founded Therapy Dogs International (TDI), a volunteer organization that focuses on testing and registering dog-handler therapy teams and promoting their therapy work. TDI currently has volunteer handlers registered in all 50 states in the United States and in Canada. In 2010, about 24,000 dog-handler teams were registered with TDI [1]. Delta Society is another animal-human service organization that trains volunteers and their pets for therapy visits through their Pet Partners® program. The social

D.A. Marcus, *Therapy Dogs in Cancer Care: A Valuable Complementary Treatment*,
DOI 10.1007/978-1-4614-3378-1_2, © Springer Science+Business Media New York 2012

nature of dogs and positive aspects of bonding that occur through dog-handler training make therapy work beneficial for both the dog and the patients visited [2].

Today, the value of therapy dogs is increasingly recognized across a broad range of medical specialties as a potential complementary therapy that adds value with minimal additional costs to treatment programs. Complementary therapy is defined as treatment that supports, facilitates, or enhances conventional treatment strategies. The sixth edition of Snyder and Lindquist's *Complementary & Alternative Therapies in Nursing* and Miller's *Handbook of Stressful Transitions Across the Lifespan* each includes a chapter devoted to the therapeutic use of animals [3, 4].

Practical Pointer: Animal-assisted interventions meet the National Institutes of Health definition of a mind-body intervention complementary therapy to facilitate the mind's ability to affect bodily functions and symptoms [5].

Animal-Assisted Therapy Versus Animal-Assisted Activities

Therapeutic interventions using trained animals are divided into animal-assisted therapy or animal-assisted activities. *Animal-assisted therapy* refers to animal-human encounters where a defined interaction will be used for a select patient or patient group, with that intervention designed to effect a specific goal. Animal-assisted therapy is a goal-directed intervention in which animals meeting specific criteria are incorporated into the treatment process for patients with selected health conditions to achieve a specific target outcome (Table 2.1) [6–11]. With animal-assisted therapy, the dog interaction is intended to produce a specific and measurable target improvement for an identified patient population, using the therapy dog interaction as complementary treatment in conjunction with other medical procedures.

Practical Pointer: Animal-assisted *therapy* provides interventions to a targeted group to achieve a specific, prespecified outcome. Animal-assisted therapy is directed by medical personnel who monitor for outcomes.

Animal-assisted activities are nondirected, casual encounters between therapy dogs and individuals with a wide range of needs. These encounters occur without an expectation of a specific improvement. Animal-assisted activities are often called *pet therapy* and generally involve a nonmedical volunteer dog handler and therapy dog interacting with people with a wide range of needs, which may include patients or nursing home residents, facility visitors, and staff members. Animal-assisted activities may be delivered by trained lay volunteers to individuals with a variety of health issues, as well as healthy individuals. Trained handler volunteers may take their therapy dogs to visit people in schools, nursing homes, hospitals, hospices, and other facilities to provide education, comfort, and companion services. Benefits from animal-assisted activities are often difficult to quantify; however, a recent review of 14 papers describing animal-assisted activities with therapy dogs reported a broad range of improvements (Box 1) [12].

Box 1 Patient Benefits from Therapy Dog Visits (Based on [12])

- Improved cardiopulmonary pressures and neurohormone levels
- Reduced stress, anxiety, and loneliness
- Improved mood and general well-being
- Improved social functioning
- Improved motivation for participation in therapy
- Increased interest in self, others, and the environment

Table 2.1 Samples of animal-assisted therapy interventions that have each been shown to achieve therapeutic goals

Reference	Study population	Target goal	Intervention	Study outcome
[6]	40 pediatric dental visits	Reduced anxiety response with dental procedure as measured by skin temperature. Increased temperature occurs with relaxation and decreased temperature with anxiety	Procedure randomly conducted with or without dog present at child's side	Significant reduction with dog visit among children reporting fear of dental visits. Among fearful children, change in skin temperature from baseline was +2.2°F while waiting for the dentist and −1.3°F during the procedure with dog present; without the dog, change versus baseline was −1.7°F while waiting and −3.6°F after the procedure
[7]	20 geriatric patients with schizophrenia on closed psychogeriatric ward	Improved mobility, socialization, and activities of daily living	Weekly 4-hour sessions with cat or dog over 1 year	Enhanced socialization and activities of daily living. Significant improvement in Social Adaptive Functioning Evaluation with animal-assisted therapy (35%, $P<0.01$) and not in control group (14%, NS). Animals served as "modeling companions" helping patients recognize how to improve their own behaviors by watching how the dog responded to others, interacted, and stayed active
[8]	35 severely depressed adults awaiting ECT treatment	Reduced psychological distress	15 min sitting in a room with a therapy dog or a room with magazines before treatment	Fear was significantly reduced ($P=0.0006$) and anxiety showed a trend toward significant reduction ($P=0.098$) with the dog visit compared with control
[9]	76 adult patients admitted to cardiac care unit or cardiac observation unit for advanced heart failure with mean left ventricular ejection fraction of 23% and New York Heart Association functional class III or IV	Reductions in hemodynamic parameters and neurohormone levels	12-min therapy dog visit versus 12-min visit from volunteer without dog versus usual care	Compared with usual care, patients receiving dog therapy had significantly greater decreases in systolic PAP (mean difference—5.78 mm Hg, $P=0.001$), PCWP (mean difference—4.31 mm Hg, $P=0.001$), and anxiety ($P<0.001$); catecholamine levels were similar between groups
				Compared with the volunteer-only group, the volunteer-dog group had significantly greater decreases in systolic PAP (mean difference—5.34 mm Hg, $P=0.002$), PCWP (mean difference—3.10 mm Hg, $P=0.02$), epinephrine (mean difference −17.54 pg/mL, $P=0.04$), norepinephrine (mean difference—240.29 pg/mL, $P=0.02$), and anxiety ($P=0.002$)
				Heart rate, blood pressure, cardiac index, and SVR were not significantly affected by the intervention
[10]	57 hospitalized children ages 3–17 with pain	Pain reduction on 0–5 pain scale	15- to 20-min visit with a therapy dog versus sitting quietly for 15 min	Significantly better improvements with dog visit versus quiet sitting for pain (34% versus 6% reduction, $P=0.006$)

ECT electroconvulsive shock therapy, *PAP* pulmonary artery pressure, *PCWP* pulmonary capillary wedge pressure, *SVR* systemic vascular resistance

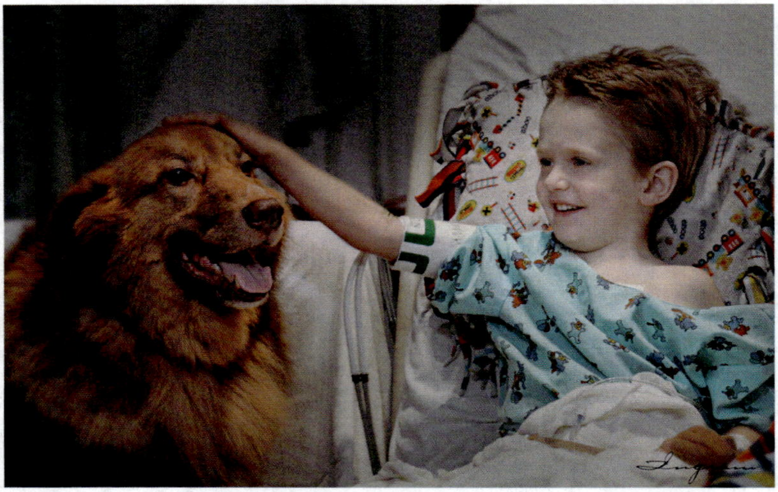

Fig. 2.1 Casual visits from Nova Scotia Duck Tolling Retriever therapy dog Cody is an example of an animal-assisted activity (Photo courtesy of Patricia A. M. Ingram of Ingram Portrait Design)

> **Practical Pointer:** Animal-assisted *activities* are untailored, nondirected encounters between the therapeutic animal and a potentially broad range of visit recipient types. Animal-assisted activities are offered with no specific outcome targeted.

Animal-assisted therapy and activities can utilize a wide diversity of animals, including pet dogs and cats, horses, and even dolphins [13] (see Fig. 2.1). In some cases, patient-owned animals may be permitted to visit their hospitalized owners; because these pets lack the certification for good health, exemplary behavior, and safety required of trained therapy dogs, these visits should be restricted to the pet's owner and should not include other patients or staff members [14]. Some long-term residential facilities may also include live-in, residential animals to provide comfort and companionship for their residents. A simple fish aquarium may also provide a useful animal-assisted intervention. A group of 62 patients with Alzheimer's disease living in specialized units had food intake during meals measured at baseline and after a fish aquarium or a photo of an aquarium was placed in the dining area [15]. There was no significant change in nutritional intake in the group with the aquarium photo in the dining room. Food intake and weight increased for most patients exposed to the aquarium (87% of patients). The average increase in nutritional intake after introduction of the aquarium was a 21% increase in food consumed ($P<0.001$). Food intake increase was noted across all meals monitored during the study. Costly nutritional supplementation also decreased, and patients viewing the fish tank gained an average of 1.65 pounds over the 16-week study ($P<0.001$).

Example of Successful Animal-Assisted Therapy for Cancer Patients

The impact of a range of animal-assisted activities was evaluated for a day hospice in the UK where most of the terminally ill patients were diagnosed with cancer [16]. The facility included a resident parakeet, a tropical fish tank, a garden pool with gold fish, and two visiting friendly Cocker Spaniels. Fifty patients and staff at the day care hospice were surveyed. Most of the 37 patients had owned a pet during their lives, while two reported a dislike of animals and another one reported having been bitten by a dog. None of the patients, however, objected to including the Cocker Spaniels at the facility as long as the dogs were well behaved. Of those seven individuals currently living with a companion pet, the pet was often considered to be their "closest companion, because it was more available than their [human] family" (p. 337).

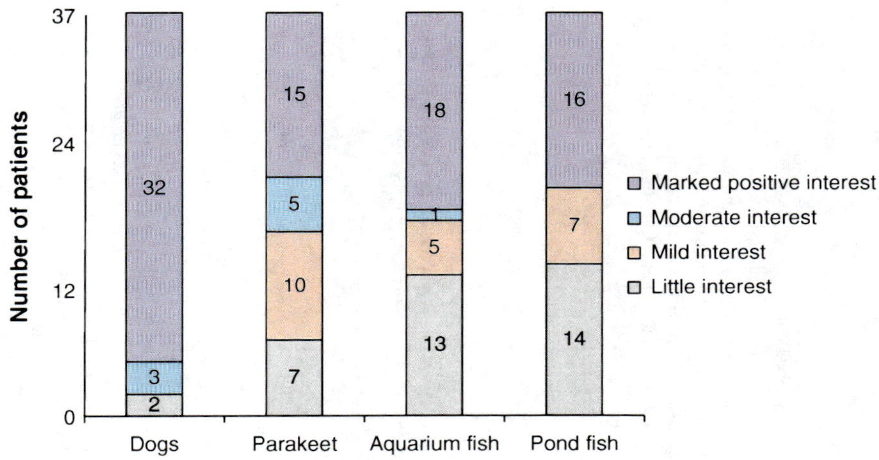

Fig. 2.2 Attitudes of 37 terminally ill patients toward animals available at a day hospice (Based on [16])

In this study, patients endorsed generally positive perceptions of each animal-assisted activity option, with substantially more positive impressions about the two Cocker Spaniels (Fig. 2.2). Staff and facility volunteers reported a range of benefits from the dog visits (Box 2). Concerns were raised about visiting dogs needing to be well mannered and clean, which are requirements for therapy dog certification (see Chap. 5). Interestingly, the author of this study noted that, following completion of this study, the facility incorporated therapy dog visits as a regular complementary medicine program at the hospice.

Box 2 Benefits from Dog Visits for Hospice Patients (Based on [16])

- Relaxation for patients and staff
- Lightening of facility mood
- More homelike, nonclinical environment
- Affection
- Attentive audience
- Social lubricant bringing people together
- Tool to facilitate positive reminiscences and sharing memories
- Aid for patients to help cope with fear of leaving their own pet when they die

Differentiating Working Dogs: Therapy Dog Versus Service Dog

The terms *service dog* (or *assistance dog* in Europe) and *therapy dog* are often confused. Both therapy dogs and service dogs undergo special training, testing, and certification and provide important service to humans; however, their roles are very different (Table 2.2).

Practical Pointer: As working dogs, service dogs and therapy dogs both provide valuable but very different types of services to humans.

Service dogs are used to help individuals with special needs or disabilities. A service dog is a dog that has been specially trained to perform specific tasks needed by the individual with a disability who has become his partner. Service dogs have been trained to help individuals with visual/hearing/motor impairments, post-traumatic stress disorder, autism, and a wide range of other disabling conditions by providing specific skills that help improve human independence. Some service dogs are also trained as medical detection dogs, for example, alerting their humans with epilepsy to impending seizures, patients with diabetes to hypoglycemia, and individuals with Addison's

Table 2.2 Distinguishing features between service and therapy dogs

	Service dog	Therapy dog
Training	Initially, about two years with a puppy raiser learning basic obedience and socialization. Adult dogs are then evaluated to see if their temperament is appropriate (not fearful, not distractible, remains focused on work, and stays unflappable in every situation). Appropriate adult dogs then receive intense skills training (opening/closing doors, unloading laundry from dryer, removing human's shoes and socks, turning on/off lights, retrieving drop items or phone) Dogs eventually receive special training to meet needs of the human with whom they will be paired	Trained to show calm, obedient behavior. Dogs generally complete at least basic obedience training and therapy dog training. Dog needs to accept clumsy handling and constraining hugs; not startle or bark when exposed to medical equipment, loud noises, people falling, or children playing; and be able to pass other dogs without interacting and food or other items on the floor without picking them up
Service commitment	"On duty" attending to their person most of the time. Dog may be performing specific tasks (e.g., giving money to cashier), monitoring the environment for potential problems, or monitoring the assigned human for changes in behavior or physiology that might alert the dog that actions are necessary	Usually works once a week to once a month for about 1 h. Most of the time, therapy dogs are simply companion dogs
Goal of dog interaction	Improve the independence of the single individual to whom the dog is assigned	To provide comfort and cheer to patients, visitors, and staff during facility visits
Expected behavior around working dog	People should avoid distracting a service dog from his work	After obtaining permission from the dog's handler, people are encouraged to interact with and pet a therapy dog
Legal standing	Dogs are permitted wherever their human might go—buses, restaurants, stores, etc.	No legal recognition of therapy dogs. Facilities may choose to allow therapy dogs into hospitals, nursing homes, hospices, schools, and libraries but only during the times when dogs are providing therapy services. Therapy dogs are not permitted at other times and have no legal right to use public transportation, go into stores or restaurants, etc.

disease to low cortisol levels. Federal laws protect the rights of individuals with disabilities to be accompanied by their service dogs in public places, as the dogs are not considered to be "pets." A service dog is considered to be on duty working most of the time every day, serving the needs of the single human with whom he is partnered.

Practical Pointer: Service dogs need to maintain focus on their human partner and required tasks for long periods of time without becoming distracted by animals, toys, or other people. During training, 70% of dogs who fail to successfully complete service dog certification do so because of behavioral problems, most commonly problems with becoming distracted [17].

Therapy dogs, conversely, are not legally defined by federal law [18]. Therapy dogs are generally pet dogs which have been trained to be obedient, social, and well mannered. Unlike a service dog that needs to maintain focus for extended periods of time on a single individual, a therapy dog often provides attention to a wide variety of individuals when making visits. The therapy dog is teamed with a handler who is responsible for the dog's care and needs during visits. The handler is the human who schedules the dog's visits, provides transportation, and attends to the dog. Unlike other volunteers who may visit nursing home residents and hospital patients, a therapy dog handler is primarily focused on the dog during visits, monitoring interactions to ensure each dog encounter is positive and safe. Conversations handlers have with patients are usually steered to focus attention onto the dog. The dog and handler are generally certified as a therapy dog team. Typically, the dog is also the handler's companion pet. When the therapy dog is working, it is expected to remain quiet, calm, and obedient. Therapy dogs must also accept attention from a diversity of strangers who may or may not be familiar with dogs; therefore, therapy dogs are trained not to react negatively to clumsy handling, restraining hugs, or other behaviors that might typically cause a dog to bark, pull away, or nip. After completing visits, the therapy dog may behave like any other companion dog, with no particular expectations of being attuned to the needs of humans in his environment.

Practical Pointer: The therapy dog *handler* is the human responsible for caring for the therapy dog during and between visits and ensuring visits are positive and safe. The handler is most often also the dog's owner.

Medical Studies Evaluating Benefits from Therapy Dog Visits

Medical benefits have been shown for incorporating dog interactions into patient care to reduce symptoms of distress and discomfort in individuals with a broad range of health conditions, including cardiovascular disease, psychiatric illness, dementia, autism, and diabetes (Table 2.3) [19–27]. These studies highlight common objective and subjective benefits from therapy dog encounters, including improvements in socialization, mood, a sense of well-being, and pain. Levels of anxiety and stress responses are typically reduced, and patients often report a reduction in their sense of isolation (see Fig. 2.3).

Limitations with Therapy Dog Studies

Despite the availability of literature evaluating the benefits of therapy dog visits, it is important to recognize that interpreting data from therapy dogs is limited by a number of factors. First, most studies have been relatively small and lack blinding. Even studies that provide comparator groups (e.g., sitting in a quiet room, talking with a volunteer, or sitting with a stuffed dog) do not permit blinding of the individual receiving the intervention or the evaluator. Furthermore, while objective changes in biological measures (including vital signs, heart

Table 2.3 Examples of therapy dog interventions over a range of medical conditions

Reference	Medical condition (sample size)	Intervention	Outcome
[19]	Children with pervasive developmental disorders ($N=10$)	While interacting with a therapist over 15 min, children were exposed to three different conditions: nonsocial toy ball, stuffed dog, and therapy dog. Each visit used only one condition which rotated among visits, with children meeting three times weekly for 15 weeks	Children exhibited a more playful mood, were more focused, and were more aware of their social environments when in the presence of a therapy dog. Children were also more likely to talk to the dog, initiating numerous conversations and verbal exchanges
[20]	Aphasia due to left hemispheric stroke ($N=3$)	Weekly 30-min speech therapy administered over 12 weeks without therapy dog followed by 12 weeks with therapy dog	Aphasia scores improved an average of 7.5 with traditional therapy and 8.3 with therapy administered with the dog present. Participants also reported greater improvement and greater motivation to work in therapy when the dog was present
[21]	Schizophrenia inpatients ($N=30$)	Random assignment to weekly 50-min therapy dog sessions for 2 months versus usual care control	Improvements with therapy dog interaction versus control, respectively: self-esteem improved 62% with dog versus 2% worse with control ($P=0.025$), self-determination improved 59% versus 2% worse ($P=0.020$), positive symptoms reduced 43% versus 4% worse ($P=0.005$), negative symptoms reduced 24% versus 8% worse ($P=0.097$), and emotional symptoms reduced 63% versus 0.9% worse ($P=0.048$)
[22]	Children with type 1 diabetes ($N=7$)	Three times weekly exercise over 12 weeks that included running a dog through an agility obstacle course versus nonexercising control group	After 3 months, insulin requirements were significantly reduced ($P<0.05$) with exercise with no change with control condition
[23]	Alzheimer's dementia in day care ($N=10$)	Two weeks baseline, 3 weeks control with stuffed dog, and 3 weeks therapy dog visits. Both control and dog visit activities were conducted with a group of patients with about 10 min of patient interaction with the stuffed or real dog three times weekly	No changes occurred after three weeks with stuffed dog interaction. Significant improvements occurred after the therapy dog intervention period for anxiety ($P=0.04$), sadness ($P=0.002$), and general alertness ($P=0.003$). Significant improvements also occurred with the therapy dog visits for motor activity ($P=0.017$) and vocal expression ($P=0.002$)
[24]	Chronic heart failure in hospital ($N=69$)	Ambulation with a restorative aide was offered with a therapy dog walking with the patient. Compared with historical heart failure population of 537 patients	7% refusal rate with walking offered with therapy dog versus 28% historical refusal rate ($P<0.0002$). Average distance walked was 235 steps when walking with dog versus 120 steps in historical control without the therapy dog ($P<0.0001$)

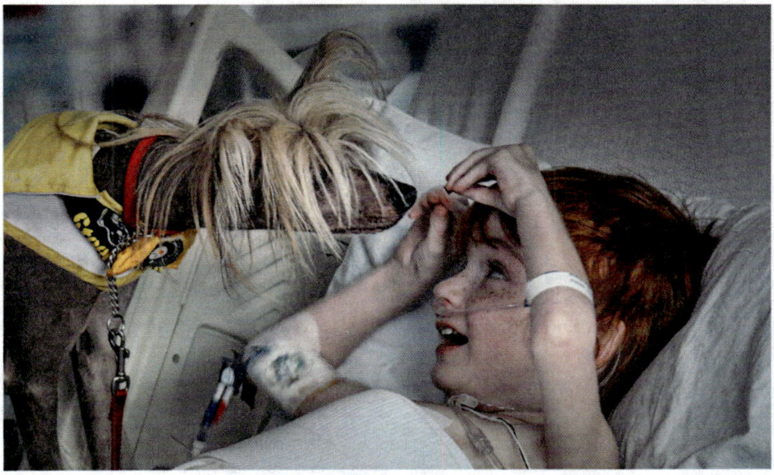

Fig. 2.3 When Chinese Crested therapy dog Ike visits patients at Children's Hospital in Pittsburgh, his handler is used to hearing, "This is the first time my child has smiled." (Photo courtesy of Patricia A. M. Ingram of Ingram Portrait Design)

pressure readings, and blood chemistries) have been evaluated in some therapy dog studies, most studies have relied on subjective measures rated by the individual or the investigator. While these limitations do not negate the findings of research studies, they do require that greater caution be used when interpreting the strength of findings and results.

Patient Benefits from Therapy Dog Visits

Typical therapy dog visits provided to a wide spectrum of patients have been shown to significantly improve a broad range of symptoms. Benefits have been reported across a wide range of patient ages, including pediatric, adult, and geriatric patients. Patients experiencing therapy dog visits verbalize a variety of positive benefits (Box 3) [28, 29]. These reports focus on psychosocial improvements related to the dog encounter. Researchers from Massachusetts General Hospital measured heart and breathing rates, pain severity, level of energy, and mood in 59 hospitalized adults (mean age 59.6 ± 15.7 years, 49.3% male) before and after a 10-min therapy dog visit [30]. Patients were evenly distributed between those with medical diagnoses (e.g., cancer, asthma, acquired immune deficiency syndrome [AIDS], cardiovascular disease, diabetes, and gastrointestinal bleeding) and those admitted for surgery (e.g., amputation, hysterectomy, aneurysm repair, venous bypass surgery, gastrointestinal surgery, and carotid endarterectomy). About half of the participants were pet owners (47.5%). Significant improvements occurred over a range of symptoms (Fig. 2.4).

Box 3 Benefits Reported by Pediatric and Adult Patients After Receiving a Therapy Dog Visit (Based on [28] and [29])

- Therapy dog visits give patients a welcome distraction from illness, symptoms, and worry.
- Therapy dogs have a calming effect.
- Snuggling with or petting a dog is comforting.
- Therapy dogs bring patients a positive "piece of home."
- Therapy dogs bring happiness to patients.
- Therapy dogs give people something to talk about with their visitors, fellow patients or nursing home residents, and staff members.

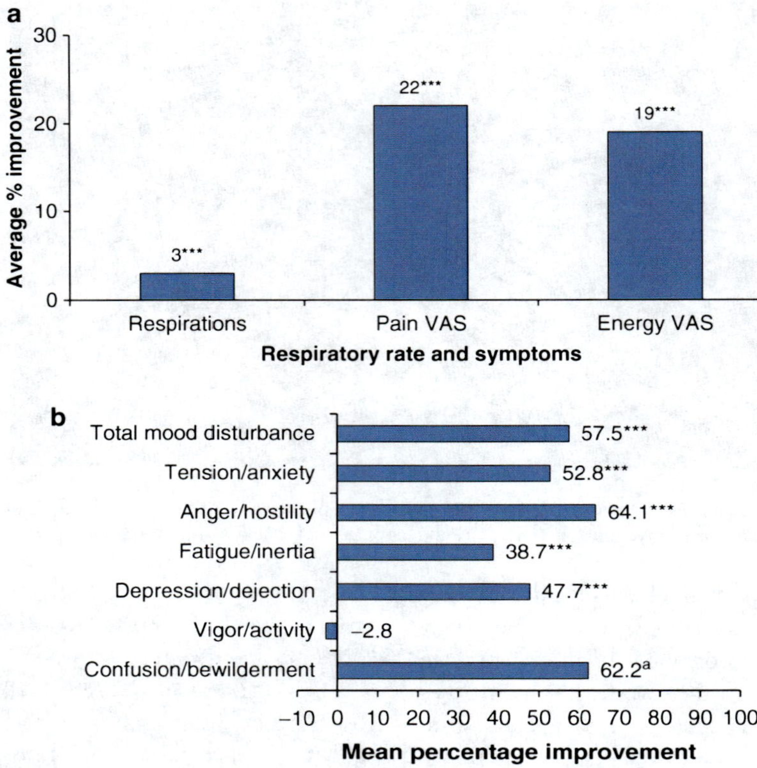

Fig. 2.4 Mean changes after 10-min therapy dog visit. Significant mean change versus baseline: [a]$P=0.06$, [***]$P\leq0.001$. (Based on [30]). (**a**) Respirations per minute and visual analogue scales (VAS). (**b**) Profile of Mood States (POMS) survey total and subscale scores (POMS is a 30-item self-report measure that assesses 6 transient mood states in which patients rate current mood on a scale from 0 [not at all] to 4 [extreme] [31]. Total mood disturbance score is also calculated)

Mood Enhancement

A meta-analysis of a total of 254 subjects evaluated in five randomized studies that included a control group concluded that animal-assisted activities and therapy effectively reduce depression (Fig. 2.5) [32]. A study not included in the meta-analysis compared outcome in depressed adult college students randomly assigned to receive therapy dog treatment or a nontreatment control [33]. Patients were divided into one of three groups: psychotherapy plus therapy dog visits ($N=9$), therapy dog visits alone ($N=12$), or a control group ($N=23$). Treatment sessions lasting 45 min occurred weekly for 7 weeks. Beck depression inventory (BDI) was measured at baseline and at study completion. At baseline, BDI scores were lower in the control group, which may have limited the ability of the control group to improve over time. In comparison to improvement among controls, reduction in BDI was significantly better among the group treated with the therapy dog intervention alone (Fig. 2.6). While six of the nine participants in the psychotherapy plus therapy dog group experienced reductions in depression scores, change in overall group score was not significant. Participants in the psychotherapy group reported that the presence of the dog helped provide a safe diversion and comfort during intense therapy moments. Researchers postulated that some of the benefits from the therapy dog visit might have been lost during the psychotherapy plus therapy dog intervention by focusing psychotherapy conversations on painful and emotionally charged issues.

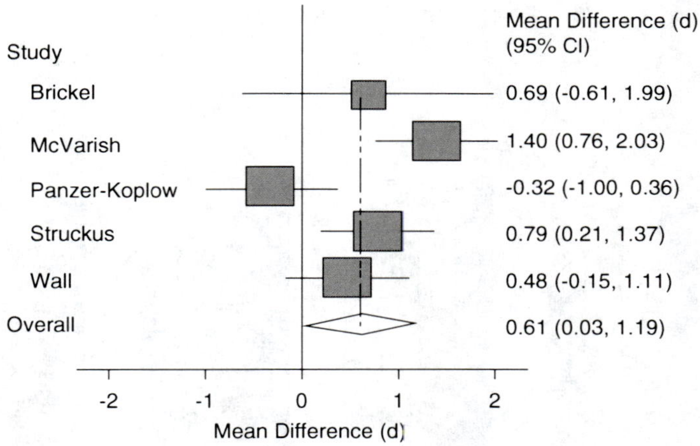

Fig. 2.5 Forest plot of standardized mean difference effect sizes for depression symptoms following animal-assisted therapy, with positive differences reflecting lower depressive symptoms in the therapy group. Box sizes are proportional to the sample size in each study (Reproduced with permission [32])

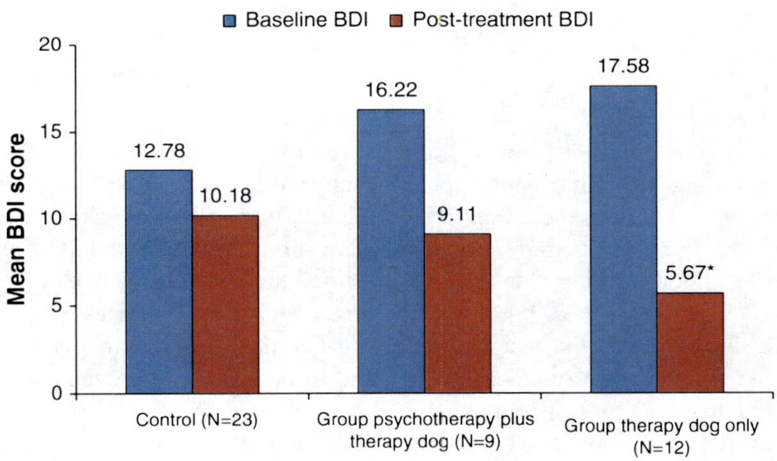

Fig. 2.6 Mood improvement with therapy dog visits for depressed college students. Beck depression inventory (BDI) scores >9 indicate depression, with scores ≥16 suggesting moderate to severe depression. Change from baseline was significantly better for the therapy dog only group versus controls: $*P<0.05$ (Based on [33])

Change in anxiety among adults hospitalized for psychiatric disorders was measured before and after a 30-min group therapy dog interaction ($N=93$) or a recreational therapy session ($N=137$) using the Spielberger State-Trait Anxiety Inventory [34]. In this study, recreational therapy included education about leisure activities plus music and art activities. Among patients with primary mood disorders, significant improvements in anxiety occurred after both interventions (Fig. 2.7). Anxiety reduction, however, was only significant after the therapy dog intervention for patients with psychotic disorders or other psychiatric conditions.

Pain Relief

Several studies have evaluated pain-relieving effects of brief therapy dog visits to general samples of pediatric and adult patients. Pain was significantly reduced in a sample of hospitalized children with pain (51% male; average age = 12.1 years, range 3–17) receiving a therapy

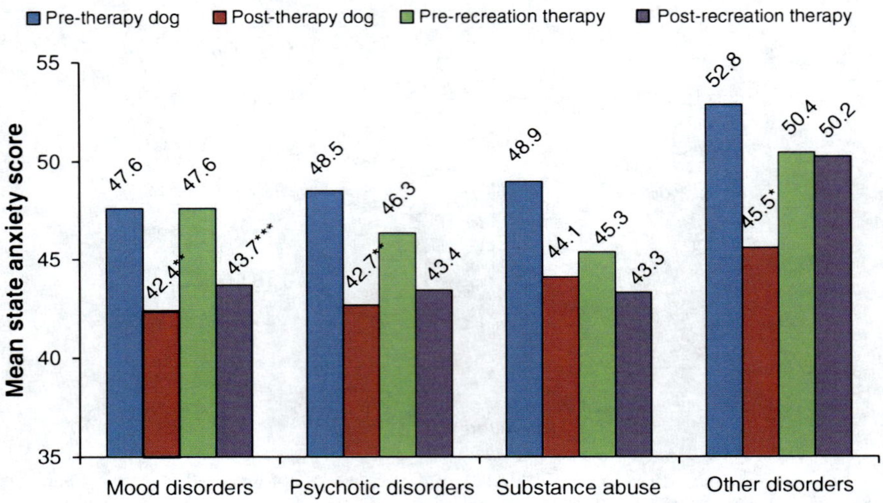

Fig. 2.7 State-Trait Anxiety Inventory scores among hospitalized psychiatric patients. Scores >40 are generally considered to correspond to anxiety. Significant improvement versus baseline: $*P<0.05$, $**P\leq0.01$, $***P=0.001$ (Based on [34])

dog visit [11]. Using an 11-point severity scale (0 = no pain; 10 = worst pain imaginable), pain decreased significantly more in the 18 children participating in a 15- to 20-min therapy dog visit compared with 39 children sitting alone quietly for 15 min (−1.6 versus −0.3, $P=0.006$). Another small, pediatric study ($N=25$) likewise showed significant pain reduction using a faces scale when children with acute postoperative pain spent 11–20 min with a therapy dog [28]. Pain relief with a therapy dog interaction was indirectly measured in adults with brain or spinal cord injuries, degenerative diseases, or severe physical disabilities living in a rehabilitation facility ($N=58$; 55% male, age range 24–60 years) [35]. Average as needed analgesic consumption was evaluated during the 3 months before and the 9 months after an 18-month-old Collie therapy dog had been added to the facility. In comparison to typical pre-intervention medications, as needed analgesic use decreased by 48% after a therapy dog had been added to facility, which indirectly suggests reduced pain severity.

Therapy dog visits have also been shown to significantly reduce pain in patients being treated for pain complaints [36]. Using an 11-point severity scale, pain reduction was evaluated in adult chronic pain patients attending a tertiary pain management clinic. Patients were surveyed before and after participating in a brief therapy dog visit ($N=235$; mean visit time = 11.1 min) or spending quiet time in the usual clinic waiting room area where magazines and a television were available ($N=83$; mean waiting room duration = 16.4 min). Significant pain reduction occurred after the therapy dog visit ($P<0.0001$) but not the waiting room control (Fig. 2.8). Clinically meaningful pain relief is defined as a decrease in pain severity ≥2 points, which corresponds to "much better" improvement [37–40]. Clinically meaningful relief occurred in 23% of pain patients after the therapy dog visit and 4% in the waiting room control. In addition, patients reporting moderate to severe pain (≥5) experience substantial pain-related interference and disability [41]. Among those patients with pain ≥5, clinically meaningful pain relief occurred for 26% visiting the therapy dog and 3% in the waiting room control. Benefits were not influenced by participant gender, comorbid mood disorder, or visit duration.

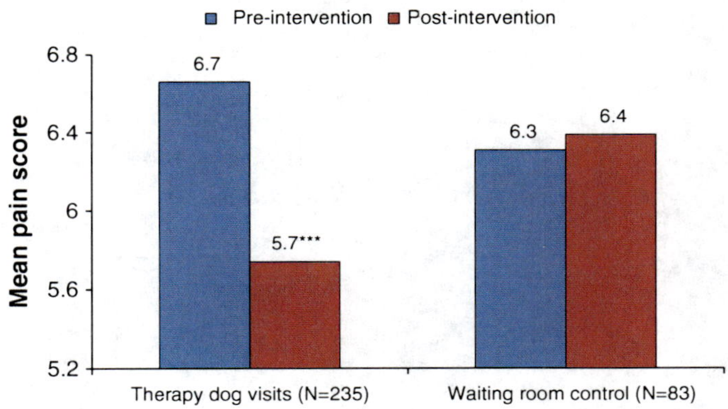

Fig. 2.8 Mean pain scores before and after therapy dog visit versus waiting room control. Improvement from baseline was significant after the dog visit, $^{***}P<0.0001$. (Based on [36])

Loneliness Reduction

A small study ($N=8$) reported that monthly therapy dogs visiting older women with dementia in a nursing home (age range 67–94 years) resulted in reduced loneliness and improved the residents' interaction and communication with the staff and fellow residents [29]. Loneliness was also evaluated in a larger study of 45 elderly residents without cognitive impairment living in one of three nursing homes [42]. In this 6-week study, residents were randomized to receive therapy dog visits once weekly, therapy dog visits three times weekly, or no therapy dog visits. Therapy dog visits lasted 30 min. Loneliness was measured using the UCLA-Loneliness Scale, which scores loneliness from 20 (never lonely) to 80 (always lonely). Loneliness was measured before each nursing home facility began receiving therapy dog visits and prior to the final therapy dog visit. There was a significant drop in loneliness among residents getting therapy dog visits, compared with those not getting visits (Fig. 2.9). Reduction in loneliness was similar between the two therapy dog groups. This study additionally highlighted that benefits from therapy dog visits persist between visits. For those residents in the once weekly group, their post-intervention assessment would have occurred a week after their last visit with the therapy dog, supporting that benefits extend beyond the time of the actual visit.

Benefits for Patient Supporters and Caregivers

Animal-assisted activities may also aid patients indirectly. Therapy dog handlers anecdotally describe positive interactions with observed changes that suggest reduced stress and improved mood when staff and patient family members receive visits from therapy dogs, even without the patient being present or engaged in the visit (Fig. 2.10). Reduced stress and anxiety in individuals interacting with patients may improve patient care. In addition, experts have recommended that interventions to help address emotional needs of carers for cancer patients be brief, due to the time demands placed on these individuals caring for seriously ill patients [43]. Brief therapy dog visits may fulfill needs for both emotional support and brevity of therapeutic intervention.

In the tertiary pain clinic study reported above, effects of therapy dog interactions were also evaluated in family and friends accompanying patients to appointments and clinic staff [36]. Therapy dog visits were completed by 34 family/friends (mean visit time = 10.2 min) and 26 staff members (mean visit time = 8.2 min), with quiet time in a waiting area assessed for six family/friends (mean time = 13.3 min) and seven staff (mean time = 19.7 min). Participants rated a variety of symptoms on an 11-point severity scale (0 = symptom is absent; 10 = symptom is extreme).

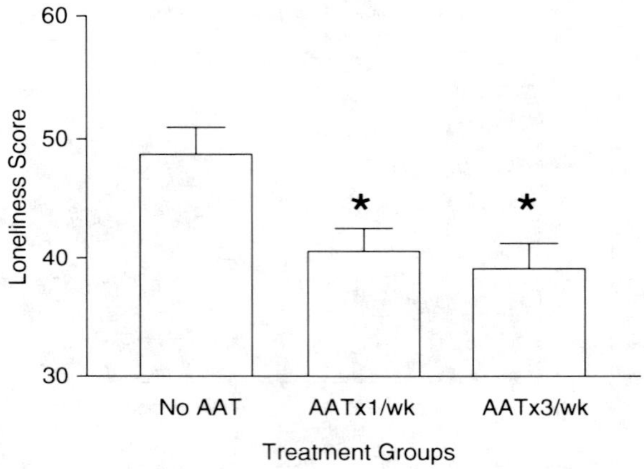

Fig. 2.9 Mean UCLA-Loneliness Scale scores in each group after 6 weeks. Animal-assisted therapy (AAT) was provided once (AATx1/wk) or three times (AATx3/wk) weekly. Differences between control group and therapy dog groups at study completion were significant: $*P=0.001$ (Reprinted with permission [42])

Case 1

Therapy dogs can help foster healthy social connections. AM was a 10-year-old-girl hospitalized at Children's Hospital in Pittsburgh for treatment of Ewing's sarcoma. She enjoyed receiving visits from the hospital therapy dogs, although some days she was too tired and would pass up dog visits. AM, however, would never pass up a visit with her favorite dog, a 217-pound Mastiff named George. Initially impressed by George's size and gentle spirit, AM developed a strong bond with George, lightening up and smiling widely as soon as she spotted him. Over the two years during which AM had periodic hospital treatments, she shared secrets with George and posted his photographs in her room. AM's mother always let George's handler, Amy Coglio, know whenever AM was admitted to the hospital, so George could be certain to make a special visit to AM. AM knew that George would be there for her as a welcome constant during the ups and downs of cancer treatment. In addition to therapy dog work, George was an active competitor in the show dog ring, ranking among the top five Mastiffs in the United States, and AM eagerly awaited reports of his success at each competition. When Pittsburgh hosted a dog show, AM was hospitalized; AM and her family, however, received permission from the doctor for AM to leave the hospital to watch George compete. George won the Mastiff breed competition, presenting AM with his winning ribbon. Through therapy dog visits, AM and her family developed strong connections with George and his handler that helped reduce feelings of aloneness and loneliness that are common during cancer treatment. George offered companionship and opened AM to new experiences to provide healthy distractions from focusing on cancer and cancer treatment.

Significant improvements were seen in a range of measured symptoms following the therapy dog visit (Table 2.4). Lack of significance for most variables among the waiting room control may reflect variability within a small sample size; however, numerical differences for most variables also favored therapy dog visits, particularly among staff members.

Therapy dog visits can provide opportunities for patient visitors and staff members to make

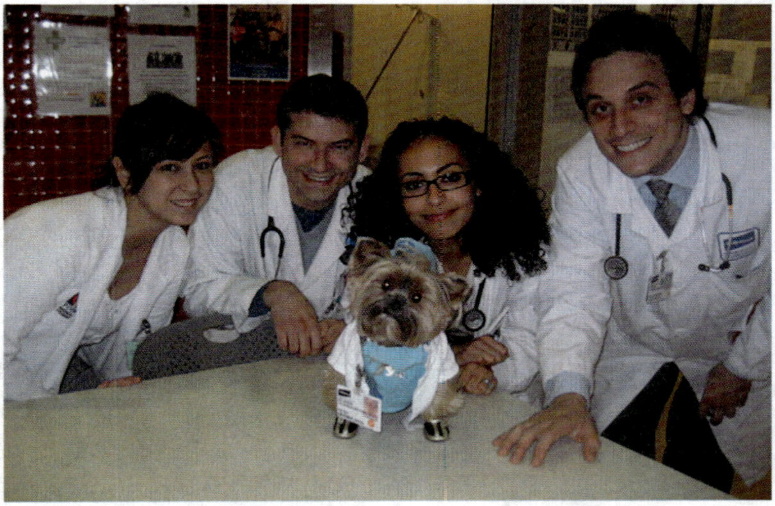

Fig. 2.10 8-year-old Yorkshire terrier therapy dog Petey brings welcome stress relief and happiness to young doctors while making his rounds

Table 2.4 Effect of therapy dog visits on nonpatients, mean (SE)

	Therapy dog visits		Waiting room control	
Symptom	Pre	Post	Pre	Post
Family and friends accompanying patients to appointments				
Fatigue	1.97 (0.41)	1.32 (0.34)**	3.00 (1.41)	1.83 (0.98)
Stress	2.65 (0.45)	1.12 (0.32)***	3.17 (1.22)	4.33 (1.67)
Aggravation	1.91 (0.46)	0.97 (0.36)**	2.17 (1.14)	2.50 (1.46)
Anxiety	2.38 (0.52)	1.18 (0.43)***	4.50 (1.54)	1.67 (0.83)
Sadness	1.59 (0.44)	0.76 (0.33)*	3.83 (1.66)	1.50 (0.96)
Irritability	1.97 (0.52)	1.09 (0.40)*	3.50 (1.29)	3.00 (1.44)
Calm	6.44 (0.55)	8.26 (0.40)***	3.50 (1.54)	4.33 (1.87)
Pleasant	7.18 (0.49)	8.71 (0.33)***	5.17 (1.68)	4.50 (1.77)
Cheerful	7.29 (0.43)	8.56 (0.35)**	4.50 (1.34)	4.17 (1.70)
Staff members				
Fatigue	1.88 (0.37)	1.12 (0.35)**	2.29 (0.92)	2.43 (0.97)
Stress	2.50 (0.41)	0.46 (0.18)***	4.14 (1.26)	3.14 (0.91)
Aggravation	1.58 (0.40)	0.27 (0.16)***	1.71 (0.68)	1.43 (0.65)
Anxiety	1.81 (0.46)	0.65 (0.2.5)**	2.43 (0.78)	2.29 (0.68)
Sadness	0.77 (0.29)	0.35 (0.17)**	1.57 (1.11)	1.29 (0.84)
Irritability	1.50 (0.36)	0.35 (0.15)***	2.86 (0.99)	1.29 (0.57)
Calm	7.00 (0.56)	8.38 (0.47)***	6.71 (0.81)	7.29 (0.87)*
Pleasant	7.65 (0.40)	9.12 (0.19)***	6.14 (1.10)	6.71 (1.06)
Cheerful	7.88 (0.35)	9.12 (0.19)***	5.86 (1.26)	6.29 (1.29)

Significant improvements compared with baseline: $^{*}P<0.05$; $^{**}P<0.01$; $^{***}P\leq 0.001$ (Based on [36])

connections with patients that are not focused on disease or health issues. The dogs can also provide a conversation topic to stimulate healthy communication. Friends, family, and caregivers for cancer patients often have unmet emotional needs [44, 45]. In a survey of 233 adult cancer patients (64% female, average age 60.3 years), having someone to share with was important for

73% of cancer patients and support from neighbors was important for 57% [45]. In some cases, family and friends can feel uncomfortable starting conversations with a loved one diagnosed with cancer. In this same survey, 43% of cancer patients reported needing help dealing with the feelings of others and 41% needed support for dealing with changes in the way others see them. In these cases, initiating conversations by discussing non-emotionally charged topics, like the visiting therapy dog, can act as a catalyst to make other conversations more comfortable.

Case 2

The unconditional love and nonjudgmental acceptance from a therapy dog can also help family and friends of cancer patients, who often need an outlet for their emotions. Seven-year-old Beagle therapy dog Charlie had been abandoned as a puppy and was found to be blind and with a puncture in one eye. Charlie was rescued, both of his eyes removed, and he was trained to be a therapy dog. Charlie visits patients on a hematology/oncology unit at Duke University. Because his eyes have been removed, Charlie's eyelids form closed slits so patients can easily see that he is blind. Charlie's handler Patricia Tirrell recalls how Charlie's disability helped one woman release needed emotions.

> *Charlie had regularly visited a lady in her 40's who was hospitalized with breast cancer. On one visit, she had a friend in the room with her, who seemed very tense and uncomfortable being in the hospital. When we walked into the room, Charlie took his usual spot on the patient's lap. Meanwhile, the patient's friend almost immediately burst into inconsolable sobbing, talking about how terrible it was that Charlie couldn't see. The patient, meanwhile, reassured her friend that Charlie was a wonderful, happy dog who was enjoying life despite the blindness.*
>
> *The patient's nurse later told me that this visit had been so helpful for this patient and her friend. The friend had been unable to share how upset she was to see her friend so sick and Charlie's visit gave this friend a chance to unleash her emotions and for these two women to start a needed conversation.*

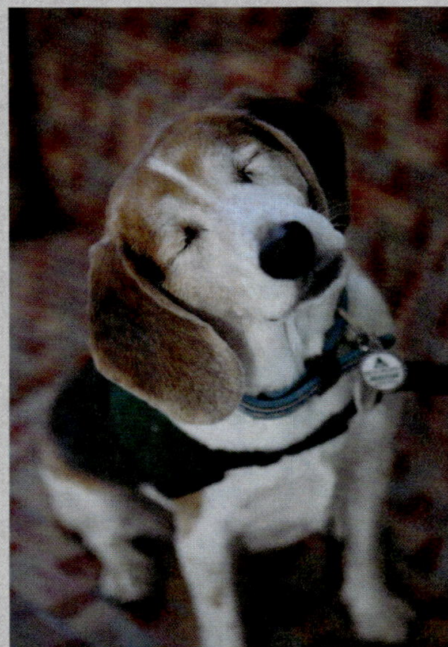

This case illustrates the ability of a nonconfrontational therapy dog visit to act as a lubricant to facilitate important conversations.

Physiological Impact from Dog Visits

Animal-assisted therapy has been critically evaluated to determine the physiology behind identified benefits. Emotional effects have been determined through subjective self-report measurements and objective markers of anxiety, such as respiratory rate, heart rate, and skin temperature. Additional markers of biological change have included measures of neurochemical and immune functions.

In addition, reduced frontal lobe activation has been documented in patients with mood disorders, showing a reduced hemoglobin oxygenation response to cognitive and physiological

Table 2.5 Median values (interquartile range) for physiological markers experiencing a significant change after a positive dog encounter or quiet reading

		Significant change reported with dog visit*		Significant change reported with quiet reading*	
Serum marker	Interpretation of change	Baseline	Post-visit	Baseline	Post-reading
B-endorphin (pmol/L)	Increase linked to pain reduction	3.1 (5.4)	8.0 (6.5)	3.5 (6.7)	5.1 (6.4)
Oxytocin (ng/L)	Increase linked to positive social bonding	2.1 (2.5)	4.0 (1.0)	2.5 (2.0)	2.9 (2.0)
Prolactin (ng/L)	Increase linked to positive social bonding	9.2 (9.1)	11.6 (10.1)	10.2 (7.1)	10.4 (6.2)
Phenyl acetic acid (pg/L)	Increase linked to positive social attachment	123.5 (4.0)	143.0 (8.0)	NR	NR
Dopamine (pg/L)	Increase linked to pleasurable sensations	86.5 (7.0)	107.0 (9.0)	NR	NR
Cortisol (mmol/L)	Decrease linked to positive social bonding and stress relief	317.0 (224.0)	309.0 (222.0)	NR	NR

Only significant changes were reported in this publication, with values representing nonsignificant changes for quiet reading not provided (Based on [49])
NR not reported as significant
*Significant pre- to post-intervention change, $P<0.01$

tasks [46]. Successful drug and nondrug treatments have been shown to improve orbitofrontal abnormalities documented on functional neuroimaging [47]. A recent case report described frontal lobe activation on functional near-infrared spectroscopy in two men with affective disorder after participation in animal-assisted therapy [48].

Practical Pointer: Research demonstrates objective biological benefits to humans from therapy dog visits, including changes in functional neuroimaging, vital signs, and levels of neurochemicals and immune markers.

Neurochemical Changes

Odendaal and Meintjes demonstrated measurable physiological benefits from brief human-dog encounters [49]. Blood pressure and serum neurochemical levels were measured in 18 healthy adults before and after a period of quiet reading and before and after a positive dog interaction. Blood pressure was significantly reduced after the dog visit, with changes occurring over a range of 5–24 min (average time = 15 min). Mean arterial pressure decreased from an average of 87.6 mm Hg before the dog visit to 84.4 mm Hg after the visit ($P<0.01$). Blood pressure was not reported for quiet reading. Significant neurochemical changes occurred with both therapy dog visits and quiet reading; however, more significant improvements occurred with the dog encounter (Table 2.5). Significant reduction in cortisol with the dog visit supports a physiological reduction in the stress response, while increases in the other markers support physiological changes linked to improved mood, social bonding, and pain reduction. Changes for the three parameters that were significant after quiet reading were substantially less than with the dog visit. The authors concluded that therapy dog visits are as relaxing as quiet reading, with additional benefits related to social bonding.

Physiological benefits have also been demonstrated in health-care providers following a therapy dog visit. [50]. Health-care workers were evaluated after a brief 5-min therapy dog visit, a 20-min therapy dog visit, or 20 min of quiet rest. In this study, reduction in cortisol over 60 min

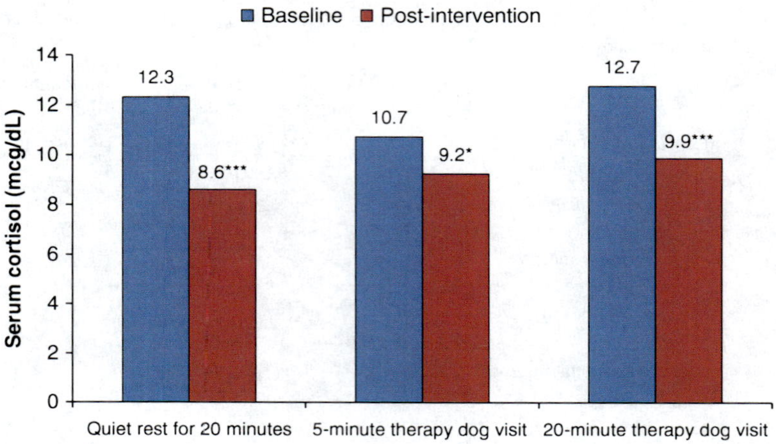

Fig. 2.11 Decreased serum cortisol 1 h post-intervention was used as a marker of stress reduction in health-care providers. Changes versus baseline were significant: $*P<0.05$, $***P\leq0.001$. (Based on [50])

after each intervention was used as a marker of stress relief. All conditions resulted in significant decreases in serum cortisol compared with baseline values (Fig. 2.11). The authors concluded that health-care providers may benefit by experiencing stress relieving changes after very brief therapy dog visits. Furthermore, physiological benefits continued after the staff person was no longer in contact with the dog.

Immune Markers

Therapy dog visits may positively impact the immune system. In an interesting study, 59 college students were randomly assigned to sit on a sofa for 18 min in one of three conditions: petting a 20-pound (9-kg) Shetland sheepdog, petting a stuffed Shetland sheepdog, or sitting quietly alone [51]. Saliva was collected before and after each intervention and evaluated for IgA. A significant increase in IgA occurred when petting the actual dog ($P<0.02$) but not the stuffed dog or when sitting quietly. Prior to study participation, each student also completed the Pet Attitude Scale, which measures attitudes toward companion animals [52]. Pet Attitude Scale scores did not correlate with the immune response, demonstrating that the physiological response was independent of the individual's attitude toward pets.

Case 3

Therapy dog visits should only be provided to individuals agreeable to meeting with a dog. Patients who express fears, allergies, or are otherwise not interested in therapy dogs should not be forced to participate in visits. Both subjective and objective benefits, however, can occur in people who are not dog owners or do not consider themselves to be dog lovers.

During a therapy dog session at an outpatient clinic, a therapist encouraged one of his patients who was having a particularly difficult day to stop in the room to see the Soft-coated Wheaten Terrier therapy dog, Wheatie. The patient entered the room and announced, "I have cats." Wheatie's handler introduced the dog, assured the lady that Wheatie loves cats, and invited her to sit down. The lady frowned, sat in a chair, looked at Wheatie, and asked, "Now what am I supposed to do?" The lady was told she could pet Wheatie if she liked and she responded with a silent look that seemed to express a sentiment that petting a dog would be a silly waste of her time. After 30 s of petting the dog, however, she

(continued)

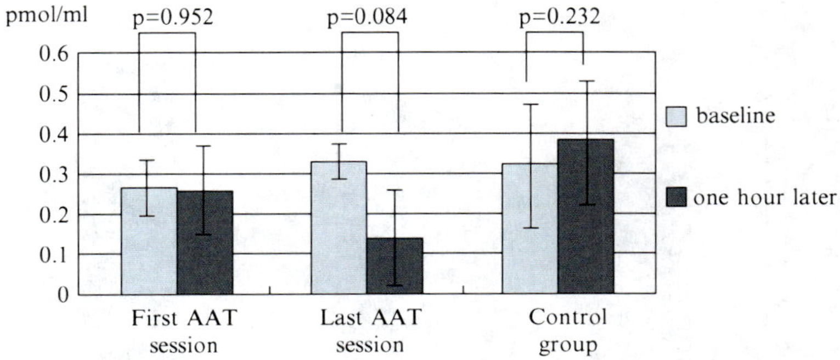

Fig. 2.12 Salivary chromogranin A levels at the beginning of the study (first animal-assisted therapy [First AAT] session), after receiving three months of biweekly therapy dog visits (Last AAT), and in a control group (Reprinted with permission from [53])

Case 3 (continued)
said, "I can't believe it. This really is relaxing." After 2 min, she announced, "It's amazing. Petting Wheatie has really gotten rid of the stress I had after seeing the doctor." After another 10 min, she was smiling, laughing, and said she was going to tell her husband they needed to get a Wheatie for their home.

Stress Response

Stress response was measured in a study evaluating the effect of every other week therapy dog visits for seniors with dementia attending adult day care [53]. Cognitive, behavioral, and stress measurements were made at the beginning of the study and after the dog had been visiting for three months. Mental stress was measured using salivary chromogranin A, a protein produced by the adrenal glands and released when the nervous system is stressed. Therapy dog sessions were provided at the same time each visit, with chromogranin A measured at fixed times before the initiation of a therapy dog visit at 1:15 PM and after visit completion at 2:15 PM to avoid circadian variability. Comparison measures were made in an analogous group at the day care center not receiving therapy dog visits. After the final visit, chromogranin A levels had dropped by 57% in seniors who visited with the therapy dog, compared with a 19% increase in residents who did not receive visits (Fig. 2.12). Changes in memory were not significant for either group (8% improvement on mini mental status examination [MMSE] with therapy dog visits versus 7% decline in controls). Behavioral improvement favored therapy dog visits (35% reduction in behavioral pathology in Alzheimer's Disease Scale [BEHAVE-AD] with therapy dog [$P=0.029$] versus nonsignificant 4% worsening in controls).

Practical Pointer: Documented reductions in stress markers, including cortisol and chromogranin A, support a positive physiological impact from brief therapy dog visits.

Ethics of Dog Therapy

Experts have explored the ethical conflicts of using dogs for human therapy. A philosophical analysis of the ethics of using pets for therapeutic interactions suggests that the social nature of dogs, as well as the positive aspects of bonding that occur through dog-handler training, support including dogs in the therapeutic process [2].

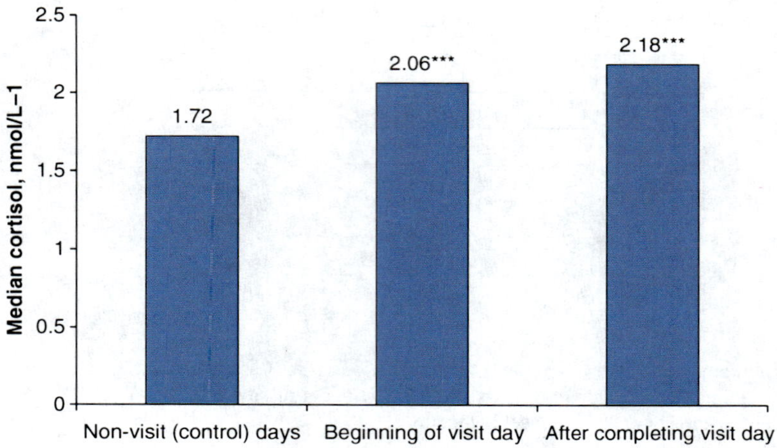

Fig. 2.13 Median cortisol levels in therapy dogs. Differences in median cortisol levels between control and therapy visit days were significant: $^{***}P \leq 0.001$. (Based on [54])

Physiological Changes in Dogs Working as Therapy Dogs

Research studies have also demonstrated measurable positive responses in dogs engaged in visits with humans. The study by Odendaal and Meintjes reported above additionally measured neurophysiological markers in the 18 dogs making visits to humans [49]. Similar to the response detected in humans, visits resulted in significant positive changes ($P \leq 0.01$) in β-endorphin, oxytocin, prolactin, phenyl acetic acid, and dopamine in the dogs, supporting that the experience would be enjoyable and associated with positive bonding experiences for the dogs. Unlike the response in humans, serum cortisol levels rose in the dogs from 366.5 to 416.0 mmol/L, although this difference did not achieve statistical significance ($P = 0.30$). Failure of dogs to experience a significant drop in cortisol during the visit, as seen in the humans, suggests that visits are not a stress reliever for dogs. Rather, the numerical increase in cortisol reinforces the understanding that therapy dog visits are work for the dog. Sitting or standing quietly for a therapy visit, maintaining a high level of obedience and calm instead of engaging in play, and accepting handling from strangers require work and effort by the therapy dog.

Researchers from the Institute for Anthropology in Austria evaluated salivary cortisol levels in therapy dogs as a marker of stress [54]. Saliva samples were collected from 18 therapy dogs on days when they were not making visits ($N = 165$ samples) and on visit days ($N = 347$ samples) during a three-month period. Nonvisit assessments were performed on three days during the period prior to the three-month visit collection and again on 3 days after the 3-month recording period had been completed. Visit assessments were performed both before and after therapy dog visit sessions. Cortisol concentrations were significantly higher during therapy days than on control days, suggesting a physiological arousal, or stress response was associated with making visits (Fig. 2.13). Cortisol was additionally increased when dogs provided more therapeutic sessions during the sampling period (Fig. 2.14). These data suggest a potentially stressful nature of therapy work for dogs, supporting limiting the number and frequency of therapy dog visits, as described in Chap. 5.

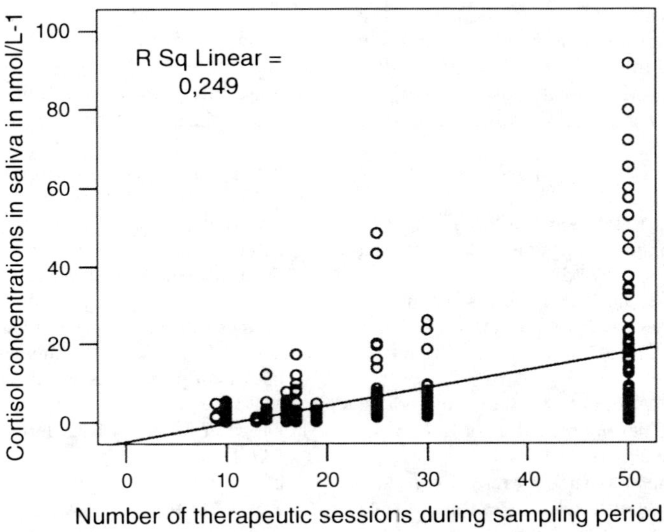

Fig. 2.14 Effect of visit frequency on cortisol levels in therapy dogs making visits over 3 months. Circles represent averages of cortisol concentrations obtained on a single day at the beginning and end of a visit. (Reproduced with permission from [54])

Summary

- Therapy dog visits produce both subjective and objective benefits for humans with a variety of medical conditions.
- Benefits from therapy dog visits are independent of patients' general attitudes toward pets.
- Benefits from therapy dog visits extend beyond the brief human-dog encounter.
- Physiological studies support that subjectively recognized improvements following therapy dog visits are linked to biological changes.
- While ethical scholars support using dogs for therapeutic visits, physiological studies demonstrate a stress response in therapy dogs that supports limiting the frequency of visits.

References

1. Therapy Dogs International website, http://tdi-dog.org. Accessed September 2011.
2. Zamir T. The moral basis of animal-assisted therapy. Soc Animals. 2006;14:179–99.
3. Snyder M, Lindquist R. Complementary & alternative therapies in nursing. 6th ed. Springer: New York; 2010.
4. Miller TW. Handbook of stressful transitions across the lifespan. Springer: New York; 2010.
5. Johnson RA, Meadows RL, Haubner JS, Sevedge K. Human–animal interaction. A complementary/alternative medical (CAM) intervention for cancer patients. Am Behav Sci. 2003;47:55–69.
6. Havener L, Gentes L, Thaler B, et al. The effects of a companion animal on distress in children undergoing dental procedures. Issues Compr Pediatr Nurs. 2001;24:137–52.
7. Barak Y, Savorai O, Mavashey S, Beni A. Animal-assisted therapy for elderly schizophrenic patients: a one-year controlled trial. Am J Geriatr Psychiatry 2001;9:439–42.
8. Barker SB, Pandurangi AK, Best AM. Effects of animal-assisted therapy on patients' anxiety, fear, and depression before ECT. J ECT. 2003;19:38–44.
9. Cole KM, Gawlinski A, Steers N, Kotlerman J. Animal-assisted therapy in patients hospitalized with heart failure. Am J Crit Care. 2007;16:575–85.
10. Barak Y, Savorai O, Mavashey S, Beni A. Animal-assisted therapy for elderly schizophrenic patients: a one-year controlled trial. Am J Geriatr Psychiatry. 2011;9:439–42.
11. Braun C, Stangler T, Narveson J, Pettingell S. Animal-assisted therapy as a pain relief intervention for children. Complement Ther Clin Pract. 2009;15:105–9.
12. Lasa SM, Ferriero G, Brigatti E, Valero R, Franchignoni F. Animal-assisted interventions in internal and rehabilitation medicine: a review of the recent literature. Panminerva Med. 2011;53:129–36.
13. Dimitrijević I. Animal-assisted therapy – a new trend in the treatment of children and adults. Psychiatr Danub. 2009;21:236–41.

14. LeFebvre SL, Golab GC, Christensen E, et al. Guidelines for animal-assisted interventions in health care facilities. Am J Infect Control. 2008;36:78–85.
15. Edwards NE, Beck AM. Animal-assisted therapy and nutrition in Alzheimer's disease. West J Nurs Res. 2002;24:697–712.
16. Phear DN. A study of animal companionship in a day hospice. Palliat Med. 1996;10:336–8.
17. Arata S, Momozawa Y, Takeuchi Y, Mori Y. Important behavioral traits for predicting guide dog qualification. J Vet Med Sci. 2010;72:539–45.
18. Ensminger JJ. Service and Therapy Dogs in American Society. Science, Law and the Evolution of Canine Caregivers. Charles C. Thomas, Publisher, Springfield: IL. 2010.
19. Martin F, Farnum J. Animal-assisted therapy for children with pervasive developmental disorders. West J Nurs Res. 2002;24:657–70.
20. Macauley BL. Animal-assisted therapy for persons with aphasia: a pilot study. J Rehabil Res Dev. 2006;43:357–66.
21. Chu CI, Liu CY, Sun CT, Lin J. The effect of animal-assisted activity on inpatients with schizophrenia. J Psychosoc Nurs Ment Health Serv. 2009;47:42–8.
22. Niewiadomska M, Radziejewska M, Horodnicka-Józwa A, Petriczko E. Agility in treatment of children with type 1 diabetes–pilot study. Pediatr Endocrinol Diabetes Metab. 2010;16:89–93.
23. Mossello E, Ridolfi A, Mello AM, et al. Animal-assisted activity and emotional status of patients with Alzheimer's disease in day care. Int Psychogeriatr. 2011;1:1–7.
24. Abate SV, Zucconi M, Boxer BA. Impact of canine-assisted ambulation on hospitalized chronic heart failure patients' ambulation outcomes and satisfaction: a pilot study. J Cardiovasc Nurs. 2011;26:224–30.
25. Rossetti J, King C. Use of animal-assisted therapy with psychiatric patients. J Psychosoc Nurs Ment Health Serv. 2010;48:44–8.
26. Matuszek S. Animal-facilitated therapy in various patient populations: systematic literature review. Holist Nurs Pract. 2010;24:187–203.
27. Muñoz Lasa S, Ferriero G, Brigatti E, Valero R, Franchiognoni F. Animal-assisted interventions in internal and rehabilitation medicine: a review of the recent literature. Panminerva Med. 2011;53:129–36.
28. Sobo EJ, Eng B, Kassity-Krich N. Canine visitation (pet) therapy: pilot data on decreases in child pain perception. J Holist Nurs. 2006;24:51–7.
29. Kawamura N, Niiyama M, Niiyama H. Animal-assisted activity: experiences of institutionalized Japanese older adults. J Psychosoc Nurs Ment Health Serv. 2009;47:41–7.
30. Coakley AB, Mahoney EK. Creating a therapeutic and healing environment with a pet therapy program. Complement Ther Clin Pract. 2009;15:141–6.
31. McNair D, Lorr M, Droppleman L. Profile of mood states manual. North Tonawanda, NY: Multi-Health Systems, Inc.; 1992.
32. Souter MA, Miller MD. Do animal-assisted activities effectively treat depression? a meta-analysis. Anthrozoös. 2007;20:167–80.
33. Folse EB. Animal-assisted therapy and depression in adult college students. Anthrozoös. 1994;7:188–94.
34. Barker SB, Dawson KS. The effects of animal-assisted therapy on anxiety ratings of hospitalized psychiatric patients. Psychiatr Serv. 1998;49:797–801.
35. Lust E, Ryan-Haddad A, Coover K, Snell J. Measuring clinical outcomes of animal-assisted therapy: impact on resident medication usage. Consult Pharm. 2007;22:580–5.
36. Marcus DA, Bernstein CD, Constantin JM, Kunkel FA, Breuer P, Hanlon RB. Animal-assisted therapy at an outpatient pain management clinic. Pain Med. 2012;13:45–57.
37. Farrar JY, Portenoy RK, Berlin JA, Kinman JL, Strom BL. Defining the clinically important difference in pain outcome measures. Pain. 2000;88:287–94.
38. Farrar JT, Young JP, LaMoreaux L, Werth JL, Poole RM. Clinical importance of changes in chronic pain intensity measured on an 11-point numerical pain rating scale. Pain. 2001;94:149–58.
39. Ostelo RW, Deyo RA, Stratford P, et al. Interpreting change scores for pain and functional status in low back pain: towards international consensus regarding minimal important change. Spine. 2008;33:90–4.
40. Salaffi F, Stancati A, Silvestri CA, Ciapetti A, Grassi W. Minimal clinically important changes in chronic musculoskeletal pain intensity measured on a numerical rating scale. Eur J Pain. 2004;8:283–91.
41. Zelman DC, Hoffman DL, Seifeldin R, Dukes EM. Development of a metric for a day of manageable pain control: derivation of pain severity cut-points for low back pain and osteoarthritis. Pain. 2003;106: 35–42.
42. Banks MR, Banks WA. The effects of animal-assisted therapy on loneliness in an elderly population in long-term care facilities. J Gerontol A Biol Sci Med Sci. 2002;57:M428–32.
43. Harding R, Epiphaniou E, Hamilton D, et al. What are the perceived needs and challenges of informal caregivers in home cancer palliative care? Qualitative data to construct a feasible psycho-educational intervention. Support Care Cancer, in press.
44. Soothill K, Morris SM, Harman JC, et al. Informal carers of cancer patients: what are their unmet psychosocial needs? Health Soc Care Community. 2001;9:464–75.
45. Soothill K, Morris SM, Thomas C, et al. The universal, situational, and personal needs of cancer patients and their main carers. Eur J Oncol Nurs. 2003;7:5–16.
46. Matsuo K, Kato N, Kato T. Decreased cerebral haemodynamic response to cognitive and physiological tasks in mood disorders as shown by near-infrared spectroscopy. Psychol Med. 2002;32:1029–37.
47. Chamberlain SR, Sahakain BJ. The neuropsychology of mood disorders. Curr Psychiatry Rep. 2006;8:458–63.

48. Iwahashi K, Fukamauchi F, Aoki J, et al. A daycare program of animal assisted therapy for affective disorder patients during psychotropic drug therapy: evaluation of the relaxation effect by fNIRS (functional near-infrared spectroscopy). Nihon Shinkei Seishin Yakuriqaku Zasshi. 2010;30:129–34.
49. Odendaal JJ, Meintjes RA. Neurophysiological correlates of affiliative behaviour between humans and dogs. Vet J. 2003;165:296–301.
50. Barker SB, Knisely JS, McCain NL, Best AM. Measuring stress and immune response in healthcare professionals following interaction with a therapy dog: a pilot study. Psychol Rep. 2005;96: 713–29.
51. Charnetski CJ, Riggers S, Brennan FX. Effect of petting a dog on immune system function. Psychol Rep. 2004;95:1087–91.
52. Templer DI, Salter CA, Dickey S, Baldwin R, Veleber DM. The construction of a pet attitude scale. Psychol Rec. 1981;31:343–8.
53. Kanamori M, Suzuki M, Yamamoto K, Kanda M, et al. A day care program and evaluation of animal-assisted therapy (AAT) for the elderly with senile dementia. Am J Alzheimers Dis Other Demen. 2001;16:234–9.
54. Haubenhofer DK, Kirchengast S. Physiological arousal for companion dogs working with their owners in animal-assisted activities and animal-assisted therapy. J Appl Anim Welf Sci. 2006;9:165–72.

3 Dogs as Cancer Detectors

Key Chapter Points

- Dogs have superior ability to detect and recognize weak concentrations of odors.
- Nasal anatomy and genome features may help explain canine sniffing abilities.
- Dogs have been reported to successfully identify several types of cancer.
- Laboratory analysis of volatile gases can be used to differentiate cancer from noncancer cells, supporting an ability to identify some cancers based on smell analysis.

Keywords

Alert • Gas chromatography • Mass spectroscopy • Olfactory • Smellprints • Volatile organic compounds

Screening for cancer by detecting biomarkers of early disease is an important aspect of cancer care. Humans have tapped into dogs' abilities to detect and identify scents for hunting and tracking, search and rescue, and police and military assistance. Dogs have also been shown to be able to detect a variety of disease conditions, including impending seizures, hypoglycemia, and cortisol changes in Addison's disease. Research has even shown that certain genotypes are linked to better scent detection ability in certain dogs and dog breeds, which may explain why some dog breeds (e.g., German Shepherds and Labrador Retrievers) and certain individual dogs have been proven to be more adept at disease recognition [1–3].

Case reports and controlled experimental studies have highlighted dogs' ability to recognize early cancer. Anecdotally, patients have reported seeking medical care after a dog consistently brought their attention to an area of their body where they had not detected a problem but that later was diagnosed with cancer. Experimental studies have shown that, with consistent training, various breeds of dogs can successfully select cancer from noncancer specimens. Studies have reported a cancer-sniffing ability of dogs for a range of cancer types with dogs sniffing cancer cells or sniffing urine, breath, or skin from patients. Identification of odor patterns or smellprints from different types of cancers may help explain the physiology

D.A. Marcus, *Therapy Dogs in Cancer Care: A Valuable Complementary Treatment*,
DOI 10.1007/978-1-4614-3378-1_3, © Springer Science+Business Media New York 2012

behind cancer-sniffing abilities in dogs. Some researchers have also postulated that dogs are able to detect changes in major histocompatibility complex components, as tumor transformation may be linked to changes in human leukocyte antigen (HLA) expression [4].

Interpreting results from canine cancer-sniffing reports must be tempered by possible unintended influences from handlers or investigators, who might inadvertently signal dogs with gestures, verbalization, or body language of which the human might be unaware [5]. In the studies described below, handlers were generally not informed about the location or the presence vs. absence of cancer in particular tested patients, reducing potential handler influence. Furthermore, the ability of mechanically detected smellprints to identify early cancers supports that the sniffing ability of dogs may indeed detect cancer in some patients.

Medical Alert Dogs

Dogs that are able to consistently identify medical symptoms or disease have been termed *medical alert dogs*. This term denotes the dog's ability to detect and alert humans to a medical condition. These dogs can be especially valuable as they are often able to detect changes that represent early markers of a disease event, prior to the human experiencing recognizable symptoms.

> **Practical Pointer:** *Medical alert dogs* have been used to recognize and alert humans to changes that occur in advance of clinically apparent symptoms for patients with epilepsy, Addison's disease, diabetes, migraine, anxiety disorders, and other medical conditions.

Both companion dogs and trained medical alert dogs have been shown to successfully recognize abnormal human physiology. For example, 65% of 212 dog owners with diabetes reported that their companion dog reacted with a noticeable change in behavior when the person with diabetes developed hypoglycemia [6]. Among individuals identifying a dog behavior that predicted hypoglycemia, 52% of patients reported that abnormal behavior in their dog was an alert to hypoglycemia for most or all of their hypoglycemic episodes. In 32% of patients, the dog had reacted to eleven or more hypoglycemic episodes. The dog reactions preceded the owner's awareness of hypoglycemic symptoms for 34% of individuals, with dog reactions occurring when the owner was experiencing early symptoms of hypoglycemia for 41%. Most dogs alerted their owners by barking or vocalizing distress (62%), licking their owners (49%), nuzzling their owners (41%), staring intently at their owners (41%), or jumping on their owners (30%).

> **Practical Pointer:** Dogs may alert humans to medical problems by displaying a variety behaviors, including barking, pawing or licking the human, or staring intently.

Companion Dogs Alerting Owners to Cancer

Dogs have also been reported to be able to detect early cancer. Published literature contains anecdotal reports of changes in behavior of companion dogs that motivated owners to seek medical attention that resulted in a diagnosis of cancer (Table 3.1) [7–9]. In each case, the dog had no previously identified experience in cancer detection. Although owners may not have suspected cancer from the dogs' behavior, the dogs' persistent annoying behavior motivated individuals to seek medical attention that identified cancer in an area consistent with each dog's attention.

Table 3.1 Anecdotal reports of companion dogs alerting owners to previously unrecognized cancer

Reference	Dog	Behavior	Outcome	Diagnosis	Outcome
[8]	Border Collie–Doberman mix	Regularly sniffing a particular mole on a 44-year-old woman's thigh, while ignoring all other moles. Behavior continued for several months, at which point the dog tried to bite off the lesion, even through the patient's clothing	Behavior motivated the woman to ask her doctor to evaluate the mole	Superficial spreading malignant melanoma	Patient's dermatologists wrote, "This dog may have saved her owner's life by prompting her to seek treatment when the lesion was still at a thin and curable stage"
[9]	Labrador Retriever	Persistently nudging a spot of presumed eczema on the thigh under the trousers of a 66-year-old man	Behavior motivated the man to seek medical evaluation	Basal cell carcinoma	Following excision, the dog no longer displayed any interest in the man's leg
[7]	Dachshund puppy	Repeatedly sniffing and poking the left axilla in a seemingly healthy 44-year-old woman when she would sit to watch television	After one month of the dog's behavior, the woman found a lump in the upper, outer quadrant of her left breast	Infiltrating ductal carcinoma	Dog continued to poke and sniff axilla postoperatively. Patient was treated with chemotherapy, radiation, and tamoxifen and died 1 year later from metastatic disease

Case 1

RM was an asymptomatic 65-year-old man who normally enjoyed interacting with his 9-month-old long-haired Akita puppy. One day, the puppy began acting strangely around RM, refusing to play and persistently sniffing and poking RM's groin. The dog would also whine, pace in circles, and then return for additional determined poking despite being corrected to stop. The puppy refused to play or otherwise positively engage with RM and would only cry, circle, and poke RM. RM's wife had epilepsy and previously had a dog who would alert her to an oncoming seizure. Sensing the Akita might be detecting a problem in her husband, she insisted they make an appointment with RM's doctor, who identified a prostate-specific antigen (PSA) of 14 ng/mL and diagnosed prostate cancer. As RM was undergoing radiation treatment, the dog's insistent poking and whining gradually decreased until the dog was again interacting normally, and RM successfully completed treatment.

Two months later, the Akita began doggedly poking RM's 65-old-wife (TM) in the buttocks and sniffing, whining, circling, and pacing. Recalling the dog's previous ability to detect cancer in her husband, TM saw her doctor later that day and insisted on an urgent colonoscopy. When her doctor asked TM what her symptoms were, she announced, "I have colon cancer. My dog told me." TM proceeded to explain that she had a "cancer-alerting Akita that insists I have a problem," which TM took very seriously as she has a family history of colon cancer. A colonoscopy was performed, revealing four polyps, one of which was precancerous and another positive for colon cancer. Following polypectomy, the Akita's behavior returned to normal. During the months since this incident, the Akita has not displayed the abnormal poking and whining behavior, and both RM and TM have remained in good health.

Dogs Trained to Alert Doctors to Cancer

In addition to anecdotal reports of cancer detection by companion dogs, doctors have also sought to train dogs to help them identify patients with cancer. For example, a Florida dermatologist collaborated with a retired police canine handler to train a dog to recognize and alert to cancer [9]. In this report, a Standard Schnauzer that had been trained for bomb sniffing was selected to be taught to recognize in vitro malignant melanoma samples. After months of training, the dog was instructed to sniff a man with several moles that had been considered to be benign by the dermatologist. The dog alerted on one mole, which was excised and diagnosed as an early case of malignant melanoma.

A later report likewise described two dogs successfully trained to alert to melanoma in a small sample of patients [10]. The dogs used in this study were a 4-year-old Standard Schnauzer and a 6-year-old Golden Retriever. Both dogs had earned obedience titles and the Schnauzer was also certified as a bomb detection dog. Both dogs underwent weeks of training involving retrieval and searching skills, followed by training to correctly identify a melanoma sample that was placed in one of several compartments within a testing box (Table 3.2). After completing training, dogs underwent test trials in which they were required to identify (1) melanoma samples that were placed on healthy individuals and (2) melanoma in actual patients. For trials using healthy volunteers, a number of bandages were placed on a disease-free control subject, with one bandage covering melanoma tissue that had been placed beneath the bandage. Each dog was tested in five trials, with a different healthy individual used in each trial. Alerting signals were the same as those used during the box test, with both dogs required to sit next to the bandage the dog identified as covering melanoma tissue and either paw at the correct bandage (Schnauzer's alert signal) or touch it with lips or tongue (Golden Retriever's alert signal). Both dogs successfully identified the melanoma-containing bandage in each trial. Dogs were subsequently presented with actual patients who each had a lesion that a dermatologist had identified as suspicious for melanoma; melanoma was verified in each patient through biopsy after completing the dog sniffing tests. The Schnauzer was presented with seven patients, correctly identifying melanoma in six of the patients (Table 3.3). The Golden Retriever searched four patients, identifying melanoma in three patients and missing the same patient who was not detected by the Schnauzer. This study confirms that, with intense training, dogs may be able to be successfully taught to identify melanoma.

Table 3.2 Dog training protocol for detecting melanoma (Based on [10])

Stage of training	Description
Retrieval training	Both dogs underwent weeks of training using perforated tubes that contained a mixture of basal, squamous, and melanoma tissues prepared by a dermatologist. Each dog was presented with a tube to sniff, which was then tossed; the dog's task was to retrieve the tube. Each dog completed about 100 trials
Search training	The Schnauzer additionally was trained with 100 search trials that involved placing a set of retrieval tubes within a 400-m^2 area, only one of which contained basal, squamous, and melanoma tissue. The dog was required to locate and retrieve the single tube containing the mixed basal, squamous, and melanoma sample
Box tests	Each dog was presented with a 68-inch × 8 inch × 8 inch (173 cm × 20 cm × 20 cm) box divided into 10 equal compartments. A melanoma sample was placed in one, randomly assigned compartment and the others were either empty or filled with bandages, gauze, latex, gloves, or rolls of tape as distractor stimuli. Alert signals were sitting next to the correct compartment and pawing it for the Schnauzer and sitting next to the correct compartment and mouthing it for the Golden Retriever

Table 3.3 Melanoma detection by two trained dogs (Based on [10])

Patient	Number of bandages placed*	Results from dog test: Schnauzer	Results from dog test: Golden Retriever	Biopsy diagnosis following dog test
66-year-old female with suspicious lesion on shoulder	21	Melanoma localized	Melanoma localized	Lentigo maligna
53-year-old male with suspicious lesion on shoulder	30	Melanoma localized	No search conducted	Superficial spreading malignant melanoma
54-year-old male with suspicious lesion on low back	14	Melanoma localized	Melanoma localized	Initial biopsy negative; subsequent step section of entire specimen revealed malignant melanoma
46-year-old male with suspicious lesion on abdomen	8	Melanoma not localized	Melanoma not localized	Superficial spreading malignant melanoma
80-year-old female with suspicious lesion on triceps	12	Melanoma localized	No search conducted	Malignant melanoma in situ
48-year-old male with suspicious lesion on low back	10	Melanoma localized	No search conducted	Lentigo maligna
68-year-old female with suspicious lesion on shoulder	10	Melanoma localized	Melanoma localized	Superficial spreading malignant melanoma

*One bandage was placed over the suspicious lesion with identical bandages covering other body locations. In some cases, bandages were visible; in others, bandages were covered with close-fitting cotton clothing

Case 2

DG was a healthy 52-year-old female whose 8-year-old English Bull Terrier began incessantly poking and licking at a spot on the posterior aspect of her right thigh. DG inspected her leg using a mirror and found a 3-mm beige spot that she believed to be a freckle or "age spot." Whenever DG would sit or lie down near the dog, the dog would again hone in on that particular spot and start licking it. Because DJ had previously observed dogs licking damaged areas on other dogs, she mentioned the dog's behavior to her family doctor, who inspected the leg and told DG not to worry. The Terrier relentlessly attended to this spot, so DG returned to her doctor and insisted on a dermatology referral.

The dermatologist likewise concurred with the family doctor that the area appeared to be benign. DG then told the dermatologist, "My dog says something is wrong and I want a biopsy." A biopsy was performed, and ten days later, the dermatologist called DG with a diagnosis of basal cell carcinoma and a request to return for more complete cancer removal. Following surgical removal, the dog no longer focused on DG's lower extremity, and the poking and licking behaviors were not repeated.

Olfactory Ability of Dogs

Dog's skill in sniffing out disease is likely to be rooted in their finely tuned olfactory system. A dog's nose contains olfactory receptor cells throughout their nasal cavity, along with an additional olfactory chamber rich in receptors called the vomeronasal organ [11]. The vomeronasal organ is believed to help dogs interpret sexual signals from pheromones and also recognize the physiological state of other animals [12]. The overall surface area of the olfactory epithelium is 170 cm^2 in dogs vs. 10 cm^2 in humans [13]. In addition, dog anatomy permits accumulation of odors, as odors remain in a pocket created by a bony subethmoidal shelf during exhalation to permit concentrating weak odors to improve identification [11]. This may help explain why dogs are able to detect odors present in low amounts.

Practical Pointer: Dogs have over 220 million olfactory receptors compared with only 5 million in humans.

Among animals, dogs seem to be particularly adept at detecting and discriminating odors, which may be rooted in unique canine anatomical and functional characteristics. For example, a recent study compared olfactory mucosa in dogs and sheep [14]. In both animals, olfactory cells formed an expanded knob covered with cilia. The number of cilia per knob was significantly higher in dogs vs. sheep (19 vs. 7, $P<0.05$). In addition, dog olfactory mucosa was thicker with a greater density of olfactory cells developing with maturation compared with sheep.

Olfactory receptor genes are shared among mammals, with the same subfamilies in dogs also present in horses, humans, and others [15]. Olfactory receptor genes have been mapped in several species, including dogs, humans, and mice. An important difference among these groups is the number of nonfunctioning genes, called pseudogenes. While 67% of human olfactory genes are nonfunctioning pseudogenes, pseudogenes represent 20% of olfactory receptor genes in mice and only 12% in dogs [16].

A review of studies investigating the ability of dogs to detect landmines concluded that [17]:

- Dogs have a lower threshold for identifying odors, making them able to recognize lower quantities of odors than can often be detected by humans and odor-detecting machines.
- Dogs have an amazing ability to separate and discriminate weak concentrations of specific target odors within a background of higher concentrations of other odors.

These abilities determined during mine sniffing might also translate into an ability to sniff out disease.

Practical Pointer: Dogs have a lower threshold for detecting weak concentrations of odors compared with other mammals and some odor-detecting machines.

Explaining the Physiology of Cancer Sniffing

Analyzing odors and gases for cancer detection is not limited to canine sniffing. A variety of laboratory studies have been performed to detect cancer based on odor or gas analysis. Chromatographic techniques and implementation of an artificial or electronic nose have been used to screen for a variety of diseases, including metabolic diseases, peptic ulceration, and infectious diseases [18–22]. Laboratory studies with similar technology have likewise identified patterns of volatile gases that have allowed differentiation of cancer from non-cancer cells for several cancer types.

Practical Pointer: An *electronic nose* is a mechanical device with sensor arrays that react to volatile gases, similar to how neural olfactory receptors react to odors. Processors within the electronic nose analyze gas patterns to interpret content.

Volatile Gas Detection in Lung Cancer

Experimental studies have detected volatile organic compounds in cultured lung cancer cells and the exhaled breath of cancer patients [23]. The occurrence of unique peaks on gas chromatography and mass spectroscopy associated with gas composition related to cancer can be used to distinguish patients with lung cancer from cancer-free individuals [24]. Alkanes, alkane derivatives, and benzene derivatives are the predominate gases identified in lung cancer patients [25]. Breath samples from 178 bronchoscopy patients (87 diagnosed with lung cancer) and 41 healthy controls were evaluated for volatile gas patterns using gas chromatography and mass spectroscopy [26]. Patients with lung cancer were identified as having increased metabolism of alkanes and nonmethylated alkanes, producing distinguishing volatile organic compound patterns. A later study by this same research group identified 30 volatile gases that helped discriminate lung cancer patients with a sensitivity of 85% and specificity of 81% [27]. The authors concluded that a volatile gas analysis could be as accurate in predicting lung cancer as chest computed tomography.

Practical Pointer: Volatile organic compounds that may alert dogs to the presence of cancer cells may include alkanes, methylated alkanes, aromatic compounds, and benzene derivatives [13].

Medical research has supported screening for early lung cancer through analysis of exhaled chemicals and odors. For example, exhaled nitric oxide and exhaled volatile organic compounds may be analyzed to screen for lung cancer [28, 29]. Concentrations of isoprene, acetone, and methanol are slightly and significantly lower in people who have lung cancer compared with healthy controls ($P \leq 0.011$ for each gas) [30].

Detecting Lung Cancer Using Smellprints

Researchers from the Cleveland Clinic compared gases in exhaled breath from 14 patients with bronchogenic carcinoma and 45 cancer-free controls using an electronic nose to determine gas patterns, termed *smellprints* [31]. Smellprints are formed based on a resistance change detected in sensors in the electronic nose, determined by the chemical diversity of gases in the sample. Gases present in exhaled breath from cancer patients included isobutane, methanol, ethanol, acetone, pentane, isoprene, isopropanol, dimethylsulfide, carbon disulfide, benzene, and toluene. A comparison of smellprint patterns showed substantial differences between cancer patients and healthy controls, whereas patterns for healthy controls and patients with noncancerous lung diseases were similar (Fig. 3.1). In this study, the electronic nose had a 71% sensitivity and 92% specificity for detecting lung cancer.

Practical Pointer: A *smellprint* is a pattern of concentrations of volatile gases that differs between individuals with cancer and without cancer. Like a fingerprint can be a unique identifier, a smellprint may be used to identify patients who are likely to have cancer.

Other studies have likewise shown that volatile organic compound smellprints from exhaled breath can distinguish among individuals with lung cancer, noncancer chronic lung diseases, and healthy controls [32, 33]. For example, a recent study from a research group in Italy evaluated 56 patients undergoing bronchoscopy for an abnormal chest X-ray with an electronic nose analysis. Bronchoscopy diagnosed cancer in 28 patients, most commonly non-small cell cancer ($N=24$) [33]. The other 28 patients were diagnosed with noncancer lung diseases (16 with chronic obstructive pulmonary disease, 5 bronchitis, 4 pleurisy, and 3 interstitial lung disease). Twenty-six of the 28 patients with an endoscopy diagnosis of lung cancer were correctly identified by the electronic nose, with six of 28 noncancer patients incorrectly identified as having cancer by the electronic nose. Caution is needed when interpreting data from electronic nose screening for lung cancer, however, as smoking history, inspired substances, and gender have been shown to influence electronic nose cancer detection [34].

Volatile Gas Detection in Breast Cancer

Volatile organic compounds identified in breath were evaluated as breast cancer predictors in a study evaluating asymptomatic women with abnormal mammograms ($N=51$ with biopsy-proven cancer and $N=50$ with negative biopsies) and 42 healthy matched controls [35]. Using five breath biomarkers, the sensitivity and specificity for predicting breast cancer in women with biopsy-proven cancer, respectively, were 94% and 85%. Using these same tests, no breast cancer was predicted in 32% of the women with

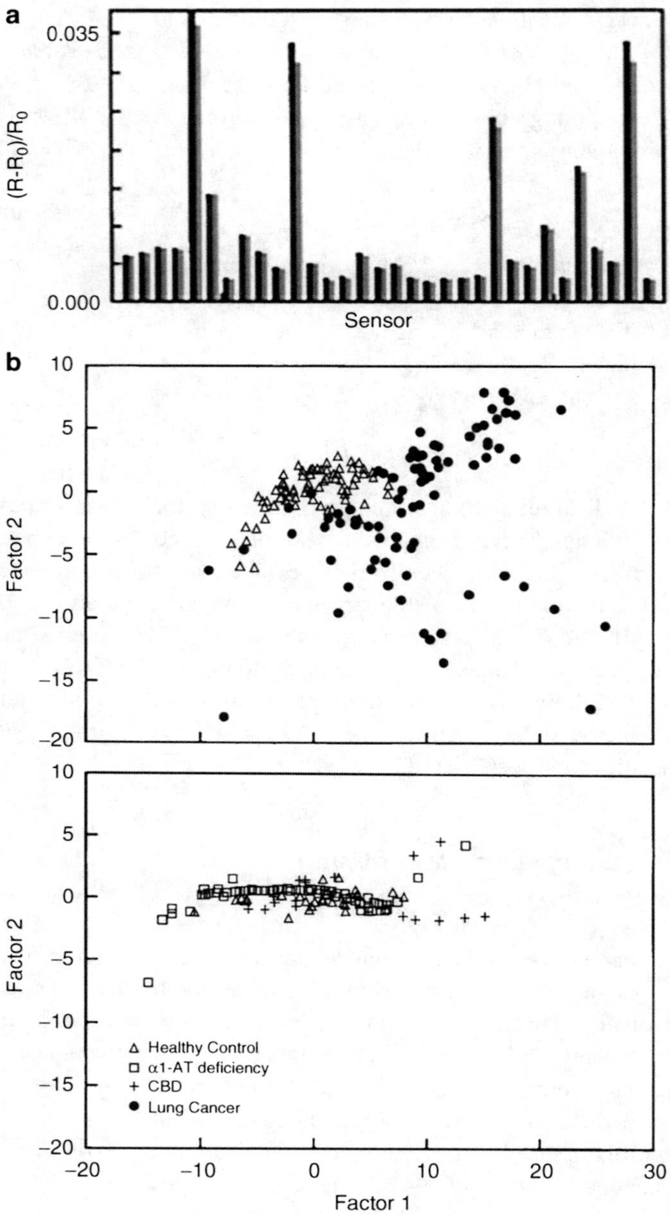

Fig. 3.1 Electronic nose derived smellprints from patients with lung cancer, healthy controls, and patients with alpha1-antitrypsin (α-1AT) deficiency or chronic pulmonary beryllium disease (CBD). Typical smellprints (**a**) are compared from a healthy control (*black bars*) and a patient with lung cancer (*gray bars*). Quantification of discrimination among samples was evaluated using a cluster analysis (**b**). Patterns distinguished healthy controls from patients with lung cancer (*upper box*); while patterns were similar for healthy controls and patients with interstitial lung disease or emphysema (*lower box*) (Reprinted with permission from [31]). (**a**) Smellprints (**b**) Cluster analysis

abnormal mammograms who were found to have no cancer on biopsy. A second study from this same group evaluated volatile organic compounds in exhaled breath from 54 women with biopsy-proven breast cancer and 204 cancer-free controls [36]. Accuracy of identifying breast cancer through gas analysis was 88%, ranging from 83% in women with stage 1 disease to 99% in those with stage 4 breast cancer.

Volatile Gas Detection in Skin Cancer

The same Italian research group evaluating electronic nose detection of lung cancer described above reported that gas chromatography analysis showed differences in patterns identified from sampling superficial skin near normal skin, benign nevi, and melanomas in 40 individuals (Fig. 3.2a) [37]. Smellprints were obtained by

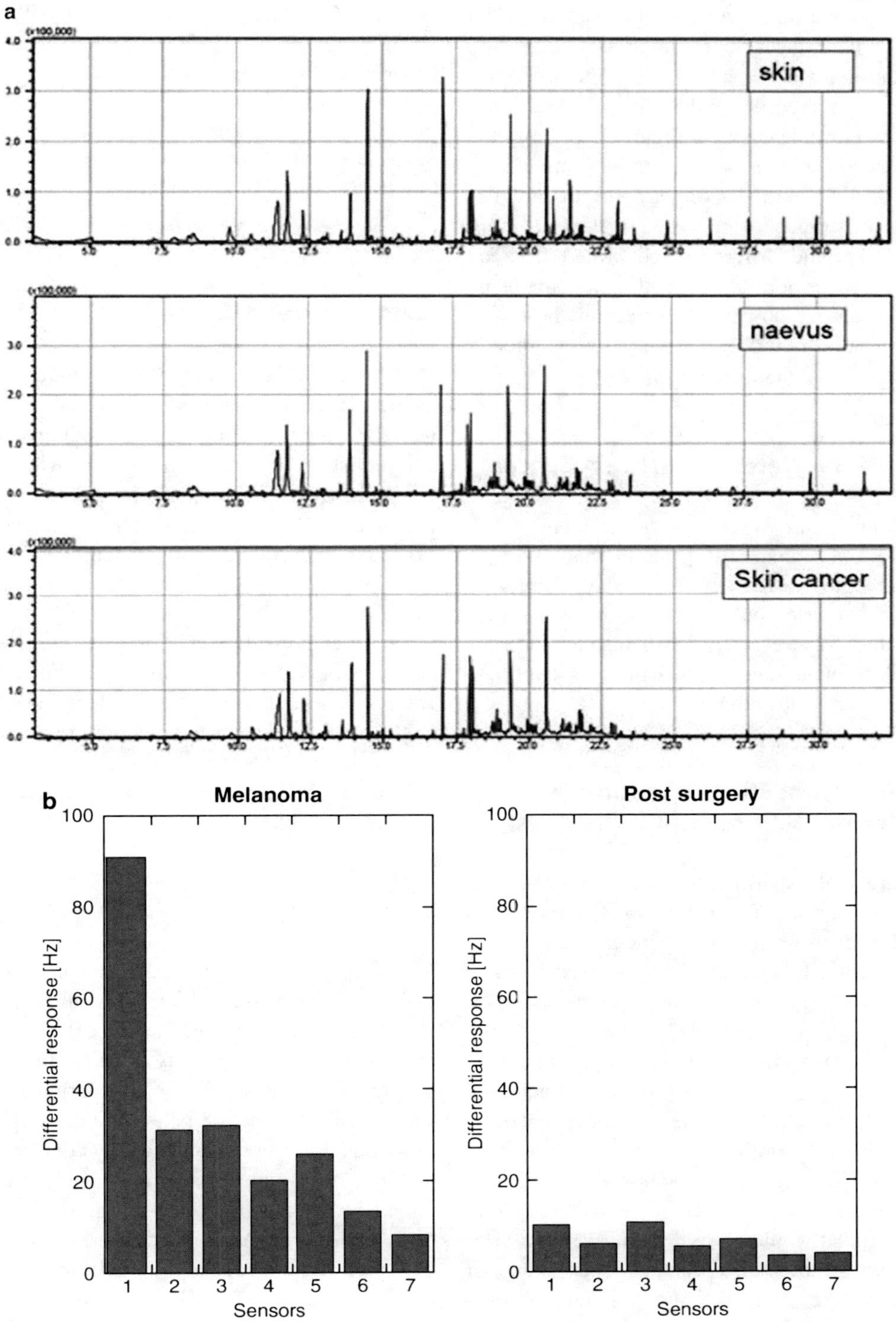

Fig. 3.2 Smellprints identified in patients with normal skin, benign nevus, or melanoma (Reproduced with permission from [37]). (**a**) Gas chromograms from normal skin, a benign nevus, and melanoma in the same individual. (**b**) Electronic nose sensor response patterns in the same individual before and after complete removal of a melanoma

exposing electronic nose sensors to air collected from skin surfaces to evaluate skin odor and calculating the difference between identified frequency shifts recorded at the site of the lesion and a nearby normal skin area. Figure 3.2b shows the difference in smellprint obtained in a patient with melanoma when the lesion was present and after complete surgical removal. The authors concluded that the differences identified between benign nevi or normal skin and melanoma using gas chromatography and the electronic nose supported studies reporting dogs' ability to correctly identify melanoma through sniffing.

Volatile Gas Detection in Brain Cancer

Electronic noses were also used to identify cultured glioblastoma cells [38]. In this study, an electronic nose originally designed to monitor air quality at a jet propulsion laboratory was shown to be able to successfully distinguish among cells from different organs (chicken heart vs. liver) and cell lines (glioblastoma vs. melanoma).

Experimental Studies Testing Cancer-Detection Abilities in Dogs

A number of experiments have been conducted testing the ability of dogs to correctly distinguish samples taken from cancer patients vs. controls. Differences among studies may at least partially reflect study design differences in the types of cancer tested, selection of dogs (breeds, gender, and ages, as well as utilizing dogs previously trained for sniffing detection vs. companion dogs), intensity of training methods, and time allowed for sample sniffing during testing sessions. In each study, dogs were trained to identify cancer by producing a specific behavior or signal that would alert the examiner to a positive identification. In order to reduce examiner bias for interpreting the dog's signals or inadvertently signaling the dog to produce a positive or negative response, examiners were blinded to the samples (cancer vs. control) during testing sessions.

Table 3.4 Canine cancer-detection trial results (Based on [39])

Dog diagnosis	Biopsy-proven diagnosis			
	Lung cancer		Breast cancer	
	Cancer	Control	Cancer	Control
Cancer identified	564	4	110	15
Cancer not identified	10	708	6	260

Lung and Breast Cancer

Researchers at the Pine Street Foundation in California have conducted the most extensive work on cancer-sniffing dogs. In 2006, researchers published findings of a study in which they had trained three Labrador Retrievers and two Portuguese Water Dogs to identify differences in exhaled breath from 27 patients with lung cancer, 25 with breast cancer, and 66 healthy controls [39]. Following 2–3 weeks of training, the dogs were presented with breath samples from 28 lung cancer patients, 6 breast cancer patients, and 17 controls in a double-blind experiment. Sensitivity and specificity for cancer detection, respectively, were 0.99 and 0.99 for lung cancer and 0.88 and 0.98 for breast cancer (Table 3.4). All five dogs performed similarly.

Bladder Cancer

Researchers from Amersham Hospital in the United Kingdom trained six dogs (three Cocker Spaniels, one Papillon, one Labrador Retriever, and one mixed breed) to identify urine obtained from patients with bladder cancer [40]. Urine samples were obtained from 108 patients with transitional cell bladder carcinoma and healthy controls, with half of the samples used for training and the remainder for post-training testing. The Spaniels and Papillon were trained and tested using freshly defrosted, liquid specimens, and the Labrador Retriever and mixed breed were trained and tested with dried specimens. During both training and testing, each dog was presented with seven urine specimens, with one from a patient with bladder cancer and the remainder from healthy controls.

Table 3.5 Accuracy of selecting one bladder cancer specimen from seven specimens over 9 tests per dog (Based on [40])

Dog	Number of correct runs (%)
Dogs testing liquid urine	
Cocker Spaniel, dog, 1.5 years old	5 of 9 (55.6)
Cocker Spaniel, bitch, 2 years old	5 of 9 (55.6)
Cocker Spaniel, bitch, 5 years old	4 of 9 (44.4)
Papillon, bitch, 7 years old	4 of 9 (44.4)
Dogs testing dried urine	
Labrador Retriever, bitch, 7 years old	3 of 9 (33.3)
Mixed breed, dog, 6 years old	1 of 9 (11.1)

Bitch is female; dog is male

Each dog was subjected to 9 test sessions during the experimental period. If dogs selected the correct specimen by chance alone, the researchers expected a success rate of 14%. Overall, the dogs correctly selected the positive bladder cancer urine on 22 of 54 occasions, for an average success rate of 41% (Table 3.5). Accuracy was higher among dogs using liquid vs. dried specimens (50% vs. 22% correct). Despite the limitations of this study, including variability among dogs and testing samples, these results do support the ability of dogs to be able to identify urine from bladder cancer patients at a rate superior to chance alone.

Prostate Cancer

Results have been inconsistent among studies evaluating patients with prostate cancer. In one study, ten dogs were independently trained by their owners to detect cancer using urine specimens from patients with breast or prostate cancer [41]. This study is limited by the lack of centralized training and variable training sessions (frequency and duration) among different dogs. Most trainers used a single training session per day 2–4 days per week, with only two dogs trained more than once daily and with training sessions occurring most days of the week. During experimental testing after the completion of training, each dog was presented with 7 urine samples, with one sample from a cancer patient and the remainder from controls. Dogs evaluating patients with breast cancer were tested with 9 cancer patients and 54 controls, with each cancer patient's urine used in two tests for a total of 18 test runs per dog. Prostate cancer dogs were tested with 33 sessions, using urine from 11 patients and 66 controls and each patient's urine used in three different test sessions. In this study, dogs were not more likely to correctly identify the breast or prostate urine samples better than by chance alone.

More recently, Cornu and colleagues reported successfully training a Belgian Malinois to identify prostate cancer odors in urine [42]. Training was reported to be a full-time job for the three individuals working with this dog, with training occurring 5 days per week over 16 months. Following training, the dog was presented with experimental runs with six urine samples (one from a patient with prostate cancer and five from controls). Urine was obtained from patients undergoing prostate biopsy, with their status as prostate cancer or control determined based on the biopsy results. A total of 33 cancer samples were used, with each sample used for only a single testing session. A total of 33 control samples were used during the experimental tests. The dog correctly identified 30 of the 33 cancer specimens as positive for cancer and 30 of the 33 controls as negative for cancer, for a sensitivity and specificity of 91% each. Interestingly, the three control subjects who were identified as false positives by the dog underwent prostate biopsy and one of these was then diagnosed with prostate cancer that had been previously undetected.

Colorectal Cancer

Breath and watery stool samples were obtained from patients with colorectal cancer (33 breath and 37 stool samples) and cancer-free controls (132 breath and 148 stool samples) [43]. Each participant was allowed to provide only one breath and one stool sample. Samples were sniffed by an 8-year-old Labrador Retriever that had been trained to detect cancer through sniffing samples. The dog correctly identified cancer in all breath and stool samples from patients with colorectal cancer, with three patients without cancer falsely identified as having a positive breath and/or stool test. These three patients were followed for 2 years, without development of cancer. The sensitivity and specificity, respectively, for the dog's diagnosis were 0.91 and 0.99 for breath samples and 0.97 and 0.99 for stool samples. The authors noted that similar tests were performed with breath and watery stool samples from patients undergoing colonoscopy who had other types of cancer (breast, stomach, or prostate), with similarly good detection rates by the dog.

Ovarian Cancer

Horvath and colleagues demonstrated that analyzing volatile organic compounds emitted by ovarian carcinomas can be a reliable method for discriminating cancer from noncancer tissues [44]. In later work, this same research group trained Giant Schnauzers to detect ovarian cancer by sniffing ovarian tissue and blood samples over 9 months [45]. Sensitivity and specificity, respectively, for testing samples from patients with ovarian cancer and cancer-free controls were 100% and 95% for tissue samples and 100% and 98% for blood samples.

Practical Pointer: Although specially trained dogs have been shown to be able to successfully differentiate cancer from noncancer samples for a variety of cancer types, success likely depends on the intensity of training, breed, and individual dog selected.

Summary

- Dog anatomy and genetic development result in enhanced ability to detect and discriminate low concentrations of odors.
- Dogs have over 50 times more olfactory cells in their nose than humans.
- Dogs are able to store smells in their nose while they sniff, making it easier to detect low concentrations of odors.
- Olfactory genes are the same for dogs and humans. In humans, however, two-thirds of possible smelling genes are no longer active or used.
- Both companion dogs and specially trained sniffing dogs have effectively identified a variety of types of cancer.

References

1. Tacher S, Quignon P, Rimbault M, et al. Olfactory receptor sequence polymorphism within and between breeds of dogs. J Hered. 2005;96:812–6.
2. Lesniak A, Walczak M, Jezierski T, et al. Canine olfactory receptor gene polymorphism and its relation to odor detection performance by sniffer dogs. J Hered. 2008;99:851–27.
3. Robin S, Tacher S, Rimbault M, et al. Genetic diversity of canine olfactory receptors. BMC Genomics. 2009;10:21.
4. Balseiro SC, Correia HR. Is olfactory detection of human cancer by dogs based on major histocompatibility complex-dependent odour components?—A possible cure and a precocious diagnosis of cancer. Med Hypotheses. 2006;66:270–2.
5. Lit L, Schweitzer JB, Oberbauer AM. Handler beliefs affect scent detection dog outcomes. Anim Cogn. 2011;14:387–94.
6. Wells DL, Lawson SW, Siriwardena AN. Canine responses to hypoglycemia in patients with type 1 diabetes. J Altern Complement Med. 2008;14:1235–41.
7. Welsh JS, Barton D, Ahuja H. A case of breast cancer detected by a pet dog. Community Oncol. 2005;2: 324–6.
8. Williams H, Pembroke A. Sniffer dogs in the melanoma clinic? Lancet. 1989;1:734.
9. Church H, Williams H. Another sniffer dog in the clinic? Lancet. 2001;358:930.
10. Pickel D, Manucy GP, Walker DB, Hall SB, Walker JC. Evidence for canine olfactory detection of melanoma. Appl Anim Behav Sci. 2004;89:107–16.
11. Alabama A&M and Auburn Universities. The dog's sense of smell. Available at www.aces.edu/pubs/docs/U/UNP-0066/UNP-0066.pdf. Accessed September 2011.
12. Døving KB, Trotier D. Structure and function of the vomeronasal organ. J Exp Biol. 1998;201:2913–25.
13. Lippi G, Cervellin G. Canine olfactory detection of cancer versus laboratory testing: myth or opportunity? Clin Chem Lab Med, in press.
14. Kavoi B, Makanya A, Hassanali J, Carlsson HE, Kiana S. Comparative functional structure of the olfactory mucosa in the domestic dog and sheep. Ann Anat. 2010;192:329–37.
15. Issel-Tarver L, Rine J. The evolution of mammalian olfactory receptor genes. Genetics. 1997;145:185–95.
16. Olender T, Fuchs T, Linhart C, et al. The canine olfactory subgenome. Genomics. 2004;83:361–72.

17. Göth A, McLean IG, Trevelyan J. How do dogs detect landmines? A summary of research results. In: McLean IG, editor. Mine detection dogs: training, operations and odour detection. Geneva: GICHD; 2003.
18. Pavlou AK, Turner AP. Sniffing out truth: clinical diagnosis using the electronic nose. Clin Chem Lab Med. 2000;38:99–112.
19. Turner AP, Magan N. Electronic noses and disease diagnostics. Nat Rev Microbiol. 2004;2:161–6.
20. Kodogiannis VS, Lygouras JN, Tarczynski A, Chowdrey HS. Artificial odor discrimination system using electronic nose and neural networks for the identification of urinary tract infection. IEEE Trans Info Technol Biomed. 2008;12:707–13.
21. Charaklias N, Raja H, Humphreys ML, Magan N, Kendall CA. The future of early disease detection? Applications of electronic nose technology in otolaryngology. J Laryngol Otol. 2010;124:823–7.
22. Popov TA. Human exhaled breath analysis. Ann Allergy Asthma Immunol. 2011;106:451–6.
23. Chen X, Xu F, Wang Y, et al. A study of the volatile organic compounds exhaled by lung cancer cells in vitro for breath diagnosis. Cancer. 2007;110:835–44.
24. Gordon SM, Szidon JP, Krotoszynski B, Gibbons RD, O'Neill HJ. Volatile organic compounds in exhales air from patients with lung cancer. Clin Chem. 1985;31:1278–82.
25. Phillips M, Gleeson K, Hughes JM, et al. Volatile organic compounds in breath as markers of lung cancer: a cross-sectional study. Lancet. 1999;355:1930–3.
26. Phillips M, Cataneo R, Cummin A, et al. Detection of lung cancer with volatile markers in the breath. Chest. 2003;123:2115–23.
27. Phillips M, Altorki N, Austin JM, et al. Detection of lung cancer using weighted digital analysis of breath biomarkers. Clin Chem Acta. 2008;393:76–84.
28. Chan HP, Lewis C, Thomas PS. Exhaled breath analysis: novel approach for early detection of lung cancer. Lung Cancer. 2009;63:164–8.
29. Horváth I, Lázár Z, Gyulai N, Kollai M, Losonczy G. Exhaled biomarkers in lung cancer. Eur Respir J. 2009;34:261–75.
30. Bajtarevic A, Ager C, Pienz M, et al. Noninvasive detection of lung cancer by analysis of exhaled breath. BMC Cancer. 2009;9:348.
31. Machado RF, Laskowski D, Deffenderfer O, et al. Detection of lung cancer by sensor array analyses of exhaled breath. Am J Respir Crit Care Med. 2005;171:1286–91.
32. Dragonieri S, Annerna JT, Schot R, et al. An electronic nose in the discrimination of patients with non-small cell lung cancer and COPD. Lung Cancer. 2009;64:166–70.
33. D'Amico A, Pennazza G, Santonico M, et al. An investigation on electronic nose diagnosis of lung cancer. Lung Cancer. 2010;68:170–6.
34. Kischkel S, Miekisch W, Sawacki A, et al. Breath biomarkers for lung cancer detection and assessment of smoking related effects—confounding variables, influence of normalization and statistical algorithms. Clin Chim Acta. 2010;411:1637–44.
35. Phillips M, Cataneo RN, Ditkoff BA, et al. Prediction of breast cancer using volatile biomarkers in the breath. Breast Cancer Res Treat. 2006;99:19–21.
36. Phillips M, Cataneo RN, Saunders C, et al. Volatile biomarkers in the breath of women with breast cancer. J Breath Res. 2010;4:026003.
37. D'Amico A, Bono R, Pennazza G, et al. Identification of melanoma with a gas sensor array. Skin Res Technol. 2008;14:226–36.
38. Kateb B, Ryan MA, Homer ML, et al. Sniffing out cancer using the JPL electronic nose: a pilot study of a novel approach to detection and differentiation of brain cancer. Neuroimage. 2009;47 suppl 2:T5–9.
39. McCullouch M, Jezierski T, Broffman M, et al. Diagnostic accuracy of canine scent detection in early- and late-stage lung and breast cancers. Integr Cancer Ther. 2006;5:30–9.
40. Willis CM, Church SM, Guest CM, et al. Olfactory detection of human bladder cancer by dogs: proof of principle study. BMJ. 2004;329:712.
41. Gordon RT, Schatz CB, Myers LJ, et al. The use of canines in the detection of human cancers. J Altern Complement Med. 2008;14:61–7.
42. Cornu J, Cancel-Tassin G, Ondet V, Girardet C, Cussenot O. Olfactory detection of prostate cancer by dogs sniffing urine: a step forward in early diagnosis. Eur Urol. 2011;59:197–201.
43. Sonoda H, Kohnoe S, Yamazato T, et al. Colorectal cancer screening with odour material by canine scent detection. Gut. 2011;60:814–9.
44. Horvath G, Chilo J, Lindblad T. Different volatile signals emitted by human ovarian carcinoma and healthy tissue. Future Oncol. 2010;6:1043–9.
45. Horvath G, Andersson H, Paulsson G. Characteristic odour in the blood reveals ovarian carcinoma. BMC Cancer. 2010;10:643.

4 Dog Therapy with Cancer Treatment

Key Chapter Points

- Therapy dog visits can improve physical and psychosocial factors in cancer patients.
- Both pediatric and adult cancer patients can benefit from complementary therapy dog visits.
- Cancer patients and the parents of children being treated for cancer usually consider therapy dog interventions to be treatment.
- Therapy dog benefits have been reported in patients undergoing diagnostic testing and during inpatient cancer care, chemotherapy, and end-of-life care.

Keywords

Chemotherapy • Compassion fatigue • End-of-life • Grief counseling • Hospice • Inpatient • Radiation • Secondary survivors • Staff

The impact of therapy dog visits has been evaluated during different phases of cancer care. Studies have been conducted evaluating patients from pediatric through geriatric age groups, patients receiving chemotherapy and radiation, and patients in hospitals and hospice facilities. Similar to benefits reported for therapy dogs visiting general medical populations (see Chap. 2), therapy dog visits have likewise been shown to produce measurable physical and psychosocial improvement when included as complementary treatment during cancer care.

As with studies evaluating benefits of therapy dogs for general medical populations (see Chap. 2), therapy dog studies with cancer management are likewise limited by small sample sizes, an inability to blind treatment when control or comparator groups are used, and subjective outcomes. In some cases, results are provided as descriptive narratives that can be difficult to quantify. In addition, some studies provided patients with options of choosing to participate in a therapy dog visit or not, with those choosing not to see the dog sometimes serving within a comparator group. Studies reporting offering a choice to receive a therapy dog visit or not, however, usually report high acceptance for meeting with the dog for most individuals who were queried. Self-selecting patients who are agreeable to dog visits likely exaggerates observed positive benefits. While this research practice limits the strength of conclusions that may be drawn from data, therapy dog visits during clinical practice are generally similarly restricted to individuals expressing an

D.A. Marcus, *Therapy Dogs in Cancer Care: A Valuable Complementary Treatment*,
DOI 10.1007/978-1-4614-3378-1_4, © Springer Science+Business Media New York 2012

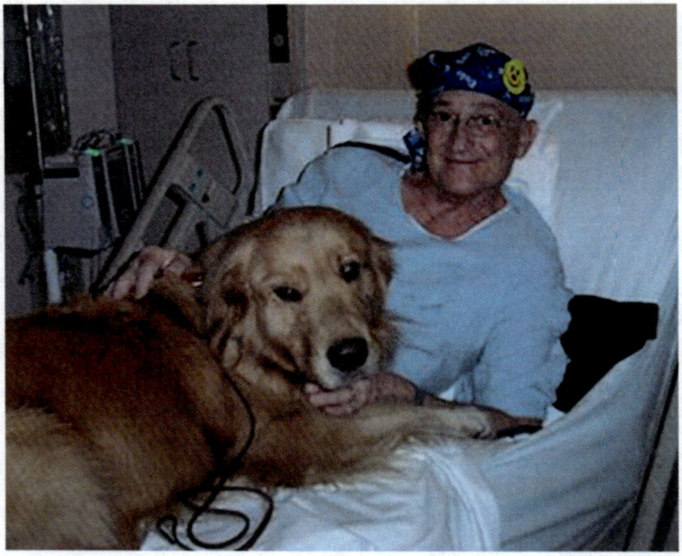

Fig. 4.1 Therapy dogs can bring smiles, comfort, and symptom reduction to patients undergoing cancer care (Photo courtesy of Kristy Everette at Pets at Duke program)

interest in receiving a visit from a dog. Despite these limitations, valuable benefits have been shown when therapy dogs are included as a complementary part of cancer care (see Fig. 4.1). Interpretations of benefits, however, must be tempered by the limitations inherent in this type of research.

Overview of Therapy Dog Impact in Cancer Care

As described in Chap. 2, therapy dog visits have demonstrated significant reduction in symptoms like pain, mood disturbance, fatigue, loneliness, and stress that are common accompaniments to cancer and cancer treatment. Therapy dog visits have also been shown to help normalize the hospital environment and improve morale for both patients and their family members [1]. In addition, animal-assisted therapy has been shown to reduce stress, anxiety, and boredom among critically ill patients, permitting the staff to affordably offer holistic treatment [2]. Therapy dog visits also make therapeutic touch feasible for critically ill patients [2].

Direct benefits from therapy dog visits for cancer patients have been documented in a number of studies. Data have been collected through prospectively conducted research and from anecdotal reports from patients, staff, and therapy dog handlers. Overall, these studies support including therapy dogs visits as complementary treatment for patients with cancer.

Prospective Research

A small, prospective study evaluated the effects of pet therapy visits from dogs and cats to 15 nursing home residents with terminal cancer [3]. In this study, 1.5-hour pet therapy sessions occurred weekly for 10 weeks. Participants were evaluated with a psychosocial questionnaire and the thematic apperception test (TAT). Baseline TAT revealed that symptoms were pervasive among this population. In addition, all patients gave responses suggesting a need for nurturing contact with others. During the pet visits, residents were noted to become more active, engage in nurturing the pets, and externalize their own concerns. For example, one resident was observed softly comforting a dog and encouraging it not to be frightened because everything would be all right. The ability of pets to help patients externalize worry and fears was linked to reduce passivity and an increased sense of self-control. Residents also enjoyed playing with the pets, which resulted

Table 4.1 Perceptions of 15 nursing home residents with terminal cancer to 10 weekly pet therapy visits (Based on [3])

Study results	Detail	Example
Reduced negative symptoms	12 of 15 residents reported pet visits lessened their fear, despair, loneliness, and isolation Twelve patients requested pets be added to the facility on a permanent basis to reduce loneliness	Pet served as a good listener "Holding the animal gave me a little life. I was able to talk to him and he listened" "When I pet an animal, he feels better and I feel better" "If I couldn't get out of bed, I'd like a little dog right there with me; then no matter what happened, I'd have my little friend"
Improved sleep	Four residents reported falling asleep faster after pet visits	None reported
No change in a minority of patients	Three residents lacked a positive response	One resident did not want to form new bonds when she perceived she would be dying soon Two patients were unable to relate positively with humans or staff, remaining distant and internally focused

in laughter. Overall, responses to the visits were positive (Table 4.1). The author of this study also made several important observations supporting benefit from pet therapy for terminally ill patients (Box 1).

Box 1 Conclusions from Observing Pet Therapy Visits with Terminally Ill Patients (Based on [3])

- Positive attributes for therapy dog visits often did not occur with human visitors.
  - Therapy dog visits encourage healthy nurturing.
    - Some patients are more able to openly give and receive affection from a therapy dog than from humans.
  - Therapy dog visits can be less strenuous for terminally ill patients than having human visitors.
- Therapy dogs are seen as accepting and nurturing.
  - Dogs do not intrude on a patient's attempts to come to terms with mortality.
  - Therapy dogs do not avoid dying patients.
- Therapy dogs can provide needed comfort and stress relief for caregivers.
  - Staff members experience burdens from caring for dying patients that might be reduced with therapy dog visits.

Anecdotal Reports

Case reports support benefits of therapy dog visits to cancer patients. For example, the book, *Moments with Baxter*, describes comfort provided to hospice patients receiving therapy dog visits [4]. A published case report describes positive impact from including a dog visit for a 13-year-old girl hospitalized with recurrent acute lymphocytic leukemia [5]. In this report, the patient was receiving chemotherapy and had been hospitalized for 42 days. Both the patient and her family had become discouraged. Planning the dog visit resulted in an improved mood and coping in the patient that the staff felt positively impacted treatment response. The visit followed protocols similar to those used for therapy dog visits to minimize infection risk. The dog visit resulted in a marked emotional response from the patient, who described happiness, joy, and peace. The dog was seen as helping bring a more homelike environment to the hospital. In addition, the dog's visit was also credited with helping foster improved relationships between the patient and the hospital staff, who also interacted with the dog during the visit.

Major oncology centers often include pet therapy as part of their complementary treatments, with anecdotal reports of benefits from therapy dog visits reported for inpatient and outpatient cancer treatment. While the strength of anecdotal data is limited, these reports can suggest areas of potential positive impact from therapy dog visits. Ellen Morrow has been taking 6-year-old

Table 4.2 Sample of interactions with 85-pound Golden Doodle therapy dog Charley and his handler Ellen Morrow

Setting	Patient(s)	Interaction
Hospital	60-year-old woman undergoing chemotherapy who received every other week visits from Charley	Charley would lie in bed with the patient, who told the handler, "I was really in a funk before you came in. After one of Charley's visits, I feel better for the whole afternoon"
Hospital	40-year-old man who had just received a cancer diagnosis	The patient's wife grabbed onto Charley and held him tightly throughout the visit, providing a source for emotional release
Hospital	Elderly man receiving end-of-life care	Patient's wife was initially sitting with her husband crying. When Charley entered the room, the wife saw Charley and stopped crying. Both wife and husband had a sweet and gentle visit with Charley. The husband enjoyed spending time with Charley and fed Charley treats. The room became more peaceful
Hospital	Young woman receiving chemotherapy	Charley joined this woman in her bed, and a calming effect was noticed. Despite being ill from her chemotherapy, the woman insisted on taking a photograph of Charley with her phone to send to her husband and children, sharing the positive connection she had made with the dog
Infusion room	Groups of patients receiving and awaiting treatment	Charley performs a series of tricks, which improves the overall mood in the room
Outpatient oncology surgery office	Charley visits the clinic every 2–3 weeks	Most patients are eager to spend time with Charley, who lightens the clinic mood. Some patients ask to have Charley stay at their side throughout the visit to help with anxiety; Charley then provides welcome support and has been called a "life line." Patients will also often begin talking with other patients at the clinic about Charley and their own dogs, facilitating healthy connections within the office community

Golden Doodle therapy dog Charley for visits for 4 years to both inpatient and outpatient oncology facilities in southern California. Table 4.2 provides a sampling of Charley's encounters. Ellen notes that Charley's visits seem to bring a gentle calmness to patients and their family members. She often hears that Charley's visits were the first time patients smiled or laughed since being in the hospital. Hospital staff also appreciate Charley's visits. During one hospital presentation, a nurse who is normally quiet and reserved surprised her team by coming to the podium to speak about the impact from Charley's visits.

Anecdotal data also support a role for therapy dogs visiting patients throughout long-term treatments. For example, including visits from German Shepherd therapy dog Pearl as part of the hospital routine was reported to serve as an important motivator to help with recovery. Pearl visited a boy in his early teens weekly during his hospitalization at Children's Hospital in Pittsburgh. Initially, the patient was confined to bed, where Pearl would join him to share petting, nuzzles, and secrets. After the boy had spent over a month in the hospital, he was able to use a wheelchair, and the boy proudly walked Pearl with the handler around the ward. When Pearl visited the next week, the patient had been successfully discharged. The nurses told Pearl's handler that they credited Pearl's visits as being instrumental in the boy's recovery, providing him with an important motivation to work hard through his therapy.

Practical Pointer: Therapy dog visits have been linked with improved mood and decreased loneliness and isolation in cancer patients.

Therapy Dog Visits When Coping with a Cancer Diagnosis

Early intervention with group psychotherapy or social support groups has been shown to help reduce distress in patients with cancer [6]. For example, a multicenter trial randomly assigned 235 women with metastatic breast cancer to supportive group therapy or a control group [7]. Pain and psychological distress were significantly reduced with the supportive group compared with the control ($P=0.04$).

In the early days of psychoanalysis, Sigmund Freud included his Chow in his therapy sessions, believing the dog's presence helped calm his patients. In 1978, Bernie Siegel, MD, developed a therapeutic intervention for cancer patients focusing on patients' drawings, dreams, and feelings, called Exceptional Cancer Patients. Dr. Siegel has also authored numerous inspirational books on healing, including *Faith, Hope and Healing: Inspiring Lessons Learned from People Living with Cancer*. Today, Dr. Siegel's cancer support groups include his two 25–30-pound dogs, Wirehaired Pointing Griffon-Terrier mix Buddy and Lhasa Apso Furphy:

> *Buddy and Furphy have very different roles in the group. Buddy is very sensitive to patients, walking around to each person and listening intently as they share their stories. He nuzzles up to people in need and gives and gets doses of love. Buddy brings a measure of calm and helps the support group bond together. Buddy's presence and attention to each person helps pull them together like a family who share a common pet.*
>
> *Furphy usually curls up under my chair and sleeps during sessions. In one session, a man who was new to the group began sharing his heart-wrenching and tragic story. Partway into the story, you could hear soft snoring sounds that grew louder and louder. The man became more and more upset until he finally exploded, accusing the group of rudeness by falling asleep when he was sharing his most personal moments. Once the other group members pointed out the snoring Furphy under my chair, the man's anger turned to laughter. The man's pain and fear just seemed to leave him and this became an important therapeutic turning point for him.*

Dr. Siegel's experience highlights the ability of therapy dogs to effectively defuse emotionally charged sessions, offer patients undivided and nonjudgmental attention, and provide a common focus to assist with developing healthy group connections and bonding.

Therapy Dog Visits During Inpatient Care

Cancer treatment can result in profound physical and emotional symptoms. A study evaluating the effect of chemotherapy on ten children and adolescents reported isolation, anxiety, pain, and boredom as common chemotherapy-related problems [8]. Isolation and loneliness were accentuated by being removed from normal daily surroundings (e.g., home and school) and experiencing physical changes (e.g., hair loss and weight change) that were perceived as barriers to maintaining normal social relationships. Boredom was accentuated by a loss of an ability to play, due to both environment restrictions within the hospital and physical limitations. Children linked cancer with loss, restrictions, and feelings of powerlessness and dependence.

Therapy dog visits can be used as an effective complementary treatment to help reduce distress related to hospital care. Researchers from the University of Missouri-Columbia and Ellis Fischel Cancer Center conducted a study evaluating the effects of 15-minute therapy dog visits for inpatients receiving nonpalliative cancer treatment [9]. Thirty patients were randomly assigned to one of three treatment conditions: a therapy dog visit during which the dog's handler was advised not to interact with the patient, a visit from a friendly volunteer, or quiet time for reading magazines. The therapy dog visit and friendly volunteer were both perceived significantly more positively than quiet time spent reading magazines, with no significant difference between the two types of visits (Fig. 4.2). Positive responses were consistently highest among participants receiving a therapy dog visit (Fig. 4.3).

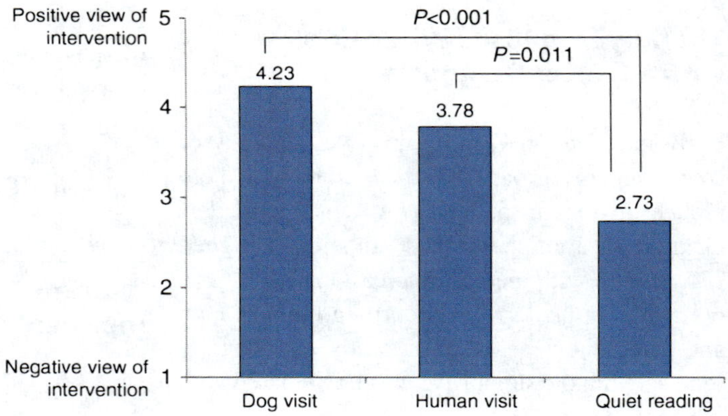

Fig. 4.2 Patient perception of interventions, using 1–5 rating scale. Average scores were obtained by evaluating responses to approximately 20 questions about the benefits of each treatment. The numerical difference between the dog and human visits did not achieve statistical significance (Based on [9])

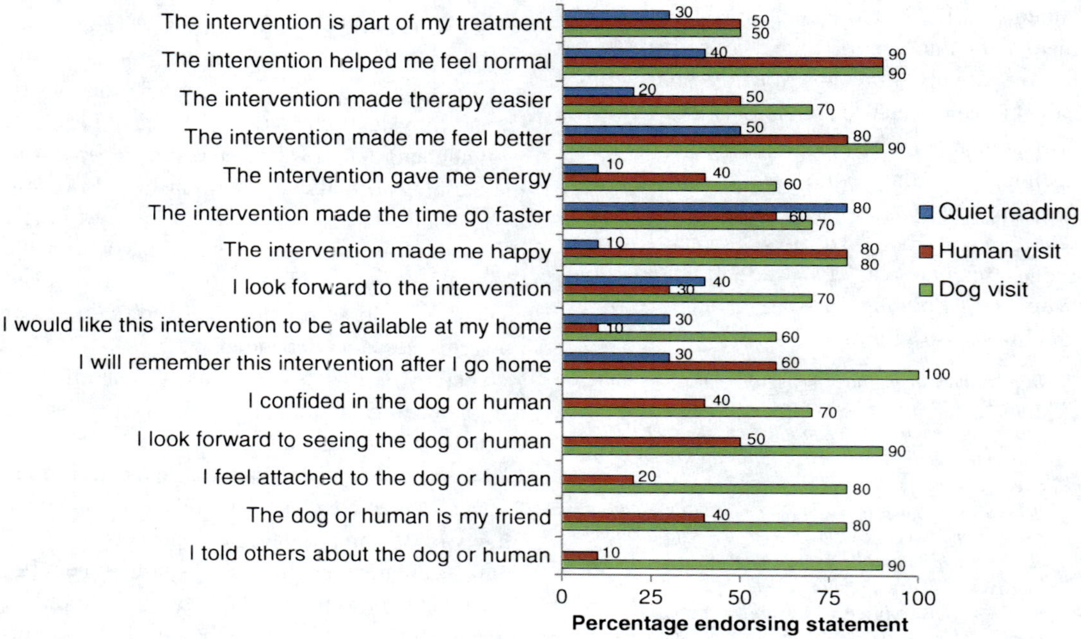

Fig. 4.3 Patients giving positive responses about interventions (Based on [9])

> **Practical Pointer:** "Patients will appreciate being viewed as human beings in need of unconditional love and attention, and not as machines that need fixing or the next medical challenge to conquer" [2, page 214].

Positive patient perceptions of therapy dog visits for cancer patients undergoing inpatient treatment may reflect a range of psychosocial benefits. Nonjudgmental and unconditional acceptance by a therapy dog can help reduce loneliness, provide a distraction from boredom, and empower patients to feel more in control of their hospital experience (case 1). In addition, dogs can also engage patients in healthy play, which has been identified as an important coping strategy for hospitalized children [10].

Case 1
SM was a 7-year-old girl with leukemia who was hospitalized for a bone marrow transplant when she told the nurses she missed her dogs and the staff arranged for visits from therapy dog Magic and his handler Tricia Larrabee. Tricia recalls how Magic lived up to his name during these visits. "The first time we met SM, she was quite ill. Despite feeling poorly, she was so happy to see Magic and asked me questions about him and told me about her dog at home. SM and her parents even invited Magic to come up onto her bed so she could really be close with him. Magic's visits seem to energize her as she enjoyed playing with him. Through our visits, Magic and SM became true friends who really connected with each other and SM told me Magic was her best friend. Magic was there for SM when she went through chemotherapy and other treatments and I know his presence was a comfort and gave support to SM, her family, and the staff."

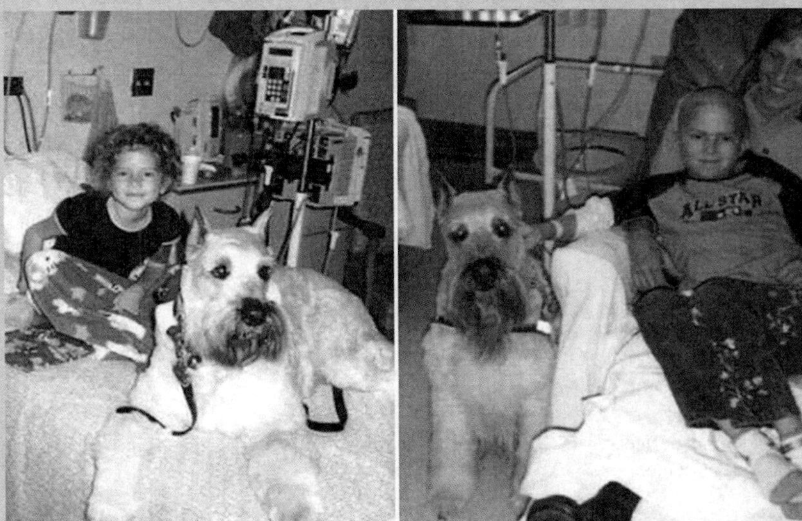

SM's first and final visits with her best friend, therapy dog Magic

Therapy Dogs for Inpatient Pediatric Cancer Treatment

A hospital-based, oncology therapy dog intervention was developed for an inpatient pediatric cancer treatment program [11, 12]. This intervention allowed children >2 years old to spend their hospital day in a room with a therapy dog. Each child was allowed to interact and play with the dog during treatments. This program was designed to improve the child's well-being and facilitate adaptation to cancer treatment. Children were excluded from participating if they were allergic to dogs, had severe neutropenia, had undergone recent surgery, or required isolation precautions. Children with problems with aggression or other behavioral problems that might interfere with interacting positively with the dog were also excluded.

Participants of this program were surveyed, with responses obtained from the parents for 16 children participating in the program and their 12 nurses (Figs. 4.4 and 4.5). Parents' impressions of the therapy dog program were overwhelmingly positive [11]:

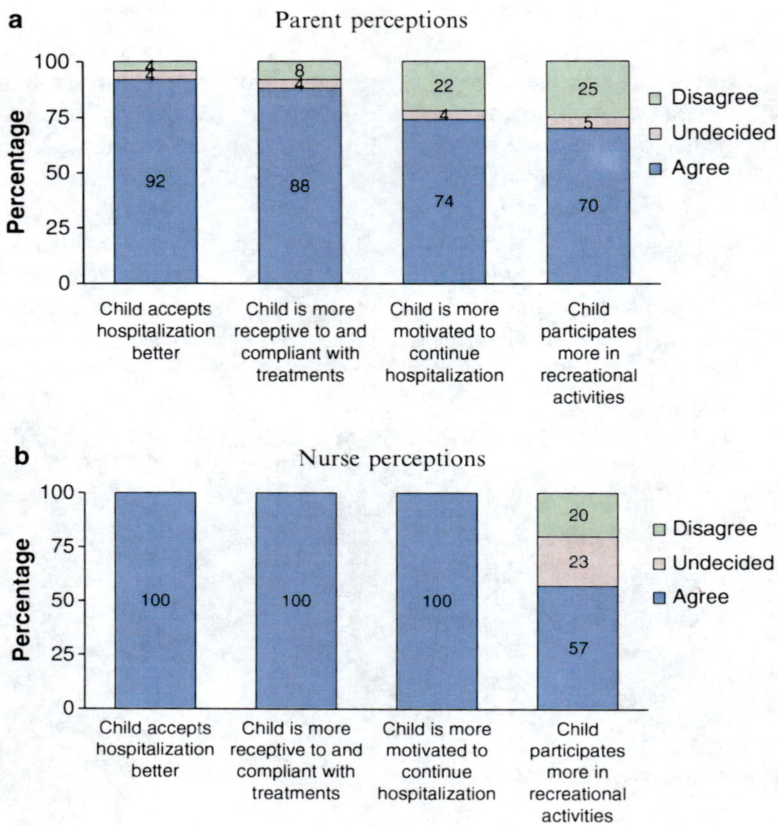

Fig. 4.4 Beneficial treatment effects from therapy dog visits for pediatric oncology patients rated by parents and nurses (Based on [11]). (**a**) Parent perceptions. (**b**) Nurse perceptions

- Ninety-six percent of parents were very satisfied with the therapy dog program.
- Most parents rated the importance of the therapy dog program to their child getting cancer treatment as important (35%) or very important (65%).
- One hundred percent of parents would recommend therapy dog visits to others.
- Availability of a therapy dog program would influence choice of a cancer hospital or unit for 92% of parents.

Furthermore, the nurses caring for children participating in the therapy dog program reported personal benefits from the therapy dogs, including being more cheerful, motivated, and positive [11]. Nurses endorsed that the therapy dogs raised the nurses' spirits and facilitated their work in addition to directly benefiting the children.

Case 2

The adolescent cancer experience is anchored in a sense of loss of control. A survey of ten youths with cancer reported that this perceived loss of control contributed to feelings of frustration and anger, as well as treatment noncompliance [13]. Therapy dog visits can help empower children to feel like they have some control over their environment.

Children hospitalized for cancer treatment regain a sense of having control when

(continued)

Case 2 (continued)
they are visited by handler Tricia Larrabee and her 85-pound Bouvier des Flanders therapy dog Magic. During visits, Tricia encourages children to put Magic through his paces by delivering a variety of obedience commands. Tricia stands behind the children as they request various tricks from Magic, using silent hand signals to facilitate a speedy response from Magic to the child's verbal commands. Children become amazed as Magic sits, lies down, shakes hands, and gently accepts a treat from the child. Tricia notes, "In the hospital, children have no control over most of what happens to them—when they're in bed, what they can eat, which treatments they get. I give them a choice to visit with Magic or not. They may choose to pet him, invite him onto their beds, just look at him from a distance, or go through his obedience commands. Children appreciate having a choice about some part of their hospital stay and their eyes brighten and faces smile when they see that even the smallest child can control my very big dog. These visits help reinforce that these children may not be able to decide everything that happens to them, but they still have some control."

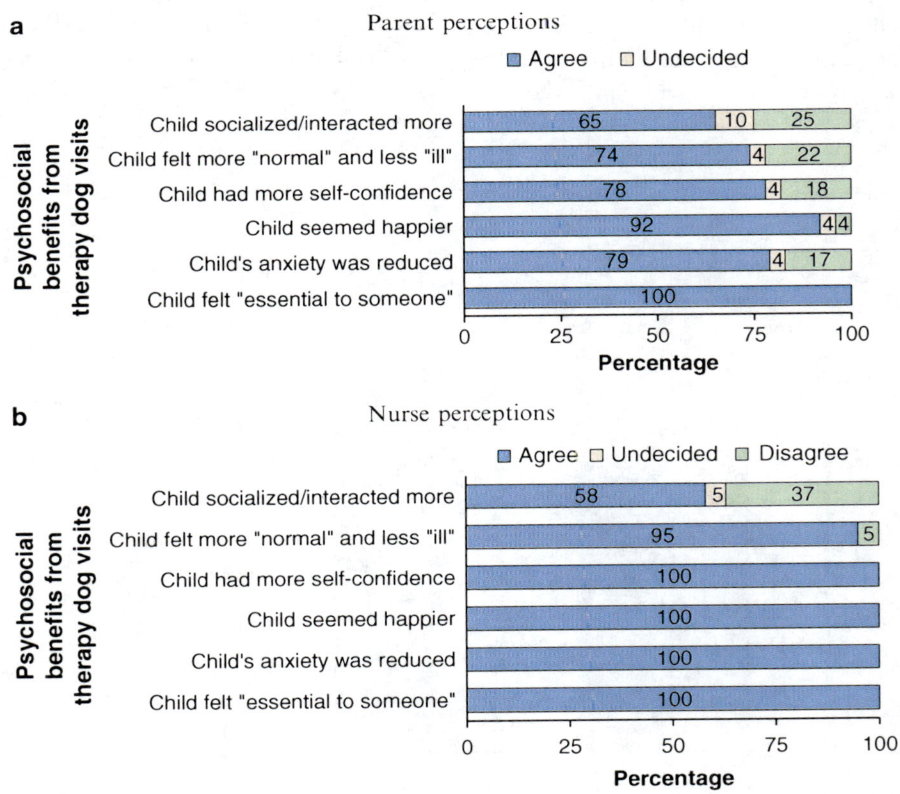

Fig. 4.5 Beneficial psychosocial effects from therapy dog visits for pediatric oncology patients rated by parents and nurses (Based on [11]). (**a**) Parent perceptions. (**b**) Nurse perceptions

Therapy Dogs Can Make a Home Away from Home

Both health-care providers and parents identify the hospital environment as a major stressor for children with cancer that negatively affects both physical and emotional health [14]. Therapy dogs can provide a more positive treatment environment. Bringing a dog into the hospital or treatment facility provides familiarity that is often comforting. For example, 138 children on pediatric hospital units, including hematology-oncology, received weekly group therapy dog visits for 20 weeks, with 5–16 children participating in each visit group (mean group size = 6.5) [15]. Children reported more positive moods after receiving a therapy dog visit compared with days when the dog had not visited (Fig. 4.6). In addition, the weekly visits improved perception of the hospital environment. On dog visit days, children were observed to be more actively involved with the dog as well as hospital personnel, with improved staff relationships.

Case 3

Lynn Ready takes 9-year-old German Shepherd-Rottweiler mix therapy dog Max to visit children staying at a Ronald McDonald House while they are undergoing specialized medical treatments at a university hospital. Family visits with the therapy dog can be helpful for the cancer patient, their parents, and siblings, who are also often negatively affected by family disruptions due to cancer management [16]. Max's visit to a 5-year-old boy undergoing radiation and chemotherapy during the previous two weeks helped shift the family's afternoon from conversations about cancer and cancer treatments to a more typical family afternoon of play. The boy, his older brother, and father enjoyed kicking a ball around, with Max playing goalie. This family has two dogs at home, and bringing Max into their temporary home during cancer treatment helped give everyone in the

(continued)

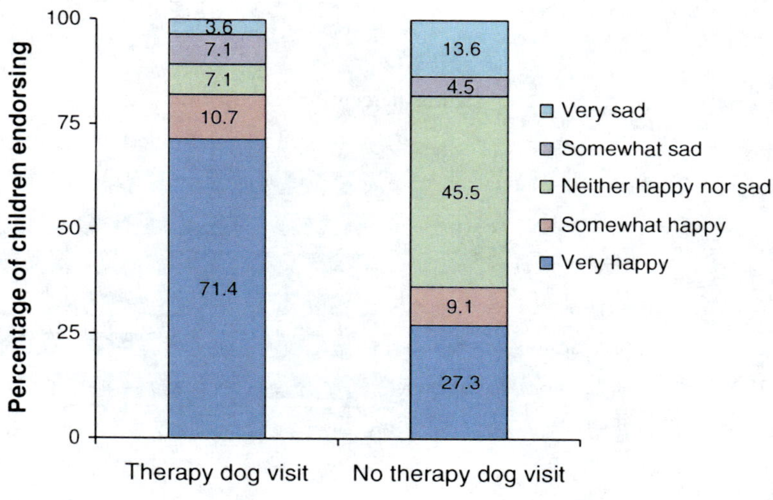

Fig. 4.6 Affect of therapy dog visits to hospitalized children. Using the standardized self-assessment manikin scale, children were asked to rate their affect after a therapy dog visit and at the same time of day on a day when the dog had not visited (Based on [15])

Case 3 (continued)
family a little taste of home and something to smile about that afternoon.

Max's visits become a special anchor for children who are long-term patients. Between Max's visits, the children have a countdown to the day for the next Max visit. One boy was particularly affected by Max. He had been very sad since coming to the hospital and had not spoken. The first words he spoke after coming to the facility were to Max, so the boy's mother dubbed Max her "miracle worker." When this boy's treatments were completed, he was upset and asked to stay at the Ronald McDonald house longer so that he could still visit with Max.

Program volunteer director Becky Magnelli comments, "Max brings a welcome warmth and peaceful energy that flows naturally to our children. When therapy dogs come to the facility, the children get to play like regular children and their parents often get down on their hands and knees too, playing with the dogs and their kids. Therapy dogs remind the children of the lives waiting for them at home after finishing treatment. When the dogs come in, there's lots of joy and laughter, and the focus on illness and hospital treatments is cast aside."

Therapy Dog Visits Before Testing or Treatment

Therapy dogs have been shown to reduce anxiety (see Chap. 2), and their anxiolytic effects may be used for patients waiting for testing or treatment sessions. Therapy dog visits were shown to reduce pretest anxiety in patients scheduled for magnetic resonance imaging (MRI) testing [17]. In this study, 28 patients spent approximately 15 min with a 5-year-old Beagle therapy dog about 30 min before their scheduled MRI. Anxiety scores pre- and post-therapy dog visits were compared and contrasted with anxiety scores measured in six individuals who waited for their MRI without a therapy dog visit. Anxiety was measured using state scores assessing current level of anxiety from the State-Trait Anxiety Inventory (STAI). After the therapy dog visit, patients experienced a 33% reduction in anxiety; there was no significant change among patients waiting for their testing without the dog (Fig. 4.7).

Practical Pointer: Therapy dog visits can reduce anxiety for patients waiting for testing.

These positive data contrast with a study in which 30 patients making frequent hospital visits for radiation treatment were assigned to spend

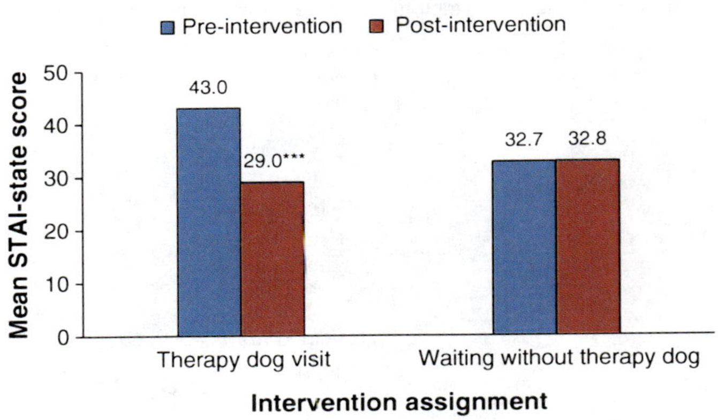

Fig. 4.7 Current anxiety level measured by state score from State-Trait Anxiety Inventory (STAI). Patients participating in a therapy dog visit experienced a significant reduction in anxiety (***$P<0.001$) (Based on [17])

15 min before their treatment sessions with a therapy dog, with a friendly human, or quietly reading for 12 sessions [18]. Typical therapy dog visits include patient interaction with both the handler and the dog, with the handler providing information about the dog, interpreting the dog's reactions for the patient, and listening to the patient talk about their dog experiences. In this study, the handler's interaction consisted of introducing the dog during the first session. For subsequent sessions, handlers were instructed to avoid conversation with the patients. There were no significant changes in mood in any of the groups with any intervention or any between-group differences. Among those patients providing information at the completion of the study, sessions were found to be helpful by 5 in 10 patients assigned to the therapy dog, 9 in 10 assigned to the friendly human volunteer, and 6 in 8 assigned to quiet reading. Seven in 10 would recommend the therapy dog to another patient, 8 in 10 would recommend the human volunteer, and 8 in 8 the quiet reading. In general, patients reported each activity provided a welcome method for reducing anxiety and providing a distraction. Some of the lack of benefit seen with the therapy dog visit may have been related to the limited handler involvement with the patient and dog during visits.

Practical Pointer: Therapy dog visits were identified as helpful for only half of patients attending radiation therapy appointments.

Therapy Dog Visits During Chemotherapy

The impact of including a therapy dog during chemotherapy visits was tested in a prospective study, in which patients were given the option of receiving chemotherapy in a room with a therapy dog or in a room without a therapy dog. Those attending treatment with the therapy dog comprised the experimental group. Patients receiving chemotherapy on alternative days when the therapy dog was not available served as the control [19]. Acceptance of the therapy dog was high, with 89 of 104 patients opting to have treatment in the room with the therapy dog. A similar group of 89 patients was recruited to serve as a control group. During the 20-minute therapy dog visit, patients could observe the dog performing obedience commands, play with the dog, and hold or feed the dog. Improvement in symptoms of distress, heart rate, and oxygenation was numerically better among patients attending chemotherapy with the therapy dog (Table 4.3). While most within-treatment changes were significant for both groups, significant differences between treatments were not tested. Patients receiving dog therapy during chemotherapy reported a significant improvement in depression (33% decrease, $P=0.01$), while depression scores were unchanged for the control group. Somatic symptoms were unchanged in those receiving pet therapy, with a significant increase in aggravation (31% increase, $P=0.01$) in controls after chemotherapy. Vital signs

Table 4.3 Changes in symptoms and signs after chemotherapy visit (Based on [19])

Outcome	Chemotherapy received with therapy dog present $N=89$	Control chemotherapy without therapy dog $N=89$
Symptoms		
Anxiety	74% Improvement***	60% Improvement***
Depression	33% Improvement**	No change
Aggressiveness	54% Improvement***	29% Improvement**
Somatic symptoms	No change	31% Worsening*
Signs		
Heart rate	Decreased from 76.3 to 69.9 beats per minute	Decreased from 77.9 to 72.6 beats per minute
Arterial oxygen saturation	Increased from 97.5% to 98.0%**	Decreased slightly from 97.4% to 97.0%

Within-treatment changes were statistically significant versus prechemotherapy values:
*$P<0.05$; **$P\leq0.01$; ***$P<0.001$

before and after chemotherapy were similar for both groups, with the exception of a 6% increase in arterial oxygen saturation with pet therapy ($P=0.004$) and a nonsignificant 4% decrease in oxygen saturation among controls. The authors considered that the improved oxygenation among patients having the therapy dog visit may have resulted from increased activity among patients interacting with the dogs compared with control patients who were generally motionless in a chair during treatment.

Practical Pointer: In one study, 86% of patients opted to have chemotherapy performed in a room where a therapy dog would be visiting. Therapy dog visits were associated with improved mood and fewer somatic symptoms during chemotherapy compared with receiving chemotherapy without the therapy dog.

Therapy Dog Visits During End-of-Life and Hospice Care

Complementary medicine can be an important component of end-of-life care. A survey of hospice residents revealed that 81% were interested in receiving complementary therapy to improve well-being and provide relaxation and pain relief [20]. Interestingly, 49% of those personally interested in receiving complementary therapy also believed that one of their supportive family members or friends would also be interested in receiving complementary therapy. Similarly, a survey of 30 hospices in Italy reported that over two in three hospice patients offered complementary therapy accepted treatment [21].

Animal therapy has been suggested as a beneficial intervention at end of life [22]. In addition, animal-assisted therapy was listed among potentially useful complementary treatments to incorporate into the intensive care setting for the management of anxiety and agitation among patients receiving mechanical ventilation [23].

Case 4

Therapy dogs can bring a sense of peace and calm at end of life. Normally exuberant 9-year-old Chesapeake Bay Retriever therapy dog Toby visits patients in a mental health facility, engaging patients in outdoor play with games of fetch and tag. On a few occasions, he has also visited patients with terminal diseases who have required quiet time with a therapy dog that Toby instinctively seems to recognize. One of Toby's regular visits was to AM, a 60-year-old woman with bone cancer. During visits, Toby would quietly rest his head on AM's lap, pushing her hand on top of his head, and sitting quietly next to her wheelchair. The impact of these brief visits lasting only a few minutes was highlighted during AM's final weeks of life when she asked to have Toby come for visits. Toby's handler was surprised to find photos of Toby placed at AM's bedside to give her comfort when Toby was not there. On visits where AM was not responding, Toby would sit close at her bedside, and the nurses told Toby's handler AM would talk about having felt Toby's comforting presence when she would briefly wake. Visits with Toby seemed to provide a distraction from AM's pain and discomfort and give her a sense of calm.

Toby also visited 55-year-old cancer patient PR during end-of-life care. Only somewhat responsive, PR was lying in his bed, grimacing, and making verbalizations, including the word "Skippy," who had been his boyhood dog. Toby rested his head on PR's bed, and the nurse lifted PR's hand to stroke the dog. During the visit, PR's face loosened, his body relaxed, and he began to smile. Toby's visit was the first time the nurse had seen PR appear calm and smile. In both cases, brief, quiet visits from Toby helped foster comfort for patients at end of life and their caregivers.

Case 5

TR was a 60-year-old man with mesothelioma admitted to hospice. TR was mainly unresponsive, but a request was made for a therapy dog visit. On TR's second day at hospice, he was visited by 25-pound, 7-year-old Beagle therapy dog Charlie and his handler Patricia Tirrell.

> When Charlie and I arrived in the room, TR's breathing was very labored, and it almost hurt to listen as he struggled to take each breath. I gently placed Charlie on the bed and Charlie stood face-to-face with TR. Charlie seemed to sense that he needed to stand very still to avoid putting pressure on intravenous tubes and catheters under the covers.
>
> As Charlie stood by TR, you could sense the tension leave TR and his breathing calm. TR's breathing became slower, less labored, and quieter. After awhile, TR started making chortling sounds that we recognized as garbled talking. Charlie moved closer to TR's face and started making a very soft sing-song Beagle speech back at TR. Charlie really seemed to be talking to TR. This was really unusual since Charlie rarely vocalizes with patients and understands a therapy dog is not permitted to bark or make noises when working in the hospital.
>
> After about 5 minutes, I took Charlie off of the bed and TR's breathing continued to stay more calm and comfortable. TR's wife stood by during the visit with tears in her eyes, and thanked me for bringing "an angel" therapy dog to help her husband.

Two days later, TR died. The positive interactions between TR and Charlie brought calm to the room and gave both TR's wife and the hospital staff a more affirmative memory of TR's final days.

End-of-Life Support for Secondary Survivors

Therapy dog visits can also provide needed emotional support to family members grieving for loved ones lost to cancer (Fig. 4.8). Research shows that caregivers and family members often experience isolation and a sense of powerlessness after a cancer death [24]. These individuals affected by cancer indirectly have been dubbed "secondary survivors" [24]. Depression after losing a family member to cancer has been reported three months into bereavement for 34% of family caregivers [25], with moderate to severe depression in 15% after 6 months [26].

Companion dogs have been shown to address important needs of people during grief, providing

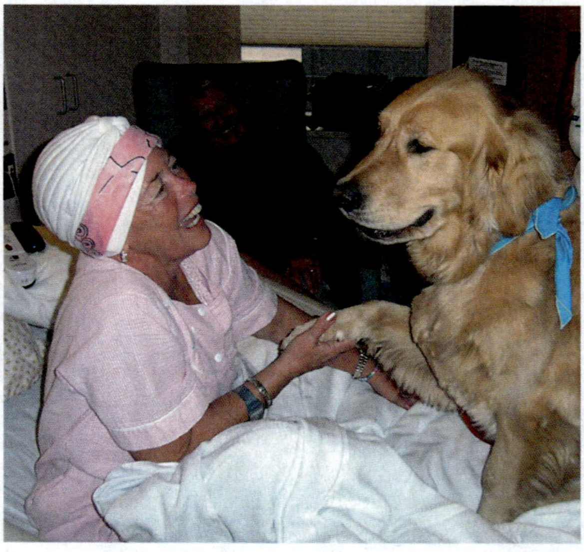

Fig. 4.8 Including dogs during family visits can ease tension, facilitate family connections, and provide positive memories of last times together (Photo courtesy of Kristy Everette of the Pets at Duke program, Duke University Medical Center)

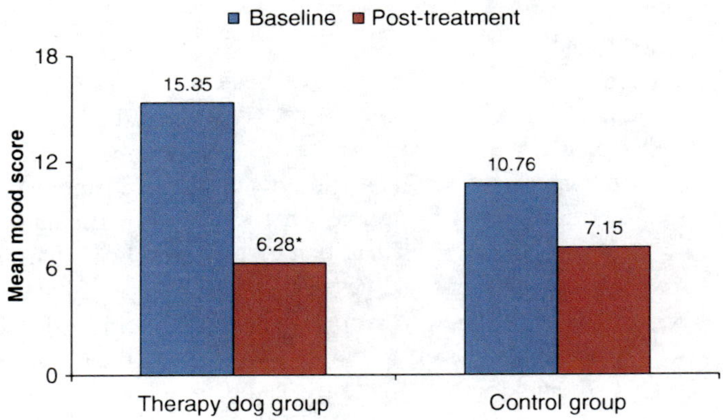

Fig. 4.9 Children's mood questionnaire scores before and after grief counseling for adolescents randomly assigned to include a therapy dog in the sessions or a control group without a therapy dog. Lower scores represent improved mood. Change from baseline to post-treatment was significant for adolescents in the therapy dog group, $^{*}P=0.02$ (Based on [28])

nonjudgmental listening, physical contact, and empathy [27]. Therapy dogs have been used to assist in the grieving process by psychologists and funeral homes. A doctoral thesis from Arizona State University describes a project addressing grief issues in 27 adolescents (mean age = 15 years) dealing with a terminally ill friend or family member or having lost a friend or family member within the previous year [28]. Adolescents attended 3 weekly one-hour treatment sessions with a child life specialist and were randomized to sessions that included either a therapy dog or no therapy dog as a control group. Mood improved 34% with the control group and 59% with the addition of a therapy dog, supporting added benefit of including a therapy dog during grief and loss counseling sessions (Fig. 4.9).

Case 6

Therapy dog visits can make healing connections during times of grief. Counselor Nancy Missildine brings Labrador Retriever therapy dog Gracie into visits with clients. Gracie has learned that grieving adults often reach for a tissue, and the dog carries tissue boxes to people as they start to cry, which deeply touches Nancy's clients. Nancy was especially moved one day when a client talked about the loss of her son. "As this lady was sharing her grief, Gracie started pacing the room, which is very unusual for Gracie. Usually with depressed clients, Gracie nuzzles into their feet. Soon, Gracie went behind the sofa and brought the grieving mother a baby doll. I was so surprised because Gracie had never pulled out a doll before and I didn't know she knew that there were dolls behind the sofa. The mother and I were both impressed by this seemingly intuitive act of understanding and empathy. During the months since that visit, Gracie has never touched the doll basket again for any other client I have seen. That simple act touched this lady and broke down barriers that would have taken a long time for words alone to do. Including Gracie and her incredible intuition during this grief visit made a profound impact in reaching someone who had been walled in by grief."

Case 7

Judith Kelly's Akita therapy dog Apple demonstrated a natural ability to identify and connect with those most in need of a therapy dog's touch. Antonio and Carmen DiGioia were from Venezuela, with limited family for support locally when Carmen received her diagnosis of stage 4 breast cancer in December 2004. Carmen was treated with surgery, chemotherapy, and radiation and remained in remission until January 2009, when metastatic disease was

(continued)

Case 7 (continued)
discovered in her liver, brain, and bones. Although Carmen was not interested in visits from a therapy dog, Apple made a special connection with Antonio. Handler Judith recalls, "When Apple first met Antonio, there was an immediate bond. Apple stood on her hind legs and gave Antonio a big kiss. Every time they met, Antonio would start their visit by bending down to get his special kiss from Apple. As Carmen neared the end of her illness, Antonio seemed to really appreciate visits with Apple. Unlike human friends and family, Apple didn't ask for updates about Antonio's wife or explanations about her condition. Apple simply focused on Antonio and his needs. These special times that were just for Apple and Antonio gave Antonio a needed break from worrying about his wife. After Antonio's wife died, Antonio continued to stay connected with Apple and even began accompanying us on our nursing home visits, acting as an interpreter for patients who didn't speak English. His continued connection with Apple seemed to help Antonio through his grieving after losing his wife."

Therapy Dogs Relieve Staff Stress

Administering cancer therapy can also take a toll on staff. Weariness that can develop in staff from repeatedly offering empathy for pain and suffering in patients has been termed compassion fatigue [29]. In an interesting study, the effect of administering chemotherapy was evaluated in nine nurses [30]. Although the nurses understood that the long-term effect of chemotherapy was intended to be positive for patients, nurses also suffered as they witnessed patients experiencing negative effects from the treatment they administered. In some cases, nurses believed patients had unrealistic expectations about the potential benefits of chemotherapy. Nurses particularly struggled in these cases and in cases where the staff had recommended more conservative treatment, but the patient had opted for aggressive chemotherapy. Administering chemotherapy was particularly difficult when the staff believed that benefit from chemotherapy was unlikely, while negative side effects were almost certain to occur. Stress developed as nurses could be torn between their role as patient advocate and as the team nurse who needed to support recommended therapy. The authors commented that nurses could suffer from a sense of "moral damage" due to conflicts between an obligation to present a positive image of chemotherapy to the patient and a personal belief that this treatment would not be helpful. Nurses were also concerned that their failure to adequately address patient fears and side effects might make patients refuse or prematurely discontinue treatment that might have been helpful. Stress was also increased when nurses were required to manage large numbers of patients.

Practical Pointer: Treating health-care providers can experience significant emotional stress related to caring for terminally ill patients and administering treatments like chemotherapy that typically result in unpleasant side effects. Therapy dog visits should also include cancer staff as a target intervention group.

Stresses inherent in treating terminally ill patients may also need to be addressed. While therapy dog visits are often included as a treatment for patients and their family members, staff may also benefit from spending a few minutes with a therapy dog to reduce stress. Benefits derived by staff may indirectly improve patient care (Fig. 4.10).

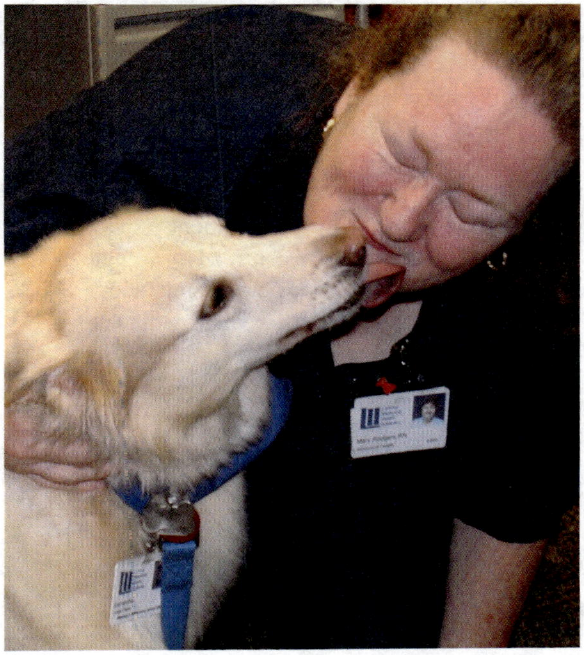

Fig. 4.10 Therapy dog Sami gives a welcome smooch to reduce staff stress

Example of Indirect Patient Benefits from Changes in Staff and Patient Visitors

How therapy dog interactions with staff might indirectly improve patient care was highlighted in an interesting study showing a social facilitation effect with increased staff-patient interactions after an 11-pound (5-kg) Miniature Poodle was added to a hospice [31]. Both staff and patients were evaluated in this study using interviews, observations, and videotaping. Evaluation of staff attitudes and nursing case notes linked staff members' level of personal happiness with their relationships with fellow staff members and patients. These data support the importance of addressing staff stress and burnout to likely improve patient care. Researchers also measured the number of staff-patient interactions in a hospice communal room, showing an increase after the Poodle had been introduced to the hospice.

Another interesting observation from this study was the change in patient-visitor interactions with the introduction of the therapy dog. Before the dog was present, interactions were observed to generally be strained and marked by tension and conversational effort. After the dog joined the hospice, patient-visitor interactions were seen as more animated and positive. In addition, researchers observed a reminiscence effect, where the presence of the therapy dog tended to promote conversations about past memories of personal pets.

Researchers noted that the staff had been concerned about problems that would be introduced to the facility related to the introduction of the therapy dog. Initially high expectations that the presence of the dog would be problematic were reversed after the dog was introduced, with the staff developing an overall favorable attitude after therapy dog visits occurred.

Practical Pointer: Brief encounters with a therapy dog can reduce staff stress, which may improve interactions and relationships among staff members and between staff and patients.

Summary

- Benefits have been shown in cancer patients receiving therapy dog visits during inpatient hospitalizations, chemotherapy, and hospice care.
- Therapy dog visits improve patients' moods, socialization, and sense of control. Physiological improvements have also been documented.
- Therapy dog visits can also reduce patient anxiety when waiting for testing appointments.
- Therapy dog encounters with staff treating cancer patients may help reduce staff stress and indirectly improve patient care.
- Therapy dogs can be helpful during end-of-life care and grief counseling.

References

1. Wu AS, Niedra R, Pendergast L, McCrindle BW. Acceptability and impact of pet visitation on a pediatric cardiology inpatient unit. J Pediatr Nurs. 2002;17:354–62.
2. DeCourcey M, Russell AC, Keister KJ. Animal-assisted therapy. Evaluation and implementation of a complementary therapy to improve the psychological and physiological health of critically ill patients. Dimens Crit Care Nurs. 2010;29:211–4.
3. Muschel IJ. Pet therapy with terminal cancer patients. Soc Casework. 1984;65:451–8.
4. Joseph M. Moments with Baxter: comfort and love from the world's best therapy dog. San Diego, CA: Sage Press; 1997.
5. Bussotti EA, Ribeiro Leão E, Nascimento Chimentão DM, Rodrigues Silva CP. Individualized care: can I bring my dog? Rev Esc Enferm USP. 2005;39:195–201.
6. Vos PJ, Visser AP, Garssen B, Duivenvoorden HJ, de Haes HM. Effects of delayed psychosocial interventions versus early psychosocial interventions for women with early stage breast cancer. Patient Educ Counsel. 2006;60:212–9.
7. Goodwin PJ, Leszcz M, Ennis M, et al. The effect of group psychosocial support on survival in metastatic breast cancer. N Engl J Med. 2001;345:1719–26.
8. de Chico Cicogna E, Nasciemento LC, de Lima RA. Children and adolescents with cancer: experiences with chemotherapy. Rev Lat Am Enfermagem. 2010;18:864–72.
9. Johnson RA, Meadows RL, Haubner JS, Sevedge K. Human–animal interaction. A complementary/alternative medical (CAM) intervention for cancer patients. Am Behav Sci. 2003;47:55–69.
10. Salmela M, Salanterä S, Ruotsalainen T, Aronen ET. Coping strategies for hospital-related fears in pre-school-aged children. J Paediatr Child Health. 2010;46:108–14.
11. Gagnon J, Bouchard F, Landry M, et al. Implementing a hospital-based animal therapy program for children with cancer: a descriptive study. Can Oncol Nurs J. 2004;14:217–22.
12. Bouchard F, Landry M, Belles-Isles M, Gagnon J. A magical dream: a pilot project in animal-assisted therapy in pediatric oncology. Can Oncol Nurs J. 2004;14:14–7.
13. Wicks L, Mitchell A. The adolescent cancer experience: loss of control and benefit finding. Eur J Canc Care. 2010;19:778–85.
14. McCaffrey CN. Major stressors and their effect on the well-being of children with cancer. J Pediatr Nurs. 2006;21:59–66.
15. Caprilli S, Messeri A. Animal-assisted activity at A. Meyer Children's Hospital: a pilot study. Evid Based Complement Alternat Med. 2006;3:379–83.
16. Murray JS. The lived experience of childhood cancer: one sibling's perspective. Issues Compr Pediatr Nurs. 1998;21:217–27.
17. Ruchman R, Ruchman A, Jaeger J, Durand D, Kelly P. Animal-assisted anxiolysis prior to MRI. Am J Roentgenol. 2001;196:A120–34.
18. Johnson RA, Meadows RL, Haubner JS, Sevedge K. Animal-assisted activity among patients with cancer: effects on mood, fatigue, self-perceived health, and sense of coherence. Oncol Nurs Forum. 2008;35:225–32.
19. Orlandi M, Trangeled K, Mambrini A, et al. Pet therapy effects on oncological day hospital patients undergoing chemotherapy treatment. Anticancer Res. 2007;27:4301–4.
20. Rahmin-Jamal S, Sarte A, Kozak J, et al. Hospice residents' interest in complementary and alternative medicine (CAM) at end of life: a pilot study in hospice residences in British Columbia. J Palliat Care. 2011;27:134–40.
21. Belletti M, Mallia L, Lucidi F, et al. Complementary therapy and support services for formal and informal caregivers in Italian palliative care hospices: an exploratory and descriptive study. Support Care Canc. 2011;19:1939–47.
22. Lander DA, Graham-Pole JR. Love medicine for the dying and their caregivers: the body of evidence. J Health Psychol. 2008;13:201–12.
23. Tracy MF, Chlan L. Nonpharmacological interventions to manage common symptoms in patients receiving mechanical ventilation. Crit Care Nurse. 2011;31:19–29.
24. Clark PG, Brethwaite DS, Gnesdiloff S. Providing support at time of death from cancer: results of a 5-year post-bereavement group study. J Soc Work End Life Palliat Care. 2011;7:195–215.
25. Holtslander LF, McMillan SC. Depressive symptoms, grief, and complicated grief among family caregivers of patients with advanced cancer three months into bereavement. Oncol Nurs Forum. 2011;38:60–5.

26. Guldin MB, Vedsted P, Zahariae R, Olesen F, Jensen AB. Complicated grief and need for professional support in family caregivers of cancer patients in palliative care: a longitudinal cohort study. Support Care Canc, in press.
27. Allen K. Coping with life changes and transitions: the role of the pet. Interactions. 1995;13:5–8.
28. Teso J. The effect of a therapy dog on the effectiveness of a child life intervention with adolescents experiencing grief and loss. Thesis approved April 2011. Available at: http://proquest.umi.com/pqdlink?did=2353103621&Fmt=7&clientId=79356&RQT=309&VName=PQD. Accessed Sep 2011.
29. Perry B, Toffner G, Merrick T, Dalton J. An exploration of the experience of compassion fatigue in clinical oncology nurses. Can Oncol Nurs J. 2011;21:91–105.
30. Saltmarsh K, De Vries K. The paradoxical image of chemotherapy: a phenomenological description of nurses' experiences of administering chemotherapy. Eur J Canc Care. 2008;17:500–8.
31. Chinner TL, Dalziel FR. An exploratory study on the viability and efficacy of a pet-facilitated therapy project within a hospice. J Palliat Care. 1991;7:13–20.

5 Adding Therapy Dogs to Your Cancer Treatment Team

Key Chapter Points

- Facility-specific guidelines need to be developed to address certification requirements for therapy dogs, practical logistics of therapy dog visits, and infection control issues.
- Policies should be developed using expertise from volunteer coordinators, risk management, infection control specialists, veterinarians, and therapy dog handlers.
- Outside agencies are used to train, test, and certify therapy dogs. Insurance is generally provided through these agencies.
- Dogs can become colonized with some human pathogens. Implementing infection control procedures and controlling dog behavior during visits reduce risks for dogs becoming colonized.
- Established programs incorporating therapy dogs as complementary treatment for cancer patients offer role models for the development of new programs.

Keywords

Certification • Infection control • Methicillin-resistant *Staphylococcus aureus* (MRSA) • Policies

Therapy dogs may be used in outpatient and inpatient settings. Facility-specific guidelines determine which areas of patient care may be included in therapy dog interventions. Before therapy dog visits are started, clear policies need to be developed to help establish the aims and procedures for therapy dog visits. Because therapy dog visits can impact a wide range of individuals, all branches of facility personnel who might be affected or have concerns about adding dog visits to a facility should be included in policy development. Policies need to be established to determine which dogs might be acceptable volunteers, the logistics of visits (including patient selection), and infection precautions. Insurance to cover mishaps during therapy dog visits would typically be provided through the organization certifying the therapy dog.

D.A. Marcus, *Therapy Dogs in Cancer Care: A Valuable Complementary Treatment*,
DOI 10.1007/978-1-4614-3378-1_5, © Springer Science+Business Media New York 2012

There are several key components to effective therapy dog programs:

- Selecting dogs with proper temperaments for patient visits
- Training handlers and their dogs before starting to make visits
  - Prior to initiating any visits, the dog-handler team should be tested and certified through recognized credentialing organizations like Therapy Dogs International, the Delta Society, or Therapy Dogs Incorporated
  - Dog-handler training is not completed with successfully achieving therapy dog certification. Handlers will need to continue to train and reinforce obedience and socialization skills in their dogs
- Orienting dog handlers to unique facility policies and providing written policy summaries for dog visits
- Requiring annual health and temperament evaluations to ensure dogs continue to be appropriate for making visits
- Establishing a relationship with a veterinary consultant who can review and approve visit policies and provide consultation when questions or concerns arise

Programs must be designed using clear policies that are understood and accepted by facility staff, the volunteer coordinator, and the therapy dog-handler teams. Careful preparation before beginning visits helps identify and correct potential problems before they occur.

Establishing a Therapy Dog Program

Similar to the development of other volunteer or facility therapeutic programs, therapy dog programs should be implemented only after facility staff have determined program feasibility, verified interest from staff and patients, resolved logistical problems, and adopted clear policies and procedures (Table 5.1). Credentialing for both the therapy dog and handler should be maintained up to date and reviewed by the program coordinator annually. In some cases, facilities may permit only a single therapy dog to visit at any particular time to avoid unwanted play between therapy dogs and excessive activity. Throughout each visit, the handler should monitor the dog for signs of stress, fatigue, or discomfort that suggest a visit should be concluded. Any incidents, including patients being frightened by well-behaved dogs, should be reported to the nursing supervisor and volunteer coordinator. In some cases, patients who have been listed as candidates for therapy dog visits are subsequently identified as noncandidates, due to patients expressing a desire not to have a dog visit or having allergies or a fear of dogs. Reporting to supervising personnel is important to avoid future unwelcome visits.

Consensus guidelines for successful dog therapy visits were published in the *American Journal of Infection Control* [1]. These guidelines were developed by an expert panel that included individuals with expertise in animal-assisted therapy and activities, infection control, public health, and veterinary medicine. Recommendations are summarized in Boxes 1 and 2.

Model Oncology Therapy Dog Program

The Pets at Duke therapy dog program has often been used as a model for developing new animal-assisted therapy and activity programs. Kristy Everette, coordinator of oncology recreation therapy at the Duke Cancer Institute, uses her expertise from the Pets at Duke program to develop guidelines other facilities can utilize to more smoothly implement successful therapy dog programs. Everette recommends establishing a multidisciplinary steering committee as an initial step for developing a new therapy dog program (Table 5.2). This committee will develop policies to be implemented by all staff and volunteers participating in therapy dog visits.

> **Practical Pearl** A multidisciplinary committee should be formed to develop therapy dog program policies.

Table 5.1 Policies needed for a variety of therapy dog program issues

Issue	Sample policy
Selecting eligible therapy dogs	Dogs should be required to have up-to-date certification from a recognized credentialing agency (e.g., Therapy Dogs International, Delta Society, or Therapy Dogs, Inc.)
	Facilities may additionally require dogs to pass temperament, behavior, and obedience skills by an examiner at the facility
	Annual health and temperament evaluations should be completed by a licensed veterinarian. State-required vaccinations (including rabies) should be maintained up to date
Screening handlers	Handlers should provide up-to-date personal references, child abuse clearance, criminal background check, and tuberculosis testing (PPD). Handlers should fulfill all facility volunteer requirements and complete facility volunteer orientation and training prior to starting to make visits. Handlers must follow all facility procedures for volunteers
Identifying dog-handler teams	Therapy dogs and their handlers should be required to wear photo identification to verify that both are serving in a volunteer capacity and are permitted in the facility. In some cases, dogs may wear bandannas and handlers may wear shirts or jackets to additionally show their volunteer status at the facility
Identifying patients	Some facilities will prescreen individuals for an interest in therapy dog visits, especially visits involving minors. In this case, parental consent is generally required
	Prior to entering any patient's room, handlers should knock and ask permission to enter; they should then ask if the individual is interested in a therapy dog visit. Individuals not interested should be thanked, and the handler should promptly remove the dog
Timing of visits	Visits should only be provided at times that do not interfere with general patient care. Visits should not occur when patients are receiving care from health-care providers, are having procedures, or are speaking with a health-care provider. Visits should not occur during meal times. Handlers may return at a more convenient time or visit the patient on a different day
Policy for companion pet visits	Many facilities restrict animal visits to certified therapy dogs and service dogs to ensure that animal visits will be safe. Some facilities may permit clean, healthy, well-behaved companion pets to visit their owners. If companion pet visits are permitted, the pet should only be permitted to visit with the pet's owner in the owner's room; the pet should not be permitted to visit with other patients or facility staff
Infection control	Dogs must be bathed and groomed before visits. Both handlers and dogs should be healthy and must be free of infectious diseases on visit days. Hand hygiene must be practiced before and after each individual patient exposure. Handlers may be required to carry a small container of hand sanitizer for themselves and patients to use before and after visits. Protocols should be followed to minimize infection exposure, such as placing fresh linens on bedding before dog visits and removing these linens at visit completion. Therapy dogs may be restricted from visiting patients who are immunocompromised, on isolation precautions, or in critical care units
Additional concerns	Dogs should not wear flea/tick collars during visits to avoid exposing patients to the chemicals contained in these collars
	Dogs displaying inappropriate or aggressive behavior during a visit should be prohibited from visiting until cleared by a veterinarian and reevaluated for appropriate behavior

Box 1 Consensus Guidelines for Therapy Dog Visits: Policies for Establishing a Therapy Dog Program (Based on [1, 2])

- Policies to be established before any visits begin:
  - *Facility requirements*
    - A facility-specific animal visitation policy should be established, with requirements explained to each dog handler before any visits are made.
  - *Selecting appropriate therapy dogs*
    - Dogs utilized should be suitable for animal-assisted activities. Suitable dogs are current family pets who have completed animal-therapy training, testing, and certification and who consistently follow their handler's commands.
    - The dog's temperament should be suitable for patient visits. Therapy dogs should not bothered by:
      - Strangers
      - Loud noises or sudden movements
      - Threatening voices or gestures
      - Crowds
      - Vigorous or clumsy petting or restraining hugs
      - Small children
      - Equipment that might be encountered during a visit (like walkers, wheelchairs, and intravenous poles)
      - Other animals
    - The dog must be in good health, with vaccinations maintained up to date.
  - *Handler requirements*
    - Both dog and handler need to complete training and certification testing for animal-assisted activities. The handler and dog should be certified as a team to ensure that they work effectively together.

Box 2 Consensus Guidelines for Therapy Dog Visits: Procedures for Therapy Dog Visits (Based on [1, 2])

- Protocol for making visits:
  - *First visit to a facility*
    - The first patient visit made by a dog-handler team at each facility they visit should be supervised by a representative of the facility's animal visitation program.
    - Dog-handler teams who are already making visits at other facilities still require facility-specific orientation, instructions, and an initial supervised visit at any new facility.
  - *Dog requirements on visit days*
    - The dog must be healthy, clean, and brushed on visit days. Dogs need annual health assessments by a veterinarian.
    - The dog must stay on a leash throughout the visit.
  - *Handler requirements on visit days*
    - The handler must also be healthy and free of infectious conditions on the day of the visit.
    - Handlers must schedule opportunities during each visit for the dog to relieve itself before beginning their visit, with additional breaks provided during the visit, as needed.
    - Handlers must wash their hands before and after seeing every patient. Handlers should carry hand sanitizer for themselves and patients to use at each visit.
    - The dog must be kept under control of the handler throughout the visit. The care of the dog should never be allocated to another person during any visit.
    - The handler should meet with staff before beginning each visit to determine which patients should and should not be visited that day.

(continued)

Table 5.2 Steering committee members for developing a therapy dog program

Therapy dog program committee role	Responsibilities
Coordinator	Spearhead, organize, and run program. Supervise other committee members and volunteers. Educate facility personnel about therapy dog program. Orient volunteers. Receive and review suggestions and complaints from staff and volunteers
Infection control specialist	Develop policies to minimize infection risk
Risk management expert	Review policies, verify insurance is available for each dog-handler team (e.g., certificates from certifying therapy dog organization), address risk concerns/complaints
Veterinarian	Provide expertise for developing program policies regarding dog training/behavioral/health requirements, review infection control policies, address dog-related concerns
Physician	Provide expertise for developing program policies, review infection control policies
Therapy dog handler	Provide expertise for developing program policies, address practical concerns about visit logistics, and verify that policies can be practically implemented during typical dog visits

Box 2 Consensus Guidelines: Procedures (continued)

Prescreening who will be visited helps respect patients who are not interested in receiving visits and ensures patients who are not able to receive visits (e.g., due to isolation precautions) will not be inappropriately visited.

- The handler must ask permission from each patient before entering his or her room.
- Visits should be avoided during patient meals, procedures, or when patients are being attended to by staff.

Everette recommends beginning therapy dog work by selecting a single medical unit that might be a candidate location for therapy dog visits. This location should be surveyed to determine interest, with the physician responsible for that unit required to provide written acceptance of an interest in pet therapy. Physicians who are not interested may be queried to determine if lack of interest is the result of misconceptions over medical risk. Following physician acceptance, all staff members working on the unit should be surveyed and any misgivings or staff fears addressed. After addressing staff concerns and approval has been given to start a therapy dog program on a unit, an in-service training session should be conducted by the coordinator with the unit staff to educate them about the logistics, benefits, and potential infection concerns with therapy dog visits. Following completion of in-service training, therapy dog visits may be initiated, with initial visits supervised by a staff member from the therapy dog team. After successful implementation in one location, the same process would be repeated to expand the program to include additional units.

Practical Pearl New therapy dog programs are often best started by restricting visits to a single unit or facility location. This allows practical aspects of program logistics to be evaluated and refined before expanded to larger areas.

Recommendations for Making Visits

Therapy dog handlers should sign in when entering a facility and sign out when leaving. Handlers should also meet with unit coordinators before patient visits are made to determine which patients are interested in visits and to review necessary restrictions.

Handlers should plan to visit a facility for a total of about 30–60 min. Each individual patient will generally spend between 5 and 15 min with the dog. Most handlers will visit a facility between once a month and once a week. More handlers will be needed for a program to provide additional visits. Research from a day hospice that added regular therapy dog visits to their facility confirmed that therapy dogs enjoy visits, but visits are work for the dogs [3]. Dr. David Phear noted, "The dogs appear to enjoy the visits and attention, but return home exhausted" (p. 338) [3]. This supports previously described data that visits are work for dogs and restrictions on visit duration and frequency are necessary (see Chap. 2).

Practical Pearl Visit expectations are generally based on total time rather than number of patients seen. After spending 30–60 min with patients, most therapy dogs are fatigued and need to end their visit.

Identifying Appropriate Dogs

Dogs may be recommended for therapy work by their owners, trainers, or veterinarians who may identify that a particular dog displays a well-mannered demeanor, social nature, and natural ability to connect with strangers (Box 3). Training a dog for therapy dog work often involves spending time walking and working on obedience commands in high traffic areas, such as busy street sidewalks or parks, to ensure the dog is comfortable and can maintain good obedience when exposed to large groups of people, noise, and unfamiliar situations. A therapy dog cannot react negatively or bark in these situations. In addition, a therapy dog must be comfortable with people of all shapes and sizes and people using equipment (e.g., crutches, walkers, wheelchairs, or other assistive devices). Including exposure of the dog to large groups of diverse people helps facilitate this comfort.

Box 3 Typical Attributes of Therapy Dog Candidates

- Consistently follows commands for sit, down, stay, and come, including with distractions (other dogs, playing outdoors, or visiting pet stores)
- Walks nicely on a leash without pulling, especially when walking by or through groups of people (e.g., on busy sidewalks)
- Enjoys being greeted by strangers (e.g., the dog should eagerly approach unfamiliar people)
- Is able to be greeted, petted, and hugged (including clumsy petting and restraining hugs) without jumping, straining, barking, or biting
- Is able to avoid sniffing or picking up interesting items (i.e., consistently follows "leave it" command)
- Tolerates crowds, activity, and noise
- Tolerates getting bathed, brushed, and having nails clipped in preparation for visits
- Greets new situations, unusual equipment, and strangers of different ages without distress

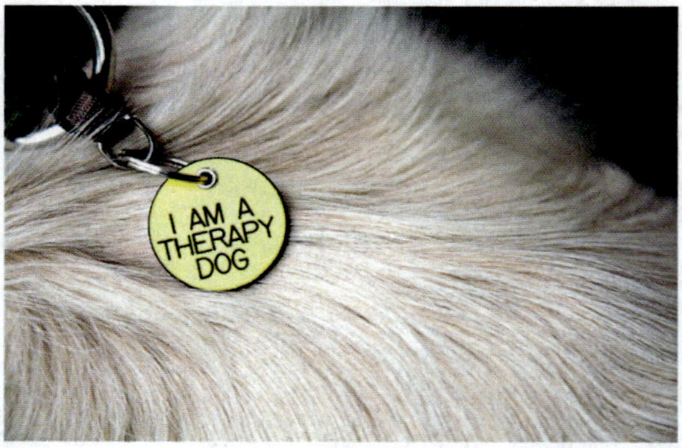

Fig. 5.1 Dogs certified through Therapy Dogs International wear a bright yellow tag (Photo by Leah Charbonneau from Charbonneau Photography)

Basic obedience training, temperament testing, and specialized therapy dog training and testing are required prior to beginning therapy dog visits (Fig. 5.1). Certification can be obtained through recognized therapy dog organizations (see Chap. 10). The American Kennel Club offers Canine Good Citizen (CGC) certification, which is intended to demonstrate that the dog has mastered basic obedience training and shows appropriate interaction with people and other dogs. CGC certification is often considered to be sufficient for therapy dogs visiting in nursing homes or participating in reading programs with children. Additional therapy dog testing is generally required to supplement CGC certification before therapy visits can be made to health-care facilities like hospitals.

Prior to making visits, therapy dogs must be evaluated and certified by examiners unfamiliar with each particular dog. Handlers will complete this testing as part of the certification process. Examination by an expert in therapy dog certification who is unfamiliar with a particular dog is essential because therapy dogs are expected to display exemplary behavior when confronted with strangers as part of their work. Assurances that a dog "normally" is well behaved or behaves perfectly at home cannot replace outside certification and credentialing.

Practical Pearl Prior to beginning therapy dog visits, verification of successfully completed therapy dog testing is needed. Certification is generally updated annually.

Breed, Size, and Age Requirements

While Golden Retrievers and Labrador Retrievers are probably the most common therapy dogs due to general obedience, outgoing demeanor, and breed popularity, all breeds or mixed breed dogs can become therapy dogs. Appropriateness for therapy work depends on the personality, temperament, and training of each individual dog rather than being related to breed. In addition, dogs of any size may be trained to be therapy dogs.

Examples of "Bully" Breeds as Therapy Dogs [4]

- Rottweiler Dillon is a therapy dog who helps abused, neglected, and at-risk children through Gabriel's Angels.
- Former Michael Vick fighting dog, Pit Bull Hector, was rescued and trained to be a therapy dog, making visits to hospitals and schools.
- Year 2006 Westminster Best In Show Colored Bull Terrier Rufus retired from the show ring to become a therapy dog, visiting injured military personnel at Walter Reed Hospital.

Individual dog temperament and size often dictate environments where dogs might be most comfortable and the activities that occur during visits. While small dogs may be placed on laps for petting, many patients enjoy petting larger dogs sitting next to their chair or bed (Fig. 5.2). In one study, seniors with dementia were offered visits from a small 11-lb (5-kg) Miniature Schnauzer, a medium 35-lb (16-kg) Schnauzer, and a large 44-lb (20-kg) Standard Poodle [5]. The longest time duration the dogs were permitted to stay with any one senior was 3 min (180 s). Seniors spent more time with and were less likely to refuse a visit from the largest dog (Fig. 5.3). This study highlights that certain populations and certain individual patients may be more comfortable with certain types and sizes of dogs. It is important to recognize that some people may feel less comfortable receiving visits from certain dogs and may require more time observing the dog at a distance before they are comfortable approaching the dog directly for petting.

Most therapy dog organizations require dogs to be at least 1 year old prior to beginning to make therapy dog visits. Younger dogs may not be adequately trained or reliable enough to successfully make visits. Many dogs first begin therapy dog work after they are several years old, when their energy level has decreased to make maintaining a quiet and calm demeanor during visits easier.

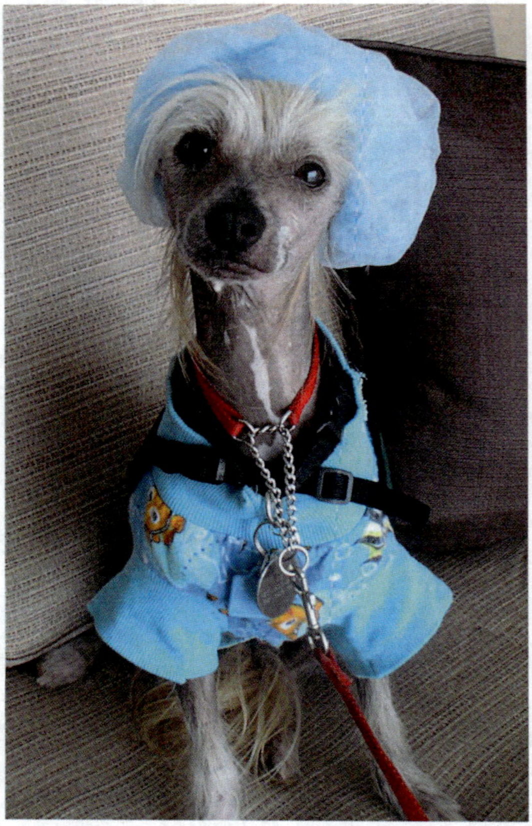

Fig. 5.2 Small dogs can be effective therapy dogs. Ten-pound Chinese Crested therapy dog Ike makes weekly early morning visits to Charlotte Regional Hospital where he spends time with children who are having surgery that day. Ike even rides on the gurney with them to the operating room

Therapy Dog Sixth Sense

Therapy dog handlers often discuss their dog's intuitive sixth sense for recognizing those most in need of the dog's attention, with dogs often preferentially gravitating to patients in need instead of the often more eager nonpatient family members [4]. Therapy dogs seem adept at quickly reading and interpreting new environments to determine how to best achieve therapeutic interventions. Like many therapy dogs, 60-lb, 5½-year-old German Shepherd Pearl has an intuitive sense about how to adjust her visits to best meet individual patient needs when visiting patients at Children's Hospital in Pittsburgh, PA, with handler Seadon Renfrow:

> *Pearl instinctively adjusts her intervention to meet the needs of her patients. Despite her size, Pearl can snuggle next to children in bed in intensive care or sit on a chair next to their beds and place her paws on the bed, carefully avoiding all the tubes that are usually connected to these children. When visiting a young girl with a brain tumor, Pearl recognized the positive energy in the room and her presence turned the room into a party atmosphere. Pearl, however, understands when it's time to present a more sedate and calming presence. When visiting this same girl shortly after the girl underwent surgery, Pearl lied calmly with the girl on her bed so the two could share some quiet loving. However Pearl interacts, you can sense that the children get a needed distraction from their pain and worry, gather some happiness, and appreciate the unconditional love they get from Pearl's weekly visits.*

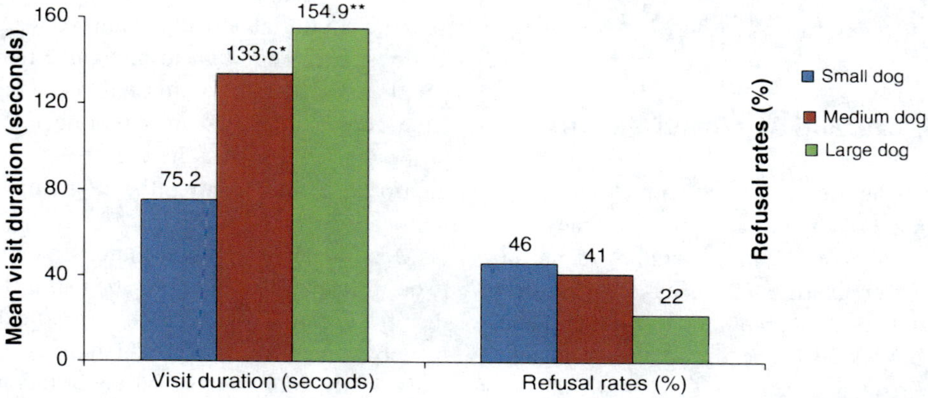

Fig. 5.3 Comparison of therapy dog visits to seniors based on dog size. Differences in visit duration between small dog and medium or large dog were significant: $*P=0.024$, $**P=0.009$. Significance was not reported for differences in refusal rates (Based on [5])

A therapy dog's ability to recognize and interpret situations that require different behavior from the dog is an important ingredient for successful therapy dog interventions.

Guidelines for Dog-Handler Teams

Therapy dog certification is generally a recognition of a specific dog-handler team. This certification covers visits made by a particular handler with a particular dog. This certification does not extend to other dogs or handlers who have not been specifically tested as a team. In most cases, handlers will bring only a single therapy dog for a visit. Occasionally, a handler may bring two dogs together; in that case, additional certification is needed to certify the handler working with the two dogs simultaneously. Therefore, this handler will likely have a certification for the handler with dog A, another certification for the handler with dog B, and a third certification for the handler with dogs A and B working together.

Volunteering has consistently been shown to improve a sense of well-being in the volunteer, as well as increase life satisfaction and improve mood [6]. Volunteers typically report that they benefit almost as much as patients from their volunteering [7]. Furthermore, volunteering has been linked to delayed mortality in the volunteer [8]. A study from Stanford University monitored 7,527 seniors for 8 years. Compared with people who never volunteered, risk of dying was 42% lower in people who volunteered sometimes and 53% lower in those volunteering frequently ($P<0.001$). After accounting for gender, age, and socioeconomic variables, risk of dying was still reduced by 34% if sometimes volunteering and 45% when frequently volunteering ($P<0.001$). After additionally accounting for medical and disability characteristics, physical activity, and social integration and support, mortality risk continued to be decreased by 19% ($P<0.05$) among those frequently volunteering. A similar 7-year study from Israel likewise linked volunteering with a reduced mortality risk, even after adjusting for age, gender, education, baseline mental health and physical health, activity level, and social engagement [9].

Handlers should limit their volunteer commitments so that therapy dog visits continue to be enjoyable and do not become tedious for either the dog or the handler. Sociologist Van Willigen evaluated the effects of volunteering on perceived health and life satisfaction by considering volunteer age, volunteer commitments, and baseline demographics, using data from the Americans' Changing Lives survey of 3,617 adults 25 years and older [10]. Analyses showed that volunteering had the same impact on improved life satisfaction in younger and older adults (Fig. 5.4a). While older adults gained increasing satisfaction with more hours spent volunteering, satisfaction peaked in younger adults volunteering about 2.5 h each week, with life satisfaction decreasing when volunteer hours increased above that point (Fig. 5.4b). Furthermore, older adults benefited more by volunteering for more than one organization, while satisfaction was reduced in younger adults volunteering for more than one organization (Fig. 5.4c). Similar patterns were shown for perceived health among volunteers, with health perceived to be better among volunteers and benefits increasing when adults ≥60 years old reported more volunteer hours and organizations. Perceived health benefits peaked in adults <60 years old when volunteering for a maximum of about 2.5 h weekly at a single organization. To maximize volunteer satisfaction and benefits, total volunteering commitments should generally be limited for the handler.

Practical Pearl Volunteer satisfaction and benefits will be maximized by limiting the number and hours spent volunteering.

Selecting Appropriate Patient Candidates for Visits

Both genders and patients who are not dog lovers or dog owners can benefit from therapy dog visits. For example, in a pediatric study evaluating therapy dogs for pain relief, similar benefit

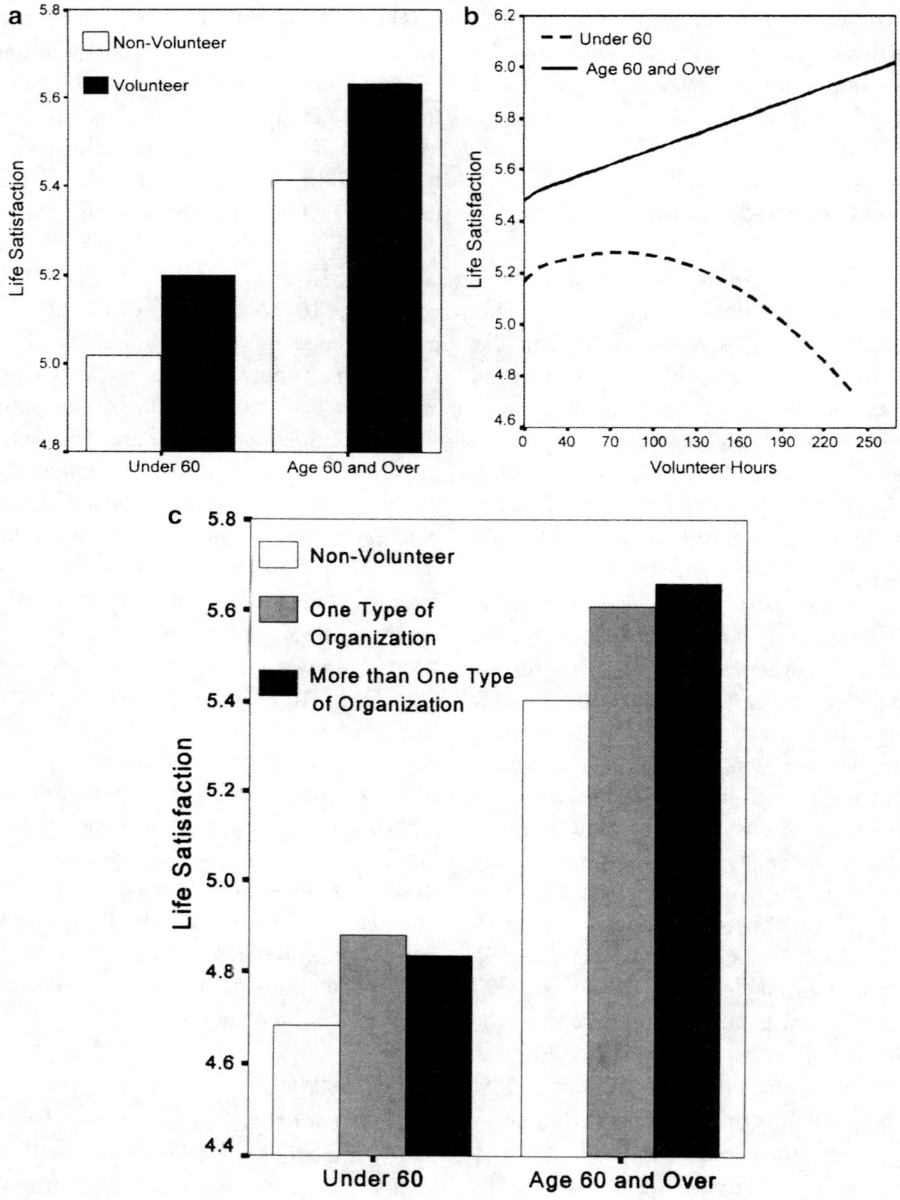

Fig. 5.4 Effect of volunteer work on life satisfaction for older and younger adults, after controlling for baseline satisfaction and demographic variables. Higher scores represent better satisfaction (Reproduced with permission from [10]). (**a**) Life satisfaction among volunteers and nonvolunteers based on age. (**b**) Life satisfaction among volunteers based on annual hours spent volunteering. (**c**) Life satisfaction based on the number of organizations for which one is volunteering

occurred for male and female patients, as well as children with and without pets in their own homes. Visits should be restricted to patients expressing an interest in a visit from a therapy dog and those who are well enough to participate in a visit. In some cases, patients' families may appreciate a visit from a therapy dog, even when the patient is unavailable or is unable to participate in the visit. During each visit, patients must be allowed to dictate the level of contact they

Table 5.3 Behaviors during the last 48 h of life. Negative symptoms were recorded during the last 48 h of life in 36% of 200 consecutive hospice patients. Frequency of individual symptoms is shown in the Table (Based in [11])

Behavior	Percentage (%)
Noisy breathing	56
Agitation/restlessness	42
Jerking, twitching, plucking	12
Confusion	9

wish to have with the dog, which may range from merely observing the dog to petting and playing with the dog.

Prior to visiting individual patients, the handler should confer with the nursing staff to ensure that patients are appropriate candidates, including patients who have previously received therapy dog visits. Changes in patient conditions, including immune compromise, development of infectious diseases, or behavioral changes, may preclude previously appropriate candidates from currently receiving visits. For example, handler Lynn Huber Jablonski was scheduled to take 7-lb Japanese Chin-Papillon mix therapy dog Boy to visit a hospice patient they had been seeing regularly. The patient had been the wife of a veterinarian, and she was particularly fond of visits from Boy. During Boy's final visit to this patient, the handler had not been informed that the patient's condition had substantially deteriorated and she had shifted into "active dying," when physiological changes occur that alert hospice workers that death is imminent. During active dying, patients often become increasingly unresponsive. Patients may also become confused, agitated, and hallucinate (Table 5.3) [11]. Confusion may occur from changes in the environment, misperceptions about unfamiliar stimuli, or biochemical imbalance [11]. A retrospective chart review of 284 consecutive hospice patients with cancer identified an agitated delirium in 20% during the five days preceding death [12]. During the visit with Boy, the patient was increasingly confused and disoriented, and when she was informed that it was time for Boy to leave, she protested and refused to loosen her grip on the dog. The nursing staff was summoned to assist Lynn in gently but firmly prying the patient's fingers from Boy's body to avoid having him become inadvertently injured. While the nurses had been aware that the patient's demeanor had markedly changed that day, failure to communicate that information to the handler resulted in the dog being placed in a potentially unsafe situation. While successfully resolved with no damage to patient or dog, this case highlights the importance of sharing essential information between staff and handlers.

Infection Precautions with Therapy Dogs

Infection control is an important concern for all patients, particularly for patients with cancer. Infection concerns are especially high in medical facilities because of the prevalence of resistant organisms. *Staphylococcus aureus* was identified as the predominant organism detected in skin and soft tissue infections in the SENTRY Antimicrobial Surveillance Program, with methicillin resistance common across continents (Fig. 5.5) [13].

Infection control with therapy dogs is, therefore, of particular importance. In general, facilities may permit visits to immunocompromised patients, if deemed appropriate by their treatment team, and infection prevention protocols are carefully followed [1, 2]. Published guidelines have recommended restricting therapy animals from visiting in critical care units or patients in isolation; this recommendation, however, is not given as a strong directive as it is supported by only limited data [1, 2]. When strict infection protocols are followed, some facilities do opt to permit therapy dog visits, with the dog leaving the facility immediately after seeing a patient in isolation to limit risks for spreading infections to other patients.

Concern about infection can limit acceptance of therapy dog programs. Of particular concern is the potential spread of infection as dogs might potentially carry germs as a vector from one patient to another. A one-year study evaluated the occurrence of infection at a children's hospital after implementing a therapy dog program [14]. After 1 year of weekly dog visits, the hospital

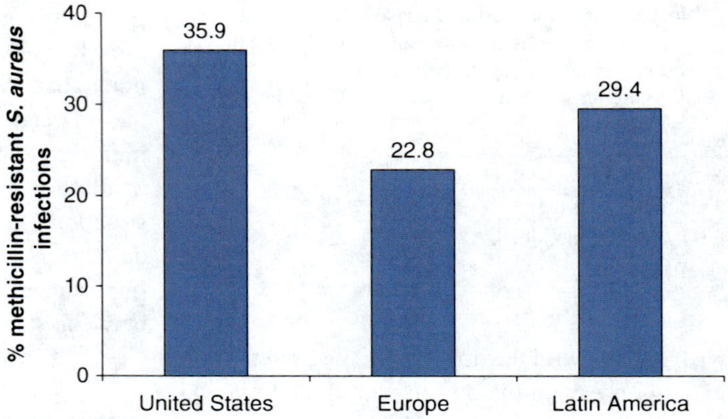

Fig. 5.5 Incidence of methicillin resistance among *S. aureus* infections (Based on [13])

infection committee concluded that there was no difference in hospital infections rate in comparison to the year prior to instituting the therapy dog program. There were also no identified instances where microorganisms or contagious illnesses had been transmitted by the dogs.

> **Practical Pointer** American College of Critical Care Medicine Task Force Guidelines [15] state:
>
> "There is no evidence that pets that are clean and properly immunized should be restricted from the [intensive care unit] ICU environment."—p. 612

Human Colonization with MRSA

Asymptomatic methicillin-resistant *S. aureus* (MRSA) colonization may be a significant source of potential infection risk. Community-acquired MRSA has been identified as a significant contributor to health-care-associated infection [16]. Asymptomatic nasal colonization with MRSA has been reported not uncommonly. Using laboratory cultures from nasal swabs obtained from 758 patients at hospital admission, 3% were colonized with MRSA and 21% with methicillin-sensitive *S. aureus* [17]. An observational study of 5,375 patients screened within 48 h of hospital admission reported MRSA in 11%, the vast majority of whom were asymptomatic carriers [18]. Another study used polymerase chain reaction (PCR) testing to identify *S. aureus* from samples taken from the anterior nares, oropharynx, palms, groin, perirectal area, wounds, and catheter insertion sites in 400 patients presenting to an emergency department [19]. Methicillin-sensitive *S. aureus* was present in 39% of patients, with 5% colonized with MRSA.

MRSA colonization is also common among health-care workers. A survey screening 100 surgical unit workers (22 doctors, 15 residents, 16 nurses, 21 medical students, and 26 nursing students) with nasal swabs indentified *S. aureus* colonization in 13% and coagulase-negative *Staphylococcus* in 63% (Fig. 5.6) [20]. MRSA was identified in two of the thirteen staff positive for *S. aureus*. A similar screening for nasal colonization reported MRSA in 15% of 105 emergency department staff members (18% of technicians were positive for nasal colonization with MRSA, 17% of nurses, and 8% of doctors) [21].

Infection Transmission Between Humans and Pets

Although infrequently reported, MRSA can be transmitted between humans and pets. A long-term care facility evaluated MRSA colonization in 11 cats and 1 dog who were added as resident pets for the facility [22]. Regular testing for nasal colonization was assessed during the first two months that the pets were present in the facility.

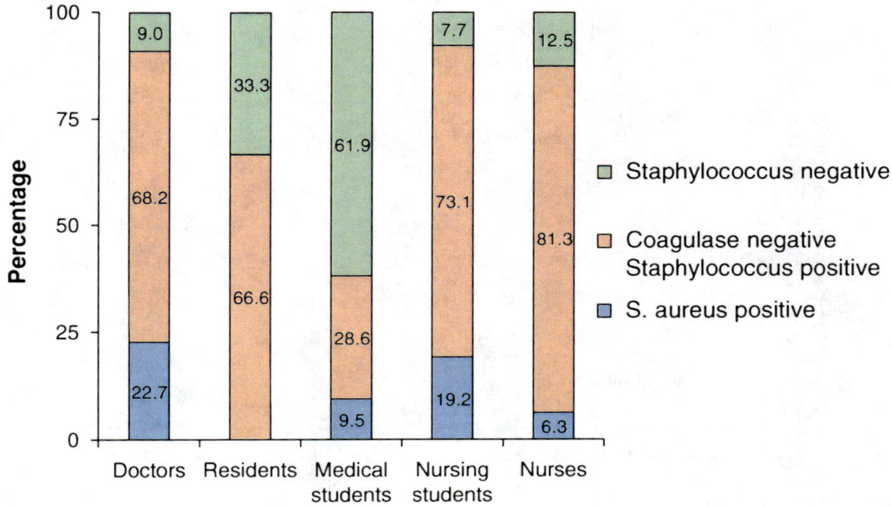

Fig. 5.6 Colonization with staphylococci in hospital staff (Based on [20])

Prior to the animals being added to the facility, three patients were diagnosed with MRSA, and the animals had access to areas that included these patients. During the 2-month evaluation, MRSA was colonized from two cats, neither of which developed clinical illness symptoms. The dog tested positive for methicillin-sensitive *S. aureus* but not for MRSA. In all cases, the bacteria transmission was considered to have occurred from human to pet, with no cases noted of the pet spreading *S. aureus* to another human. Companion dogs and cats have also been identified as possible sources of MRSA [23]. These data verify that interspecies transmission is possible and support enforcing strict precautions when therapy dogs might be exposed to patients with MRSA or other contagious infections.

Possible spread of infections from patient to patient through the therapy dog as a vector has also been evaluated. Researchers at Ontario Veterinary College of the University of Guelph collected nasal swab and fecal samples from therapy dogs every 2 months for 1 year [24]. Dogs were divided into those who would be providing therapeutic visits in hospitals or long-term care facilities ($N=96$) and those to be used in non-health-care settings, such as schools or group homes ($N=98$). Baseline testing occurred prior to the first visit. MRSA was not detected at baseline in any dog, with a single positive test identified after making visits in seven dogs visiting health-care facilities and two dogs visiting other facilities (Fig. 5.7); no dog tested positive for MRSA colonization on more than a single test. *Clostridium difficile* was identified in no dogs scheduled to visit health-care facilities and nine non-health-care dogs at baseline. During the following year, *C. difficile* was recovered from 50 fecal samples from 39 other dogs (23 visiting health-care facilities and 16 visiting other facilities). Only 1 of the 16 dogs that had not been exposed to health-care facilities had two consecutive positive test results, whereas three dogs visiting health-care facilities had three consecutive positive test results, and three others had two consecutive positive test results. None of the dogs from which *C. difficile* was recovered had diarrhea in the 2 months preceding or the 2 months following sample submission. Therefore, rates of acquisition of MRSA and *C. difficile* were 4.7 and 2.4 times higher, respectively, among dogs visiting human health-care facilities compared with rates among dogs involved in other animal-assisted interventions. Visit behaviors were identified that substantially increased risk for developing colonization. Among dogs that visited human health-care facilities, those that licked patients or accepted treats during visits were

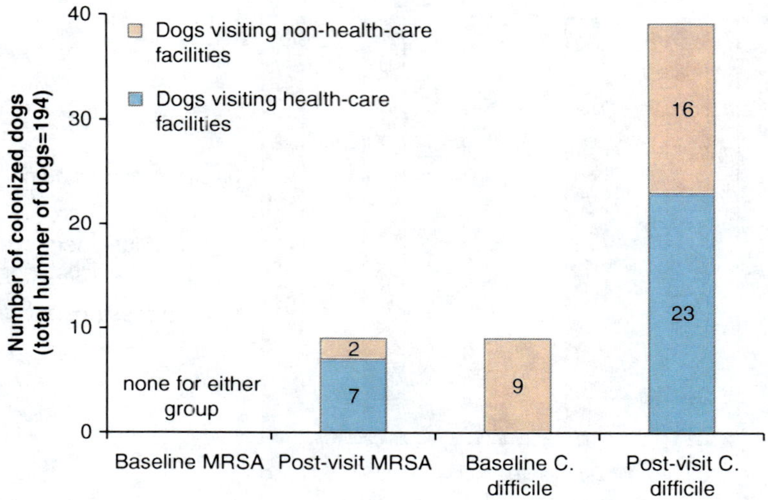

Fig. 5.7 Prevalence of MRSA and *C. difficile* in 194 dogs (96 visiting health-care facilities and 98 visiting non-health-care facilities). There were no dogs colonized with MRSA at baseline; nine dogs who would visit non-health-care facilities and no dogs who would visit health-care facilities were colonized with *C. difficile* at baseline (Based on [24])

more likely to be positive for MRSA and *C. difficile*. In a subsequent study, this same research group tested therapy dog forepaws and hair coat before and after visits to acute and long-term health-care facilities [25]. Neither MRSA nor *C. difficile* was detected prior to visits. Of the 26 dogs tested, one dog acquired *C. difficile* on its paws after visiting an acute care facility. The authors postulated that this dog may have acquired *C. difficile* when walking through the hospital or when "shaking paws" with patients. In addition, MRSA was isolated from the investigator's hands after petting one dog that had visited a long-term care facility. This dog was repeatedly placed on patient beds and had been kissed on the head by two patients. These data suggest that awareness of possible infection spread and appropriate precautions to minimize risk be included in therapy dog policies.

> **Practical Pointer** Therapy dogs are more likely to become colonized by MRSA and *C. difficile* if they are placed on patient beds without fresh linens, lick patients, or accept treats from patients during visits.

Minimizing Spread of Infection Between Dogs and Humans

Policies for reducing infection spread with therapy dog visits include permitting visits only when both dog and handler are healthy, requiring bathing before visits, observing strict hand washing procedures, placing fresh gowns on patients and linens on beds before dogs place feet or lie on patient bedding, and limiting behaviors that might increase dogs acting as an infection vector (e.g., licking patients, shaking paws, and accepting treats from patients). The World Health Organization recommends hand hygiene before and after direct patient contact, after contact with contaminated materials, and after contact with inanimate objects or medical equipment close to a patient [26]. Handlers should wash their hands/use hand sanitizer before and after entering each patient's room and between patients if more than one patient is in a particular room. When hand sanitizer is used, hands should be thoroughly rubbed together on both surfaces and between the fingers until the hands become dry; this typically takes about 20–30 s [26]. Hand washing with soap and water for 10 s will also effectively reduce many germs [27]; however, 30 s was shown to be necessary to eradicate vancomycin-resistant *Enterococcus* (VRE) contamination on hands [28]. Handlers additionally should carry hand sanitizer for patients to use before and after visiting with the dog.

Diet can also affect infection risk in therapy dogs, with risk minimized by limiting the dog's consumption of raw meat, particularly for dogs allowed to visit immunocompromised patients. A relationship between shedding Salmonella and other pathogens with the consumption of raw meat was evaluated in 200 healthy therapy dogs, with fecal specimens collected and analyzed every 2 months for 1 year [2]. Among the 200 dogs, 40 dogs ate raw meat at some point during the study. The incidence rate of Salmonella shedding in the raw meat-fed dogs was 0.61 cases/dog-year, compared with 0.08 cases/dog-year in dogs that were not fed raw meat ($P<0.001$). Dogs consuming raw meat were significantly more likely to test positive for Salmonella at least once during the year than dogs not eating raw meat (odds ratio [OR] 22.7; 95% confidence interval [CI] 3.1–58.8; $P<0.001$). Raw meat consumption was also significantly associated with shedding *Escherichia coli* (OR 17.2; 95% CI 9.4–32.3). There were no associations between *C. difficile*, MRSA, or VRE and raw meat consumption.

Box 4 Tips for Minimizing Infection Risks with Therapy Dog Visits

- Restrict visits to handlers and dogs who are both free of infectious symptoms or conditions.
- Avoid feeding therapy dogs raw meat diets.
- Observe strict hand washing before and after patient contact.
- Use hand sanitizer on dogs' paws before and after patient contacts.
- Prohibit patients from giving food or other treats to dogs during visits.
- Discourage licking and kissing behaviors.
- Curtail subsequent visits on that same day following visiting a patient with MRSA, VRE, or *C. difficile* infections.
- Bathe dog immediately after visits and before subsequent visits to health-care facilities.

Visiting Patients in Intensive Care or Isolation

The value of including therapy dog visits for critically ill patients in intensive care units is being increasingly recognized by health-care providers. The American College of Critical Care Medicine guidelines provide a grade B recommendation for including therapy dogs in intensive care settings to promote a more patient-centered medical experience [15]. A recent review of therapy dogs visiting critical care patients conducted by nurses at Wright State University concluded that therapy visits from specially trained pets, like therapy dogs, and their handlers can help meet both physical and emotional needs for many patients in intensive care [29]. The ability of therapy dogs to provide unconditional love without expecting anything in return from the patient was seen as particularly valuable for these patients.

Practical Pearl "Animal-assisted therapy is invaluable on a critical care unit, as it enables the nurse to affordably treat the patient's body in a holistic manner, and may be the only available complementary therapy to offer therapeutic touch to socially and emotionally isolated people" [29; page 214].

Many facilities prohibit therapy dogs from visiting patients in critical care units or patients in isolation. Some facilities do allow visits when strict protocols are followed to ensure the safety and well-being of both the patient and the therapy dog. Facilities may allow visits to patients with compromised immune systems if the treatment team considers visits to be appropriate and strict precautions are followed to avoid spreading infections to these patients [8]. The handler may need to wear a clean gown, gloves, and/or mask, as appropriate for particular patients. In addition to changing the patient's gown and bed

Case 1

Including therapy dog visits as a complementary intervention for more critically ill patients can help provide needed physical contact and emotional connections [29]. Impact from a therapy dog visit is highlighted by the case of JB, a college senior studying biology and psychology when he was diagnosed with acute myeloid leukemia. JB initially approached his treatment like a dispassionate scientist, focusing on white blood cell counts and other numbers that might show positive progress. During his long hospitalization, however, JB began to recognize his important psychological needs from coping with cancer and cancer treatment:

> *Pretty soon I began to feel lonely. My immunocompromised body could never be touched, and masks and contact gowns were a normal occurrence. I had to tell my mother she couldn't kiss or touch her child, and my scientific and empirical approach to the cancer slowly lost its value. This is when I began to understand the importance of the mind, keeping things positive, and controlling your own destiny.*
>
> *When I found out about pet therapy from the recreation therapist on the cancer ward, I wanted to give it a try. I wasn't sure what was involved, but I was interested nonetheless. When the day came to see the therapy dog, I learned that just being around the dog was all that was involved. They helped the dog—a beautiful black Lab—jump onto my bed. He just circled and settled next to my stomach. The dog was simply living, experiencing the moment with his senses. I closed my eyes, put my hand on his chest, and began to breathe deeply. A huge sense of peace overcame me as I lied there with the dog in my hospital bed. My mind cleared, and I forgot there were people in the room. I forgot about the IV's in my chest and arms. I began to understand the power of the moment and simply living. Spending time with the dog helped me achieve a sense of peace I hadn't been able to find before.*

Being able to include therapy dog visits provided JB with both physical contact and an emotional connection that helped provide comfort and a sense of peace. Establishing policies to make these visits safe and feasible for patients in intensive care or isolation can help address unmet patient needs.

linens before a visit and following appropriate hand hygiene techniques, additional precautions may be needed, as determined by individual facility infection control personnel. For example, when therapy dogs visit a room that includes a patient in isolation, the dog should also avoid walking directly on flooring in the room. Smaller dogs can be carried into the room and held by the handler during visits; for larger dogs, fresh linens should be placed on the floor to make a clean path for the dog to walk to and from the patient, with the linens removed after the visit has been completed. To avoid inadvertently carrying difficult to treat organisms between patients, only a single isolation patient may be visited by a dog on a given day. Following that visit, the dog and handler should leave the facility without additional contacts with other patients, visitors, or staff.

In many cases, patients in isolation will be prohibited from having direct contact with a therapy dog. When these patients have expressed an interest in a visit, handlers may conduct visits at a distance, keeping the dog outside of the patient's doorway where the patient can observe the dog, which might perform tricks, such as raising a paw to wave at the patient. Handlers might also leave visit cards that include a cheerful message, their dog's photograph, and the dog's name for patients to keep as a visit memory.

Box 5 Suggested Policies for Visiting Approved Patients in Isolation

- Before the visit:
  - The handler should verify with the staff that visiting a particular patient has been approved.
  - A staff member should accompany the handler during the visit to assist with special isolation procedures.
  - The handler must wash her hands before making a visit.
  - The handler must wear an isolation gown, gloves, and possibly a mask, as deemed appropriate by the staff member.
  - A fresh gown should be placed on the patient, and a clean top sheet put on the patient's bed before the visit.
  - The patient must wash his or her hands.
- During the visit:
  - The dog should enter the room without touching the patient's floor (either being carried or walking on clean sheets a staff member has placed on the floor).
  - The dog should remain on the handler's lap or on the clean linens that were placed for the visit.
  - The dog should avoid shaking paws, kissing, or licking behaviors.
- After the visit:
  - The staff should remove extra linens and place them in the laundry.
  - The handler should dispose of all isolation gear outside of the patient's room.
  - The patient should wash his or her hands.
  - The handler should wash his or her hands and the dog's paws.
  - The handler and dog should exit the hospital. No more visits should be made on a given day after visiting a patient in isolation.

Example of a Typical Therapy Dog Visit During Cancer Care

For most animal-assisted activity visits with a therapy dog, the primary goal is to allow the dog to interact with individuals in need, with the handler acting as a facilitator for the interaction. Visits will vary depending on the energy and health of the patient, facility visited, and size and personality of the dog. In some cases, patients will be entertained by watching a dog perform a series of obedience commands and tricks, while other visits focus on cuddling.

Lynn Huber Jablonski visits hospice patients with her Pekingese therapy dog Shen Li, who was identified by the trainer in her early obedience classes as an excellent therapy dog candidate (Fig. 5.8). While each visit is different, the following visit described by Lynn clearly illustrates the role of the handler. "The room was packed with a large group of very tired-looking family and friends clustered around the patient in her bed. The nurses told me that the patient had recently lost her husband and then her beloved pet–a small, white dog. The patient was not

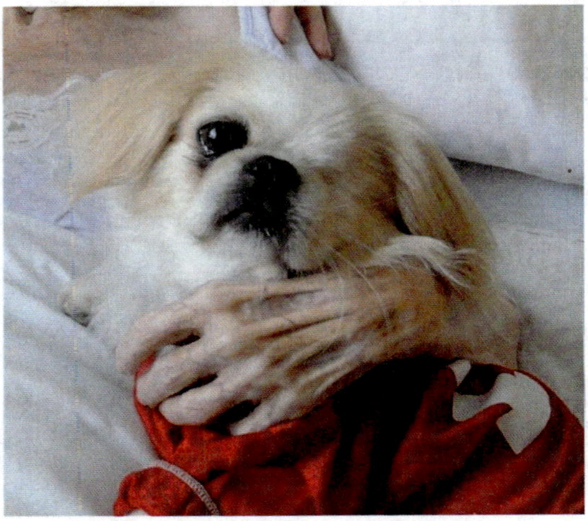

Fig. 5.8 Ten-pound Pekingese therapy dog Shen Li who had lost an eye to trauma was an ideal therapy dog candidate because of her excellent obedience, even temperament, outgoing disposition, and acceptance of strangers and restraining hugs

expected to live for more than a few more days and for the last few days had only communicated by squeezing her hand. She had not shown any response to her family for the last two days. When I placed Shen Li next to this lady, Shen Li snuggled tightly into the woman's armpit. The patient threw back her head and exclaimed, 'Puppy!' and began to rapidly pet Shen Li's soft fur. After a few minutes, her hand fell back on the bed and I gently returned her hand onto Shen Li's soft back. The patient again began to pet Shen Li. For 45 min, I helped place the patient's hand onto Shen Li and she petted my dog. During this time, her family and friends remained close around the bed and I think they gathered some comfort seeing their loved one connect with this little dog."

This visit typifies many therapy dog visits, with the focus on helping the patient make a connection with the therapy dog. The handler's attention was centered on the dog's safety and needs and ensuring the patient was able to make a connection with the dog rather than involving conversations with the many visitors in the room. The day following this visit, the patient died. By focusing on the patient, this visit brought comfort to a dying patient and a lasting memory of peace and joy to her grieving family and friends.

Successful Programs Caring for Cancer with Therapy Dogs

Therapy dogs have been used in cancer care in a range of capacities, including both inpatient and outpatient programs. The following programs offer a range of visit options that might be included within a cancer treatment center. The success of each program depends on careful organization, the development of procedures and policies for visits, and appropriate expectations of outcomes related to therapy dog interventions.

Cancer Caring Center at the University of Pittsburgh

At the University of Pittsburgh Medical Center, the Cancer Caring Center has partnered with Animal Friends shelter to provide a therapy dog program for children coping with cancer in themselves or a parent. Animal Friends trains and certifies therapy dog-handler pairs and maintains an active group of therapy dog-handler volunteer teams who make visits throughout a wide range of facilities. The Cancer Caring Center therapy dog program was designed to provide three group therapy dog sessions for each participant, with time spent interacting with the dog (Fig. 5.9), story time with the dogs, and pet-related activities during three 1½-hour sessions provided one Saturday each month. Staff from the Cancer Caring Center, staff from Animal Friends, and therapy dog handlers are present throughout each session. The goals of the program are to offer children respite from cancer concerns, bonding with the dog, and time to make a positive memory. Children and their parents were surveyed about how well they were coping with cancer before and after participating in this program.

In 2008, 17 new children participated in this program. Three of the children had cancer, with cancer in a parent in the remainder. Responses to pre- and post-intervention surveys are shown in Fig. 5.10. In order to accommodate the schedules and health issues of the children participating and their families, this program was subsequently changed to allow children to attend as many or as few therapy dog sessions as they preferred. Furthermore, some children and families opted to continue to attend pet therapy sessions after cancer recovery.

Pets at Duke

The Pets at Duke program is part of oncology recreation therapy provided at the Duke Cancer Institute at Duke University in Durham, North Carolina. Pets at Duke started in 1994 with one therapy dog-handler team visiting hematology/oncology patients for about an hour each week. Additional teams, facilities, and visit times were added, and today, dogs make visits two days each week to separate facilities for adult, pediatric, and radiation oncology patients. Pets at Duke

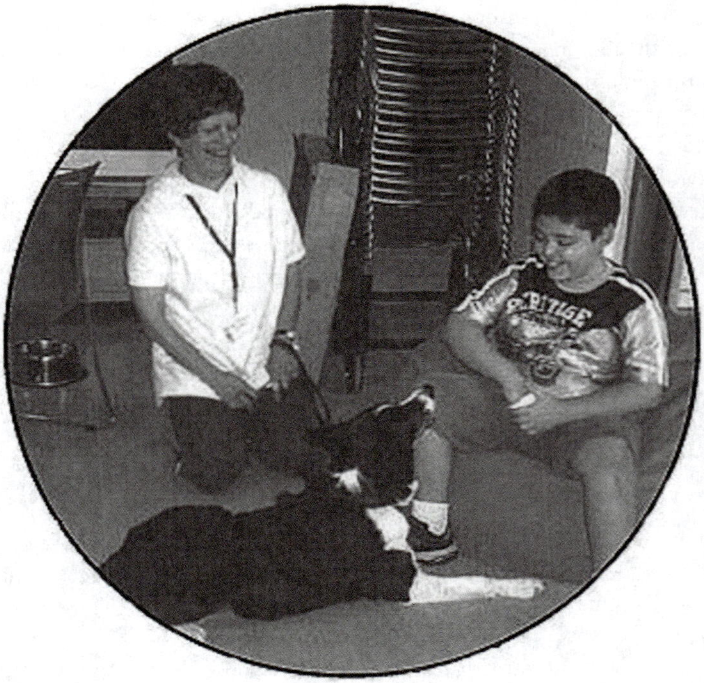

Fig. 5.9 A 10-year-old participant whose mother was diagnosed with cancer gives ice chips to Border Collie therapy dog Birdie, enjoying some nurturing time during a Cancer Caring Center pet therapy visit (Photo courtesy of Ann Cadman, Animal Friends)

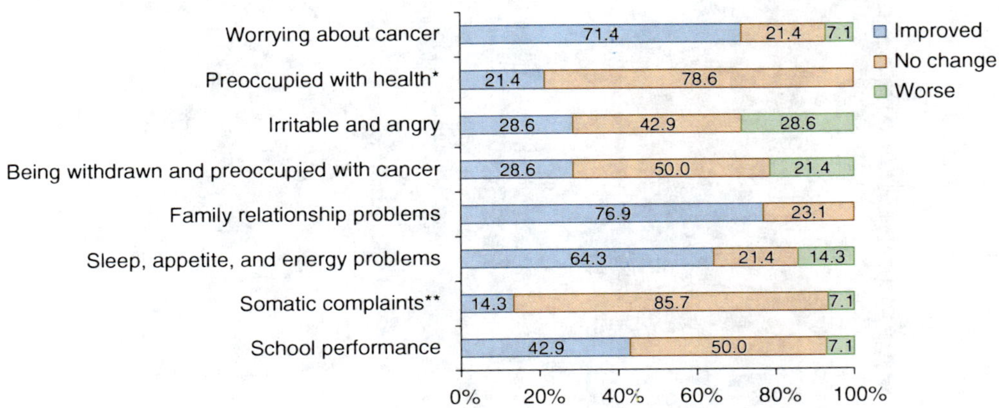

Fig. 5.10 Cancer Caring Center pet therapy program outcome. Fourteen participants completed both pre- and post-therapy dog intervention. *Children with no change in being preoccupied with health experienced a midrange of preoccupation both pre- and post-intervention. **Children with no change in somatic complaints reported few somatic complaints at the beginning or end of the program

expanded to include Duke-affiliated community settings in 2010, with therapy dogs making weekly visits to adult patients and their families staying at a temporary residence. Weekly visits have also been added at two inpatient hospice facilities affiliated with Duke. (See Fig. 5.11.)

Prior to volunteering as part of the Pets at Duke program, human volunteers must complete hospital volunteer requirements and orientation. Therapy dog certification, current health and vaccination records, and veterinarian approval are also reviewed. Before candidate therapy dog-handler teams begin making visits, they are first evaluated by a therapy dog program staff member, and then interactions with patients for both the handler and dog are assessed during supervised visits.

The Pets at Duke program is coordinated by recreation therapists, with competency-trained staff and adult volunteers acting as facilitators during visits. Prior to visits, facilitators identify appropriate patients to be visited. During visits, a staff member is available to address potential risk management issues, and another facilitator is assigned to greet each therapy dog-handler team and accompany them on visits. In order to

Case 2

A 62-year-old man with a lower extremity sarcoma was admitted to the Duke Cancer Institute awaiting below-the-knee amputation. The man had no obvious support network and had had no outside visitors. When the surgeon spoke with the patient about his upcoming surgery and care, the man offered minimal responses. The Pets at Duke program sent Gus, a Golden Retriever therapy dog, to visit the man. While the man had shared very little with his human health-care providers, he poured out his concerns to Gus, telling Gus how scared he was about losing his leg and feeling like he could not go on living. Being able to verbalize his concerns and needs to the therapy dog provided an opening to connect the patient with a limb loss specialist. The patient's health-care team shared with the Pets at Duke program staff that they believed Gus' visit had made an important difference by opening doors to support services the patient might not have otherwise accepted.

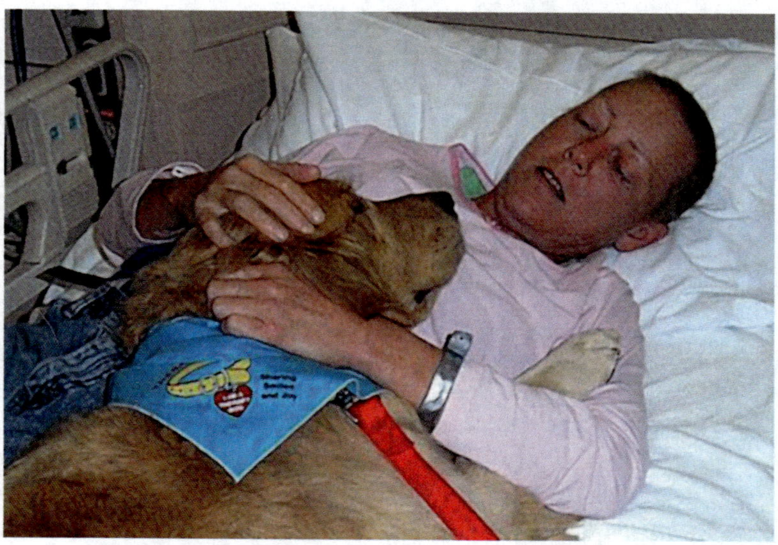

Fig. 5.11 Golden Retriever therapy dog Gus serves as a pet therapy volunteer in the Pets at Duke program, having visited over 7,000 cancer patients (Photo courtesy of Kristy Everette of the Pets at Duke program, Duke University Medical Center)

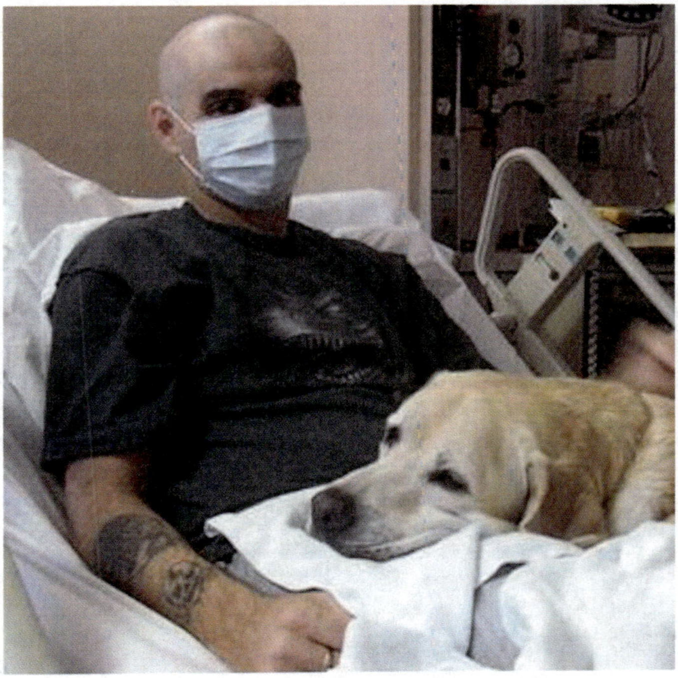

Fig. 5.12 Facilitators help ensure that proper infection controls are followed to minimize infection risk (Photo courtesy of Kristy Everette of the Pets at Duke program, Duke University Medical Center)

minimize infection spread, therapy dogs in the Pets at Duke program are only permitted to meet with patients for whom visits have been scheduled. The facilitator uses a low traffic route to patient areas to help minimize contact with hospital visitors and others, while the dog and handler are traveling to the patient area where visits will occur. Both the handler and facilitator are trained to discourage public interaction with the therapy dogs, and the dogs wear vests with the words, "Pets at Duke, Therapy Dog in Action," to alert the public that the dogs are there to visit patients. The facilitator also announces the presence of the therapy dog before the team enters elevators to make certain other elevator riders are comfortable with a dog. Once visits begin, the facilitators have a background presence, allowing patients to primarily focus on interacting with the dog. Facilitators also ensure that proper precautions are followed, including placing a fresh sheet over the patient's bed before visits, making certain the patient has used hand sanitizer before and after visits, and ensuring all necessary infection precautions are followed (Fig. 5.12). Facilitators take a supply cart on visits that includes hand foam, sanitizing wipes that can be used to clean chairs, and fresh sheets to place on beds. If the therapy dog encounters a patient on contact isolation (i.e., MRSA or VRE), no additional visits are permitted that day, and the facilitator escorts the therapy dog-handler team from the facility using a low-volume route expected to have minimal visitors to avoid additional contact of the dog with others.

Facilitators also carry a camera and portable printer on their supply cart so they can take photographs during visits to leave as a token for patients. For many patients, the dog visit is a positive experience they enjoy sharing with others, and photos from these visits are placed in patient rooms where they serve as conversation material with both staff and visitors. In some cases, a shared love of dogs helps foster connections between patients and their health-care providers. Visitors often ask patients about the dog, which can remove some of the heaviness from conversations that might otherwise focus on disease discussions. For some families, these photographs become cherished memories, capturing times of pleasure during an otherwise difficult end of life.

> **Case 3**
> AM and her husband were both in their 70s and had spent a lifetime together after being high school sweethearts. Dogs had also been a part of their lives. When AM was admitted to Duke's intensive care unit for end-of-life care, a therapy dog visit was requested from Pets at Duke. When the therapy dog was placed in AM's bed, AM responded with a smile and the husband displayed a welcome sense of relief. The husband asked the therapy dog facilitator to photograph the visit, with the pictures serving as a reminder of the last time he and his wife were smiling together.

Angel Foundation's Kids Kamp

Angel Foundation is a Minnesota-based 501 (c) (3) organization founded in 2001 to help families affected by cancer. Angel Foundation has provided emergency financial assistance, education, and support to more than 15,000 individuals affected by cancer since its founding. The organization's Facing Cancer Together program provides support for families facing a parental cancer diagnosis through activities that offer education, promote family resilience and communication, and reduce a family's distress and sense of isolation. Therapy dogs are used as an integral part of the Kids Kamp program—three days of fun, support, strength building, and learning for children and adolescents 5–18 years old who have a parent diagnosed with cancer.

Boxer therapy dog Buster and his handler Dori Weisbrod became the first therapy dog-handler team to join Kids Kamp (Fig. 5.13). Spending time with Buster became a popular part of the three-day program. Because Buster readily made strong connections with participating children, his role was expanded to include opportunities for interaction during the camp, with continued connections outside of the camp program (Table 5.4). In 2011, Buster passed away from cancer, although the important work he started continues with other therapy dogs participating in Kids Kamp.

Buster and other therapy dogs have been used to facilitate the achievement of program goals (Table 5.5). In addition, team members have noted that the presence of the therapy dog often enhances positive interactions between children and staff and fosters an improved ability of

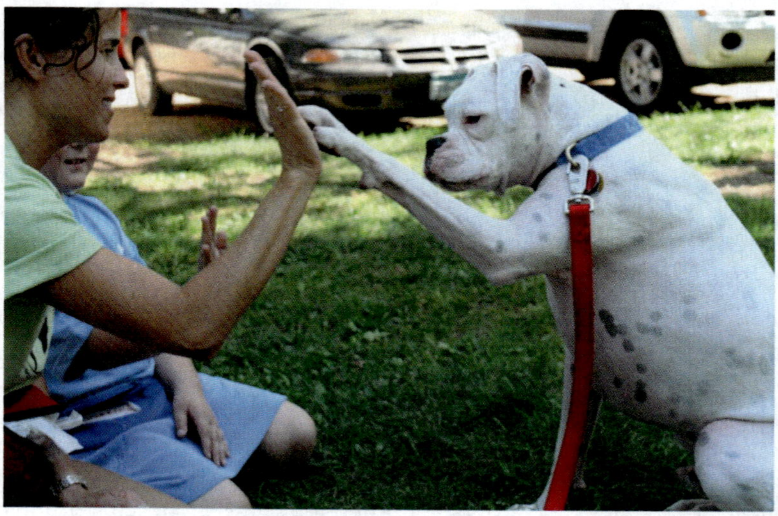

Fig. 5.13 Angel Foundation therapy dog Buster with handler Dori Weisbrod during Kids Kamp

Table 5.4 Kids Kamp roles for therapy dogs include contact during the three-day camp plus additional opportunities to make and maintain connections with therapy dogs, like Buster, after the camp is completed

Therapy dog role	Logistics	Example from Buster's visits
Nonjudgmental listener	The therapy dog is available to children participating in group activities if they are feeling upset, sad, lonely, etc. Children may also have one-on-one visits with the dog and handler to "talk" with the dog about how they are feeling	Children felt safe that they could share all of their feelings with Buster Staff noted, "The children tell Buster everything" "Buster makes you *feel heard*"
Social connection	Therapy dogs receive and respond to mail, e-mail, and Facebook messages	Children could opt to send messages to Buster through "give your problems to Buster" mail and online initiatives Children joining Buster's "fan club" will receive birthday cards and other messages periodically from Buster
Playmate	The therapy dog can fill the need for play and fun, especially when the parent is limited by fatigue	Buster naturally engaged children in healthy play, providing positive reinforcement for play through his attentiveness and engagement

Table 5.5 Using therapy dogs to accomplish program goals for children coping with a parent with cancer

Target goal	Therapy dog intervention	Examples
Improved communication	Therapy dog provides opportunities for verbal communication with dog and others Therapy dog can provide safe venue for expressing fears, anger, and concerns	Conversation between children and other children or adults was often initiated during time petting Buster Children felt safe sharing emotions with Buster; one child was heard telling Buster, "The reason I like Buster is he never says to me 'you're going to be okay.'" "He just listens" Children often shared emotions by writing letters or drawing pictures for Buster
Reduced isolation	Therapy dog interactions provide healthy opportunities for nurturing	One boy commented, "Buster is a friend to me, so I'm going to be a friend to him and get him water." Then he said, "Buster deserves better than to drink water from the floor, so I'm going to hold his water dish up for him to drink"
Reduced distress	Petting Buster provided stress relief and mood improvement	Children generally became calmer after spending time with Buster The family of one participant added a companion dog to their home because of the positive benefits achieved by their daughter after spending time with Buster
Improve expression of emotions	Therapy dogs are a nonjudgmental resource with whom feelings can be shared	One girl commented, "I can tell Buster feels the same way I do sometimes"
Improved self-esteem	Therapy dogs provide unconditional love and acceptance	Children enjoyed sharing their achievements with Buster, e.g., birthdays, report cards, or time spent helping at home Buster would send children a "High 5 From Buster" card to reward their accomplishments Children would carry Buster's "business card" in their pockets and brag to their friends about being in his fan club. One parent shared that her boy carried Buster's business card with him for months at school until the card became wrinkled; the boy was so excited when Buster gave him a new card to replace the old one

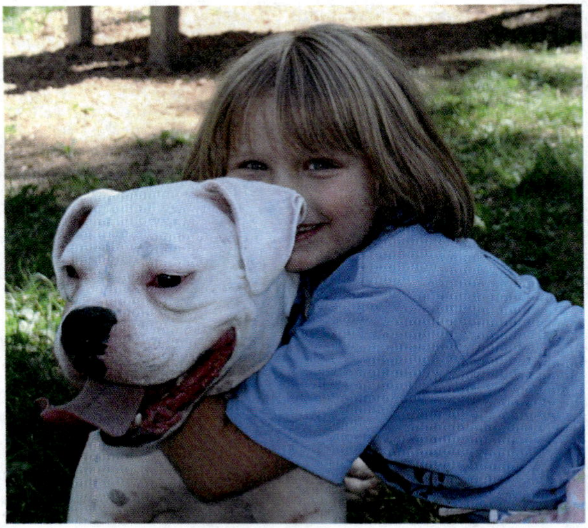

Fig. 5.14 When a parent has cancer and is going through treatment, he or she may be too ill, too fatigued, or too sensitive to the touch to hold a child or to play and interact as much as a parent and child would like. Therapy dog Buster was an important member of the Kids Kamp team, bringing children joy and, through his patience and charm, reassuring children that their parents' love, like his, was unconditional (Photo courtesy of Deborah Erickson, Angel Foundation)

children to benefit from other interventions. For example, when children participate in a group in which the dog is present, staff have noticed that children tend to be more attentive, focused, and better listeners. One boy attending the program was particularly energetic and had difficultly staying focused and on task. When Buster arrived, the boy quickly became calm, patient, and focused, which allowed the staff to work on other activities with the boy while Buster was at his side. The staff helped the boy teach Buster tricks, which nurtured healthy connections between the staff and the boy. While the therapy dog intervention is only a small part of the Kids Kamp program, including therapy dogs enhances the ability of children to benefit from a broad range of intervention opportunities (Fig. 5.14).

Summary

- Therapy dog certification by recognized agencies is recommended to verify the appropriateness of individual dogs for making therapy visits.
- An individual therapy dog will typically spend about 30–60 min in total time visiting patients during a visit, with an individual dog usually visiting a facility weekly or monthly. Most patients will spend about 5–15 min with a dog during a visit.
- Asymptomatic colonization with MRSA has been reported in 3–11% of patients on hospital admission and up to 15% of healthy healthcare workers.
- Pathogens can be spread from patients to therapy dogs. Therefore, procedures need to be routinely used to minimize infection risk during therapy dog visits. Specific policies are needed to address whether dogs will be permitted to see patients in intensive care or isolation.
- Certain visit behaviors increase risk for therapy dogs becoming colonized with MRSA and *C. difficile*, including allowing dogs to sit or lie on patient beds without fresh linens, lick patients, or accept treats from patients during visits.

References

1. LeFebvre SL, Golab GC, Christensen E, et al. Guidelines for animal-assisted interventions in health care facilities. Am J Infect Contr. 2008;36:78–85.
2. Lefebvre SL, Reid-Smith R, Boerlin P, Weese JS. Evaluation of the risks of shedding Salmonellae and

other potential pathogens by therapy dogs fed raw diets in Ontario and Alberta. Zoonoses Public Health. 2008;55(8–10):470–80.

3. Phear DN. A study of animal companionship in a day hospice. Palliat Med. 1996;10:336–8.
4. Marcus DA. The power of wagging tails: a doctor's guide to dog therapy and healing. New York: Demos Health; 2011.
5. Marx MS, Cohen-Mansfield J, Regier NG, et al. The impact of different dog-related stimuli on engagement of persons with dementia. Am J Alzheimers Dis Other Demen. 2010;25:37–45.
6. Cattam M, Hogg E, Hardill I. Improving quality of life in ageing populations: what can volunteering do? Maturitas. 2011;70:328–32.
7. Selli L, Garrafa V, Junges JR. Beneficiaries of volunteering: a bioethical perspective. Rev Saude Publica. 2008;42:1085–9.
8. Harris AH, Thoresen CE. Volunteering is associated with delayed mortality in older people: analysis of the longitudinal study of aging. J Health Psychol. 2005;10: 739–52.
9. Avalon L. Volunteering as a predictor of all-cause mortality: what aspects of volunteering really matter? Int Psychogeriatr. 2008;20:1000–13.
10. Van Willigen M. Differential benefits of volunteering across life course. J Gerontol B Psychol Sci Soc Sci. 2000;55:S308–18.
11. Lichter I, Hunt E. The last 48 hours of life. J Palliat Care. 1990;6:7–15.
12. Morita T, Tei Y, Inoue S. Impaired communication capacity and agitated delirium in the final week of terminally ill cancer patients: prevalence and identification of research focus. J Pain Symptom Manag. 2003;26:827–34.
13. Bassetti M, Nicco E, Mikulsak M. Why is community-associated MRSA spreading across the world and how will it change clinical practice? Int J Antimicrob Agents. 2009;34 Suppl 1:S15–9.
14. Caprilli S, Messeri A. Animal-assisted activity at A. Meyer children's hospital: a pilot study. Evid Based Complement Alternat Med. 2006;3:379–83.
15. Davidson JE, Powers K, Hedayat KM, et al. Clinical practice guidelines for support of the family in the patient-centered intensive care unit: American college of critical care medicine task force 2004–2005. Crit Care Med. 2007;35:605–22.
16. Otter JA, French GL. Community-associated methicillin-resistant *Staphylococcus aureus* strains as a cause of healthcare-associated infection. J Hosp Infect. 2011;79:189–93.
17. Davis KA, Stewart JJ, Crouch HK, Florez CE, Hospenthal DR. Methicillin-resistant *Staphylococcus aureus* (MRSA) nares colonization at hospital admission and its effect on subsequent MRSA infection. Clin Infect Dis. 2004;39:776–82.
18. Parvez N, Jinadatha C, Fader R, et al. Universal MRSA nasal surveillance: characterization of outcomes at a tertiary care center and implications for infections control. South Med J. 2010;103:1084–91.
19. Schechter-Perkins EM, Mitchell PM, Murray KA, et al. Prevalence and predictors of nasal and extranasal staphylococcal colonization in patients presenting to the emergency department. Ann Emerg Med. 2011;57:492–9.
20. Vinodhkumatadithyaa A, Uma A, Srinivasan M, et al. Nasal carriage of methicillin-resistant *Staphylococcus aureus* among surgical unit staff. Jpn J Infect Dis. 2009;62:228–9.
21. Bisaga A, Paquette K, Sabatini L, Lovell EO. A prevalence study of methicillin-resistant *Staphylococcus aureus* colonization in emergency department health care workers. Ann Emerg Med. 2008;52:525–8.
22. Couglan K, Olsen KE, Boxrud D, Bender JB. Methicillin-resistant *Staphylococcus aureus* in resident animals of a long-term care facility. Zoonoses Public Heath. 2010;57:220–6.
23. Heller J. Methicillin-resistant staphylococci in companion animals. Vet Rec. 2001;169:68–9.
24. Lefebvre SL, Reid-Smith RJ, Waltner-Toews D, Weese JS. Incidence of acquisition of methicillin-resistant *Staphylococcus aureus, Clostridium difficile*, and other health-care–associated pathogens by dogs that participate in animal-assisted interventions. J Am Vet Med Assoc. 2009;234:1404–17.
25. Lefebvre SL, Weese JS. Contamination of pet therapy dogs with MRSA and *Clostridium difficile*. J Hosp Infect. 2009;72:268–9.
26. Pittet D, Allegranzi B, Boyce J. The World Health Organization guidelines on hand hygiene in health care and their consensus recommendations. Infect Contr Hosp Epidemiol. 2009;30:611–22.
27. Sickbert-Bennett EE, Weber DJ, Gergen-Teague MF, et al. Comparative efficacy of hand hygiene agents in the reduction of bacteria and viruses. Am J Infect Contr. 2005;33:67–77.
28. Noskin GA, Stosor V, Cooper I, Peterson LR. Recovery of vancomycin-resistant enterococci on fingertips and environmental surfaces. Infect Contr Hosp Epidemiol. 1995;16:577–81.
29. DeCourcey M, Russell AC, Keister KJ. Animal-assisted therapy. Evaluation and implementation of a complementary therapy to improve the psychological and physiological health of critically ill patients. Dimens Crit Care Nurs. 2010;29:211–14.

6 Incorporating Companion Dogs into Cancer Rehab: Emotional Support

Key Chapter Points

- Attachment to pets provides support and reduced isolation and stress for cancer patients undergoing treatment.
- Pets enhance their owners' sense of good health and social engagement.
- Pet owners tend to be more involved in neighborhood activities than individuals without pets.
- Dog owners report their relationship with their dog often helps them connect with neighbors and their community.

Keywords
Civic engagement • Pet • Stress • Social capital • Support

Therapy dogs can provide moments of positive interaction and benefit for cancer patients and their caregivers. Companion dogs may also offer therapeutic assistance for their owners with cancer or owners affected by someone with cancer. Studies suggest that interacting with a well-behaved companion dog may be therapeutic, resulting in both emotional and physical benefits [1]. Living with a pet has been linked to improved social contact and interactions [2], as well as better mood for single women [3].

The decision to add a companion dog to a household requires careful consideration and planning, particularly when a household is affected by health concerns. Practical tips to help decide if a companion dog should be added and how to successfully add a dog are discussed in Chap. 9.

Emotional benefits from companion dogs are similar to those described for therapy dog encounters, with dog owners reporting that a companion dog can provide consistent friendship, support, and a nonjudgmental listening ear. The responsibility that owners feel for their dogs can also provide motivation for patients to maintain a positive attitude and active lifestyle.

D.A. Marcus, *Therapy Dogs in Cancer Care: A Valuable Complementary Treatment*,
DOI 10.1007/978-1-4614-3378-1_6, © Springer Science+Business Media New York 2012

Case 1

RH was an otherwise healthy 57-year-old English teacher who developed breast cancer. She was treated with surgical resection, followed by five months of chemotherapy and then 42 radiation treatments. After surgery, her doctor encouraged RH to maintain her activity level through cancer treatment. At the time of her diagnosis, RH was working on completing agility titles with her Soft-Coated Wheaten Terrier, Gráinne. Agility is a sport for dogs where the dog runs through an obstacle course, directed by a human handler. Accuracy and speed are measured, so both the dog and handler need to stay mentally alert and move swiftly around the course.

When I was first diagnosed with cancer, focusing on Gráinne's agility was the highlight of my week and helped me stay brave. I thought, "I may have cancer, but I can't give up on Gráinne's training and competitions." I had made a commitment to finish Gráinne's agility work and I couldn't let cancer interfere with that. When I'd come home from each 6-hour chemotherapy treatment plus 2 hours of driving, I'd change my clothes, jump in the car with Gráinne, and go to agility training. We also competed in trials during those months with my head covered in caps and scarves.

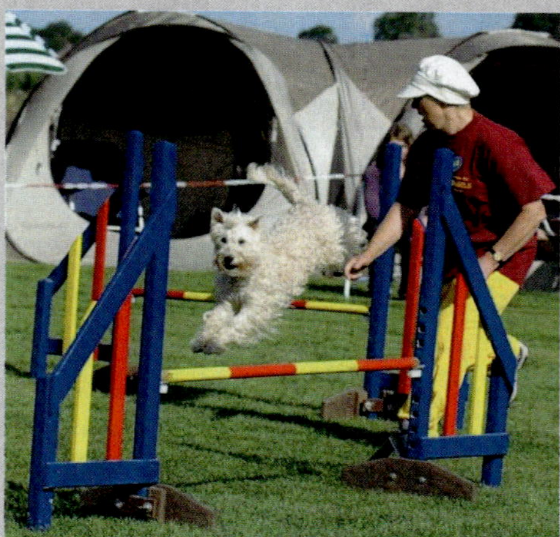

My husband knew Gráinne was getting ready to retire from agility trials, so he brought a second Wheaten puppy to our home when I started chemo. Having my terriers to take care of helped me through those months of treatment. Raising a new puppy is hard work, and I had a dear friend who helped with my puppy Diarmuid while I was at treatment. But long treatment sessions didn't keep me from spending time with my dogs every day. Except for four days when I was in the hospital for surgery, I never missed a single daily dog walk during my months of treatment.

My Wheaten Terriers were literally my whole life those 14 months. My doctors encouraged me to stay active to help reduce treatment side effects, like fatigue and nausea, and I had very few symptoms throughout treatment. I really credit my terriers for my positive attitude, my ability to stay active, and having very few treatment side effects.

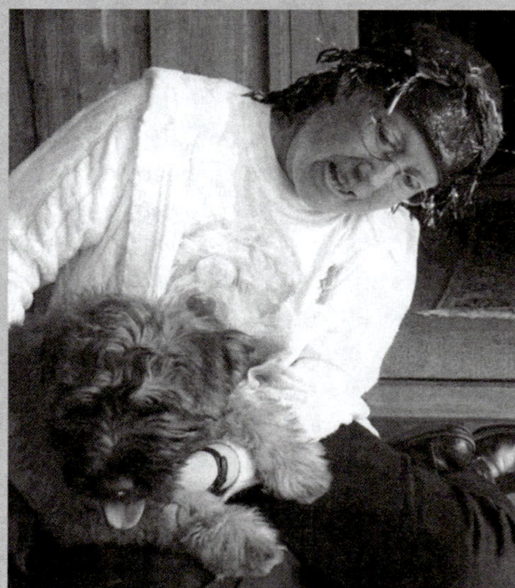

Overview of Companion Dogs' Role During Cancer Treatment

Companion dogs can provide support and comfort to patients undergoing cancer treatment, which many patients view as fostering a positive attitude and healing. Researches from Mayo Clinic surveyed 309 cancer patients receiving chemotherapy [4]. Chemotherapy was being performed without curative intent for 61% of study participants. Among this sample, 170 participants were pet owners, most commonly of dogs (72%). Most patients described strong attachment to their pet (Fig. 6.1). Two in three chemotherapy patients endorsed that their pet contributed to better personal health and stress reduction (Fig. 6.2). Only 6% of patients expressed concern about being close to a pet (e.g., having concerns about increasing infection risk) while undergoing cancer treatment.

Dogs Relieve Stress

As described in Chap. 1, high stress is common among cancer patients, with stress postulated to negatively impact cancer progression. Stress management techniques have been endorsed as

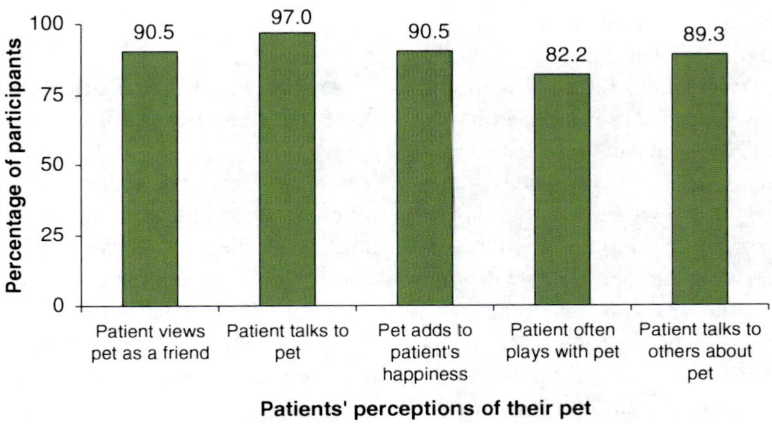

Fig. 6.1 Reported attachment to pets (Based on [4])

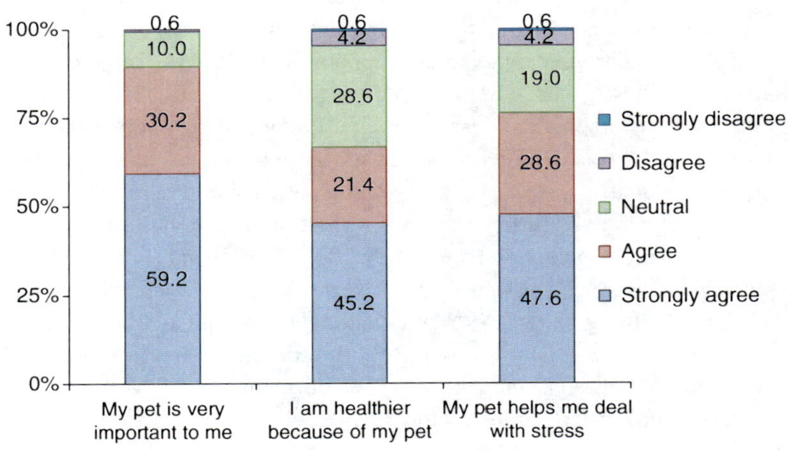

Fig. 6.2 Reported benefits of pet ownership for chemotherapy patients (Based on [4])

complementary therapy for both male and female patients with cancer, with benefits shown for reducing perceived stress and anxiety, improving quality of life, and positively impacting immune markers [5–7]. In addition, experimental studies support that spending time with a dog can also be an effective stress relieving therapy.

Cardiovascular Reactivity Decreases with Companion Dogs

Systolic blood pressure was reported to be lower among pet owners in one large study (N=5,741) [8], while other studies have failed to report this link [9, 10]. While effects on overall blood pressure have been inconsistent, companion pets did effectively reduce cardiovascular reactivity to stress exposure in a study in which 120 healthy married adults were exposed physical stress (hand immersion in ice water) and mental stress (performing math calculations) [11]. Stress response was measured before and after exposure to the stressor under three separate conditions: (1) when the subject was alone, (2) when the spouse was in the room with the subject, and (3) when the subject was accompanied by his or her pet dog or cat for pet owners or a supportive friend for individuals not owning a pet. Data were analyzed separately for dog and cat owners, with similar results obtained; therefore, analyses were presented with dog and cat data combined into a single pet category. In this study, baseline heart rate and blood pressure were significantly lower in pet owners ($P<0.001$). In comparison with the other conditions, cardiovascular reactivity was lowest when stress occurred with the pet present (Fig. 6.3). In addition, cardiovascular parameters also recovered to baseline after stress fastest when the pet was present.

In a related study, individuals with hypertension and high-stress jobs were treated with lisinopril; half of the participants were also assigned to a group required to get a pet dog or cat (N=24), and half served as the non-pet control group (N=24) [12]. Vital signs and plasma renin were measured during stressful tasks (performing math calculations and delivering a speech) at baseline and 6 months after starting lisinopril and acquiring a pet for the pet group. For the pet group, the pet was present and allowed to roam freely during post-intervention testing. The authors did not report how many individuals had selected a dog and how many had selected a cat as their pet and analyses were performed for new pet owners as a total group. As expected, before stress, blood pressure decreased in both groups after adding lisinopril (Table 6.1). Cardiovascular reactivity to stress was significantly lower among those patients who also acquired a pet. In addition, accuracy during math calculations at baseline testing was 74% for both patient groups. At 6-month follow-up testing, math accuracy was essentially unchanged at 75% in the lisinopril only group, improving to 92% for patients who had acquired a pet.

Therapy Dog Visits Reduce Stress for Patients and Their Caregivers

When dogs cannot be added to a household, stress relief might still be achieved by utilizing therapy dog visits. These visits can provide stress reduction for both patients and their caregivers, who often also experience psychological distress. A recent review of randomized trials favored including supportive interventions to help reduce psychological distress among informal caregivers of patients with terminal disease [13].

The ability of dogs to reduce stress for patients and their support network was evaluated in outpatients attending a chronic pain clinic (N=235), friends and family accompanying patients to their appointment (N=34), and clinic staff (N=26) after a brief therapy dog visit [14]. Responses were compared to control measures conducted with 83 patients, six family or friends accompanying patients, and seven staff who spent a similar amount of time in a quiet waiting area without the dog. Participants were asked to rate stress severity before and after the therapy dog visit or waiting in the quiet room on an 11-point scale (0 = no stress, 10 = worst stress imaginable). Mean visit duration (range) with the therapy dog was 11.1 ± 7.4 min (1–45 min) for patients, 10.2 ± 5.6 min (1–25 min) for family and friends, and 8.2 ± 5.1 min (1–25 min) for staff. The time

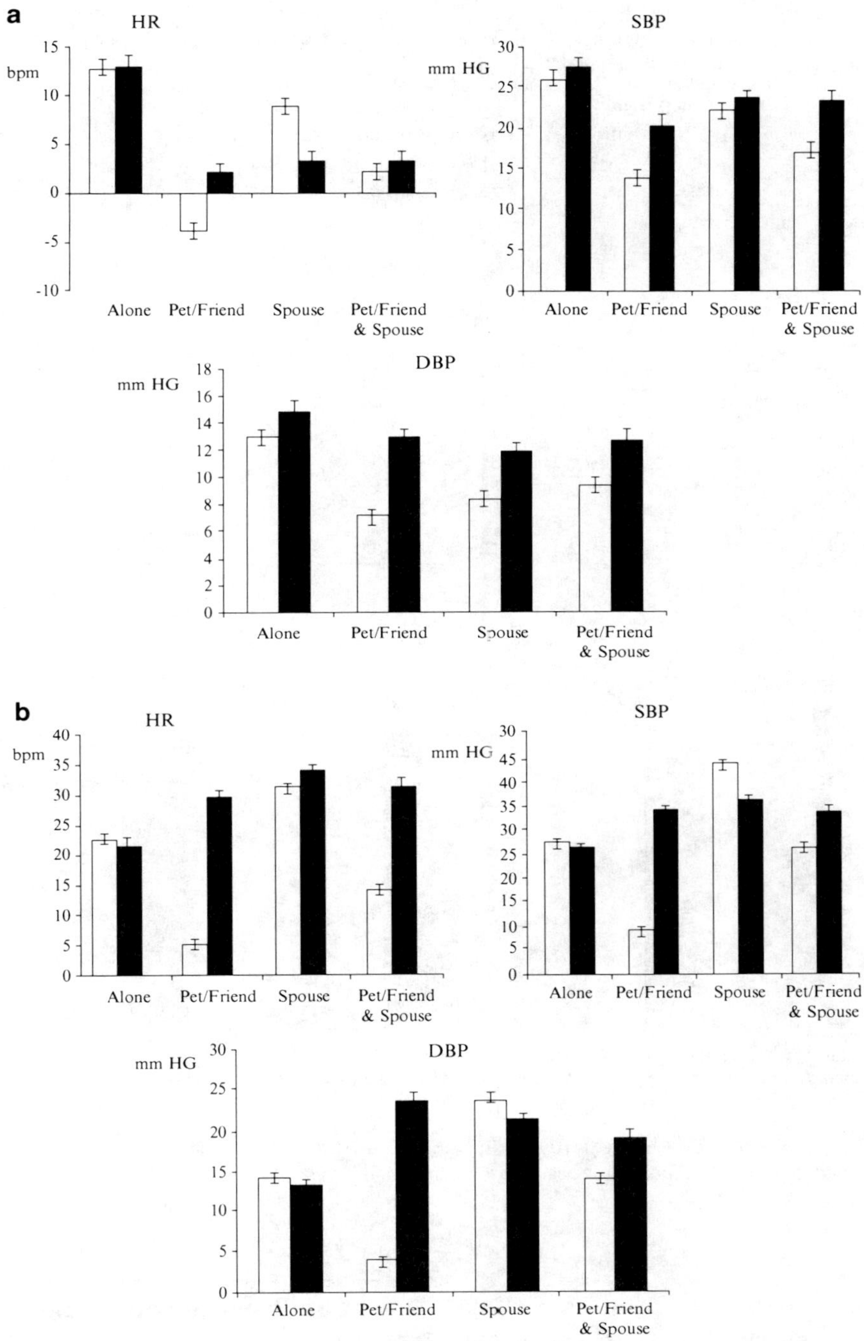

Fig. 6.3 Cardiovascular stress response to physical and emotional stressors. Pet owners are shown with the *white bars* and non-pet owners with *black bars*. During the second condition (pet/friend), the subject's pet dog or cat was present in the room during the stress condition for pet owners; non-pet owners were accompanied by a supportive friend during this condition. bpm, beats per minute; DBP, diastolic blood pressure; HR, heart rate; SBP, systolic blood pressure (Reprinted with permission [11]). (**a**) Physical stress: cold pressor test. (**b**) Mental stress: performing math calculations

Table 6.1 Effect of including the addition of a pet to a hypertension prescription for stress response. Differences in reactivity after the intervention were significantly lower in the group treated with lisinopril plus a pet compared with the lisinopril alone group: ***$P<0.001$ (Based on [12])

	Lisinopril alone				Lisinopril plus acquiring pet			
	Pre-intervention		Post-intervention		Pre-intervention		Post-intervention	
	Before stress	After stress	Before stress	After stress	Before stress	After stress	Before stress	After stress
A. Reactivity with math stress								
SBP	162	179	121	139	163	180	122	130***
DBP	104	116	82	95	105	115	83	90***
Heart rate, beats per minute	73	89	71	88	73	87	71	78***
Plasma renin, ng/mL	7.2	9.3	12.2	15.8	7.3	9.4	12.3	13.5***
B. Reactivity with speech stress								
SBP	163	182	120	139	164	183	118	126***
DBP	105	120	81	99	103	118	80	89***
Heart rate, beats per minute	72	93	70	93	70	91	69	79***
Plasma renin, ng/mL	7.1	10.2	12.0	16.0	7.2	10.3	12.1	13.7***

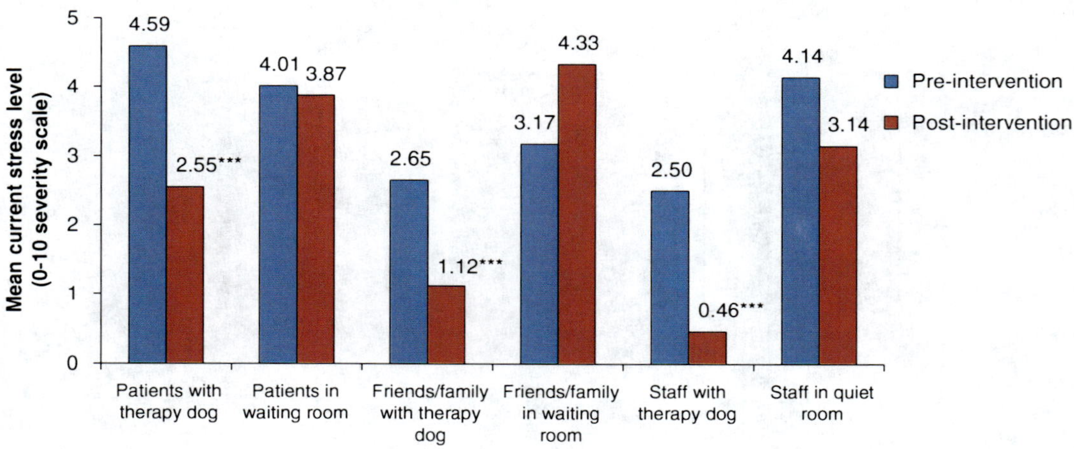

Fig. 6.4 Self-reported stress levels using 0–10 severity scale (0 = no stress; 10 = extreme stress). Stress reduction after the brief therapy dog visit was significant for each participant group: ***$P<0.0001$ (Based on [14])

for the waiting room survey between pre- and post-survey completion was 16.4 ± 6.5 min (5–40 min) for patients, 13.3 ± 5.2 min (5–20 min) for family and friends, and 19.7 ± 6.0 min (14–30 min) for staff. Significant reductions in average stress level occurred after spending time with the dog for each group, with no significant improvement among controls (Fig. 6.4).

Dogs Can Provide Emotional and Social Support

In an article in the *Journal of the American Medical Association*, David Spiegel, MD, argues that an important part of cancer treatment includes facilitating a supportive environment for cancer patients, as chronic stress and social isolation

Case 2

In *The Power of Wagging Tails*, the ability of a companion dog to serve the emotional needs of a cancer patient was highlighted by the story of a Border Collie-mix dog named Lucky D. When Lucky D's owner heard her daughter had been diagnosed with cancer, both she and her daughter were understandably upset. While the daughter sat on the sofa, Lucky D quietly brought her one of his toys and dropped it on her lap. He returned to his toy stash for another and then another until the daughter was loaded with every toy he owned. Lucky D then joined the woman on the sofa while she sat quietly crying. Soon, Lucky D reached over and began licking the tears from her face. Lucky D's owner recalled, "[Lucky D's] simple, unselfish acts of love and devotion were a bigger comfort to [my daughter] than all the words anyone might have said [16]."

have been linked to poor outcome [15]. Companion dogs often provide an important source of nonjudgmental acceptance and foster healthy emotional connections that can add important ongoing support to patients' human support networks.

Cancer Patients May Feel Emotionally Isolated from Human Support Network

Cancer patients can feel isolated from family and friends. Cancer patients can often achieve an outlet for sharing feelings through peer support groups. Support groups have been shown to fill an important role for many cancer patients by providing an arena in which patients experience unconditional acceptance and can safely express their emotions [17]. A survey of nine peer support groups for patients with cancer described support groups as providing a unique community for patients with cancer that provided both information and unconditional acceptance that were often difficult to achieve from family and friends [17]:

> "[The cancer support groups provided patients] safety and non-judgmental acceptance, which were reported to have facilitated open and honest expression of feelings, allowing them to cry, to be angry or moody, or to be vulnerable."—p. 2569

Companion and therapy dogs may also provide an additional resource offering unconditional acceptance. Research shows that cancer patients do not always want to share difficult emotions with their medical staff [18]. In these cases, patients may more easily unload emotions on a dog. Psychologist Gavriele-Gold described healing encounters during therapy sessions when patients who were unable to connect with him were able to open up to a therapy dog to begin a healing process [19]. In these cases, the therapy dog provided a consistently nonjudgmental resource that immediately inspired trust and acceptance and facilitated patients being able to release emotions to begin a healing process.

Case 3

After her yearly mammogram, DH was diagnosed with ductal carcinoma in situ at age 42. Her mother had died from breast cancer at age 41 and her older sister, two aunts, and two cousins had also been diagnosed with breast and ovarian cancers. Initial lumpectomy for DH was complicated by inadequate tumor resection and a lower extremity deep venous thrombosis. After completing anticoagulant therapy, DH underwent repeat lumpectomy followed by radiation therapy.

Although family and friends offered DH hope and encouragement through her treatments, she particularly appreciated the support she received from her 7-year-old Labrador Retriever mix, Sonia.

(continued)

Case 3 (continued)

I was very lucky during my cancer treatment to have a devoted family and friends. When everyone was busy, Sonia was the one who was always there for me. She seemed to understand if I needed her to just sit next to me or if she should try to make me laugh. Being there for me was the only thing she focused on. Sonia was also the one I really felt safe to be myself with. People work hard at trying to cheer you up and sometimes you just need to let down and cry. When I'd cry around other people, I'd worry about upsetting them and they'd feel the need to make things better for me. Sonia seemed to understand and just let me be myself. Sonia was so nonjudgmental—she didn't try to change me. During my cancer treatment, I loved her for that more than anything else. She let me cry when I needed to, and being able to cry on someone who didn't feel the need to make it better really made all the difference.

This case illustrates both the nonjudgmental perception of support from dogs and the ability of dogs to help fill in emotional support gaps that often occur as patients undergo months of cancer treatments.

Companion Dogs as Social Capital

An interesting survey examined the role of pets as "social capital" [2]. This study investigated whether living with a companion pet might increase social contact and interaction, contribute to a sense of community, and foster reciprocity of favors among neighbors. In this survey, 339 adults living in three suburbs were evaluated, 59% of whom owned a pet. Dogs were the most commonly owned pet (63% of pet owners), followed by cats. This study linked pet ownership and dog ownership specifically with a better perception of overall health and increased engagement in one's neighborhood (Figs. 6.5 and 6.6). While 41% of pet owners reported that they got to know their neighbors through their pets, this was true for half of dog owners, who often engaged with neighbors during dog walks (Fig. 6.7). After adjusting for potentially confounding influences from age, gender, educational status, and family members, pet owners were 74% more likely to have a high social capital scale score compared with non-pet owners ($P=0.04$; Fig. 6.8). In addition, pet owners were

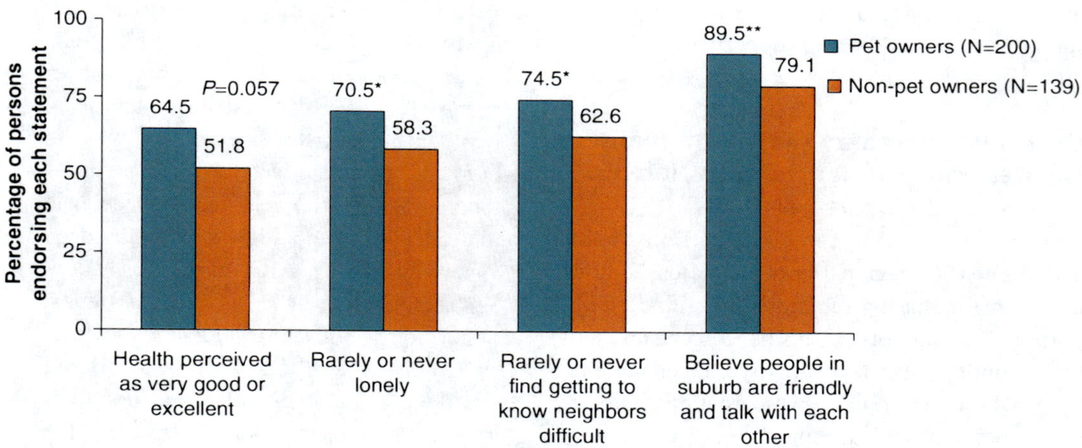

Fig. 6.5 Differences in health and social capital outcomes based on pet ownership. After adjusting for age, between-treatment differences were significant, favoring pet owners: $*P<0.05$, $**P<0.01$ (Based on [2])

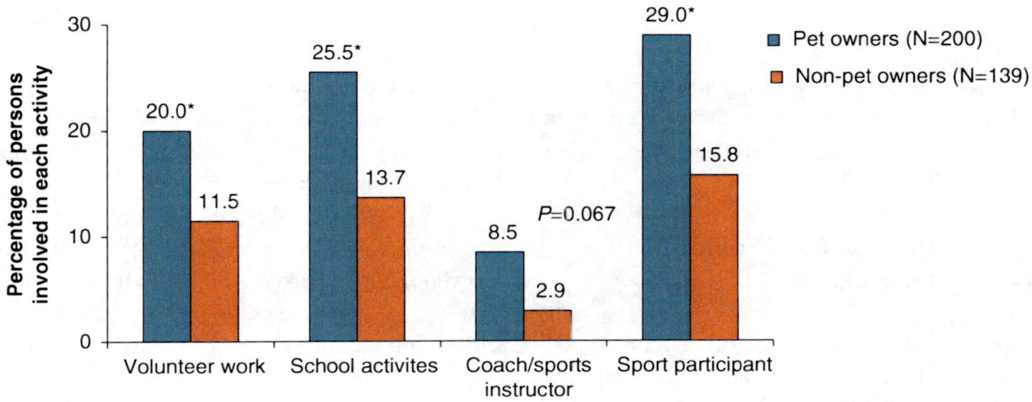

Fig. 6.6 Differences in involvement in suburban activities based on pet ownership. After adjusting for age, between-treatment differences were significant, favoring pet owners: $*P<0.05$ (Based on [2])

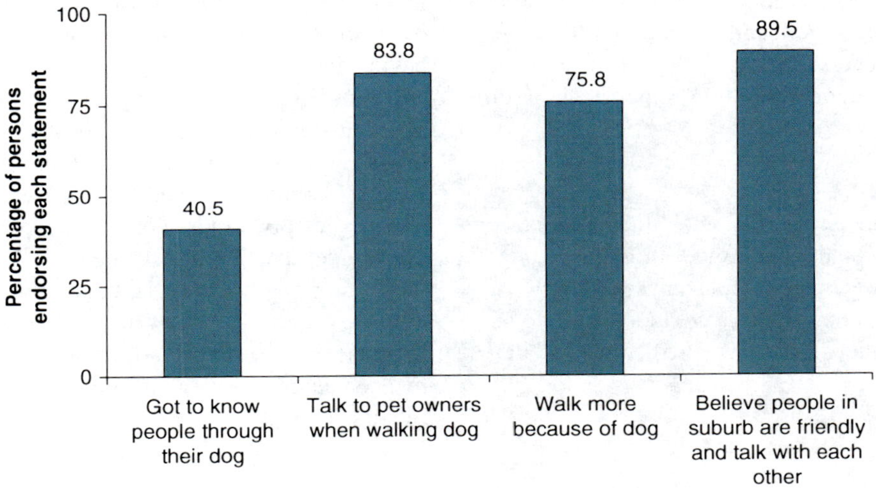

Fig. 6.7 Social engagement associated with dog ownership (Based on [2])

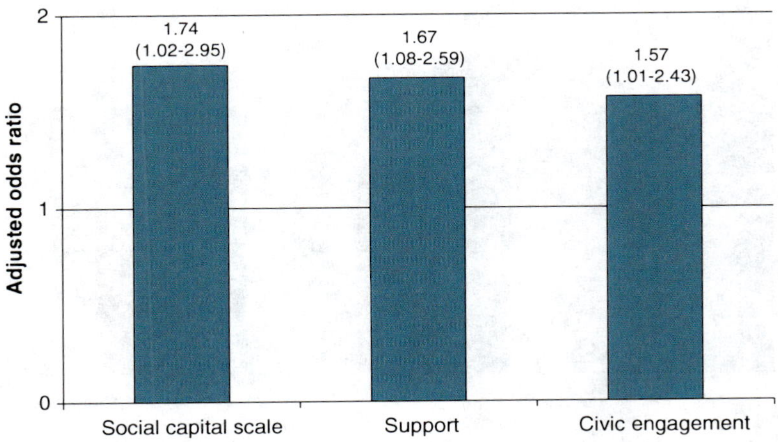

Fig. 6.8 Odds ratio (95% confidence intervals) for social capital associated with pet ownership, adjusted for age, gender, education, and children. The social capital scale includes community support; perceptions of neighborhood friendliness, sharing, and networking; and civic engagement. Odds ratios >1 favor pet owners over non-pet owners (Based on [2])

67% more likely to find social support from their neighbors ($P=0.02$) and 57% more likely to be civically active ($P=0.04$; Fig. 6.8).

Companion Dogs Can Provide Unwavering Support

Companion dogs are also often appreciated because of their consistent and persistent support. While research shows cancer patients want support throughout their cancer journey, most patients report receiving support at the time of diagnosis and their initial treatment, with support diminishing significantly over time [20].

Researchers from the National Cancer Institute published data evaluating support at baseline (an average of 51 days postbreast cancer diagnosis) and 5 months later. The percentage of women receiving very helpful emotional support decreased significantly over time ($P<0.001$; Fig. 6.9) [20]. Notably, continuing to receive helpful emotional support at 5-month follow-up was significantly linked with better health-related quality of life and perceived health competence, reinforcing the importance of emotional support. Dogs may offer a constancy that helps provide ongoing needed support.

> "Pets are non-judgmental, unconditionally loving, loyal, and usually nonthreatening. Compared with interpersonal relationships, interactions with a pet are more likely to be experienced as more predictable, stable, and secure [21]."

Experts have concluded that therapy dog interactions can likewise fulfill unmet attachment needs, even for individuals who may not have companion pets [21]. Animals were seen as having an ability to provide "...a safe haven and constitute a source of support, comfort, and relief in times of need [21]." In comparison to human relationships, relationships with pets were generally perceived as more consistently and predictably secure, positive, supportive, and noncompetitive, with pets perceived as being more emotionally available. In addition, pet relationships were also viewed positively because they lacked the expectations and disappointments that occurred with human interpersonal relationships.

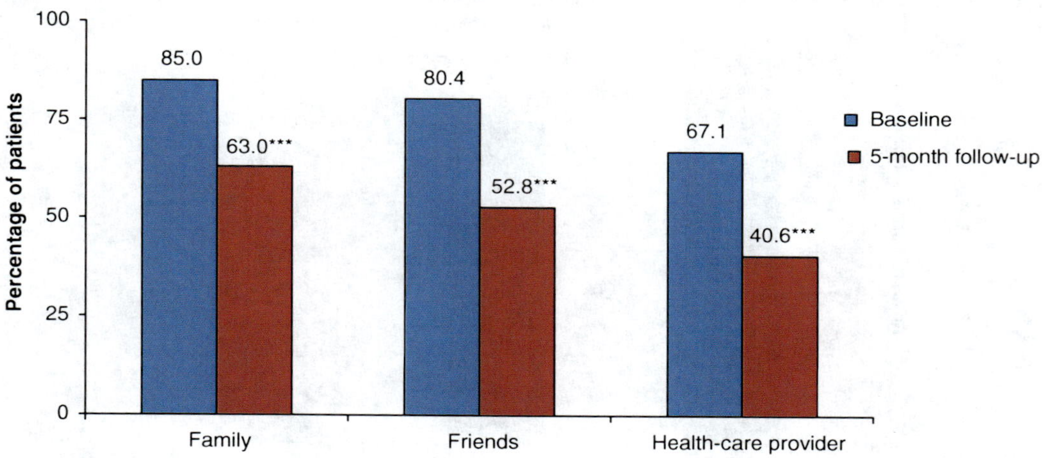

Fig. 6.9 Amount of very helpful support received by breast cancer patients at initial diagnosis and 5 months later. Differences versus baseline were significant: ***$P<0.001$ (Based on [20])

Psychologist Raymond B. Hanlon, MS, Describes Steadfast Support Patients Can Receive from Dogs

For some people, more so than their family, friends, or work, a dog has been the one stable, positive constant in their lives. Dogs provide unconditional, nonjudgmental love and support consistently during both good and bad times. This consistency is difficult for a human to duplicate. When people see a therapy dog, their previous positive experiences with dogs help them anticipate a caring encounter that can reduce their level of distress.

This is not to suggest that human-to-human emotional or social support is less valuable or essential. There is considerable scientific research that establishes the importance and value of human emotional support in times of distress. The difference lies, perhaps, with the consistency and quality of the support that humans are able to provide. When humans are in a situation to provide support to another, their capacity to provide the desired support may be confounded by circumstance or personal issues the supportive individual is experiencing. Human support requires the individual to bypass confounding variables at play in the moment to provide the desired support. This is accomplished sometimes in some situations, and, when it does occur, the resultant support to the recipient individual can be powerfully healing and validating. Unfortunately, this is not a consistent and predictable scenario. With a therapy dog, or family pet dogs, the inconsistency of response and confounding variables of human support are supplanted by the dog's instinctive loyalty and desire to please his owners and handlers. Obviously, a dog does not have cognition and judgment such that it may consider, "I did not get my biscuit today; should I offer my loving support?" Instinct has developed over centuries of domestication of dogs and the extraordinary relationships between dogs and their owners or handlers. Ironically, the primitiveness of this simple dog instinct, by comparison to the extraordinarily complex and highly evolved human brain, may be the difference in the consistency and unconditional response of the dog in support situations.

When one looks at the history of relationships between dogs and humans, the hypotheses suggested here are not too far of a reach, primarily due to the domestication of the dog and the relationship dogs and humans have fostered over centuries. Some evidence traces the dog and prehistory human relationship back some 26,000 years ago, with discovery in Chauvet Cave in southern France of bare footprints of an 8- to 10-year-old that are followed alongside by paw prints hypothesized to be a wolf or dog. Most of us are aware of extraordinary stories of dogs risking their own lives to rescue others, or dogs finding their way home after being lost hundreds of miles away. Consider the extensive literature of dogs and humans, some fictional, some real, such as Jack London's *White Fang*; James Herriot's prolific stories and novels surrounding his experience as a veterinarian and love and curiosity of dogs and animals; David Wroblewski's *Edgar Sawtelle*; and the extraordinary true story made into a movie of the dog Hachiko (nicknamed Hachi) who maintained his loyalty to his master long after the master's death by continuing to go to and wait at the master's old train stop every day for years after his master's death, only discontinuing as a result of his own death from old age. The literary and true stories of dogs and humans repeatedly reveal an interdependency established through love and loyalty and, from the dog more so than the human, love and loyalty that is essentially unconditional. It makes good sense, and is increasingly revealed by scientific research, that dogs can offer comfort, pleasure, and affection and that these qualities of interaction can prove to be supportive and validating to humans who desire support in times of difficulty.

Case 4

After ignoring a breast lump for years, 53-year-old BB was diagnosed with stage 3, triple-negative breast cancer in January of 2010. Although she was initially scheduled for eight chemotherapy treatments, because of the size of tumor, the doctors decided to perform her double mastectomy after finishing the third treatment. All lymph nodes were negative, and BB was rediagnosed as having a rare phyllodes tumor. Postoperatively, BB completed 33 radiation treatments.

During BB's surgical recovery and cancer therapy, her pack of dogs (13 Dachshunds and one Miniature Schnauzer) were a source of comfort.

> *You might have thought having all the dogs in the house would be too much noise and activity when you're not feeling well. Actually, my dogs turned out to be ideal companions during recovery. When I was going through treatments, my normally rowdy pack of dogs seemed to instinctively understand I needed them to be close, but calm. They would lie on the couch right next to me and cuddle. Unlike my human visitors, my dogs could keep me company and not expect me to say a word. When I was recovering, it would sometimes be so hard when people would come to visit because there were many times I didn't have the strength to talk and human visitors just wore me out. My dogs could provide comfort without expecting anything in return at a time when I really had little to give back.*
>
> *Every night while I was so sick and on meds, I could only be comfortable lying on my back. My Dachshund Ruste would quietly lie on my chest when I was in bed, remaining still and steadfast all night while I slept. It was such a comfort knowing he was there with me. There were some nights I wondered if I would wake up in the morning, and having Ruste watching over me kept me from being so scared.*
>
> *Having my dogs to depend on me also helped keep me positive—I knew I had to get well for them. My son and husband tended to the dogs' needs when I was in the hospital and first home, but I had made a commitment to care for my pack of dogs that I intended to keep.*

Two years after her initial diagnosis, BB remains cancer-free and continues to stay surrounded by Dachshunds. She decided to give back by helping homeless dogs as a foster parent for the Dachshund Lovers of Texas rescue organization. In addition, because she missed her own dogs so much when she was hospitalized, she is currently training one of her Dachshunds to become a therapy dog and is eager to start therapy dog work as a cancer survivor.

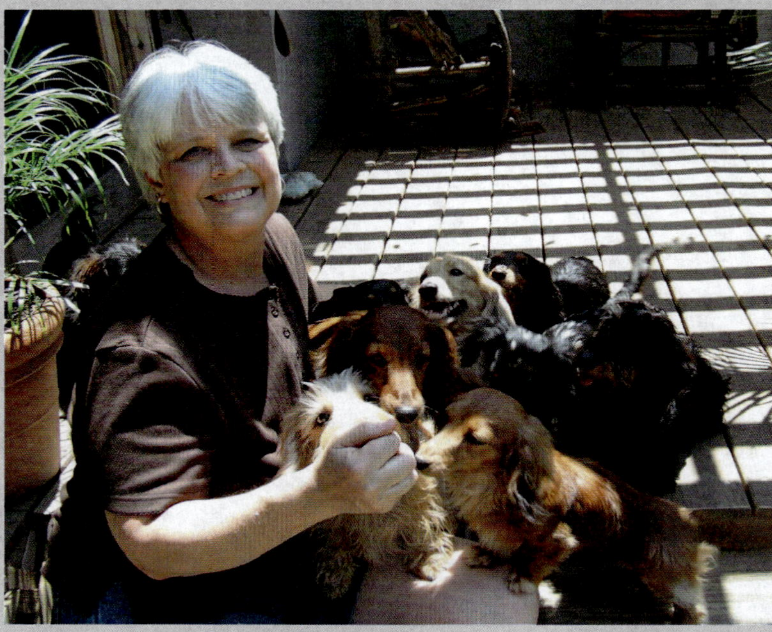

Summary

- Pet ownership provides social capital, facilitating people's ability to connect and engage with neighbors and their community.
- Owning a pet has been linked to reduced negative physiological responses to stress.
- Pets can offer social support that differs from that provided by human companions.
- Dogs can offer consistently available support and comfort throughout cancer treatment and recovery.

References

1. Friedmann E, Son H. The human-companion animal bond: how humans benefit. Vet Clin North Am Small Anim Pract. 2009;39:293–326.
2. Wood L, Giles-Corti B, Bulsara M. The pet connection: pets as a conduit for social capital? Soc Sci Med. 2005;61:1159–73.
3. Tower RB, Nokota M. Pet companionship and depression: results from a United States Internet sample. Anthrozoös. 2006;19:50–64.
4. Larson BR, Looker S, Herrera DM, et al. Cancer patients and their companion animals: results from a 309-patient survey on pet-related concerns and anxieties during chemotherapy. J Canc Educ. 2010;25: 396–400.
5. Kang DH, McArdle T, Park NJ, et al. Dose effects of relaxation practice on immune responses in women newly diagnosed with breast cancer: an exploratory study. Oncol Nurs Forum. 2011;38:E240–52.
6. Loprinzi CE, Prasad K, Schroeder DR, Sood A. Stress management and resilience training (SMART) program to decrease stress and enhance resilience among breast cancer survivors: a pilot randomized clinical trial. Clin Breast Cancer. 2011;11:364–8.
7. Traeger L, Penedo FJ, Benedict C, et al. Identifying how and for whom cognitive-behavioral stress management improves emotional well-being among recent prostate cancer survivors. Psychooncology, in press.
8. Anderson WP, Reid CM, Jennings GL. Pet ownership and risk factors for cardiovascular disease. Med J Aust. 1992;157:298–301.
9. Parslow RA, Jorm AF. Pet ownership and risk factors for cardiovascular disease: another look. Med J Aust. 2003;179:466–8.
10. Wright JD, Kritz-Sliverstein D, Morton DJ, Wingard DL, Barrett-Connor E. Pet ownership and blood pressure in old age. Epidemiology. 2007;18:613–8.
11. Allen, et al. Cardiovascular reactivity and the presence of pets, friends, and spouses: the truth about cats and dogs. Psychosom Med. 2002;64:727–39.
12. Allen K, Shykoff BE, Izzo JL. Pet ownership, but not ACE inhibitor therapy, blunts home blood pressure responses to mental stress. Hypertension. 2001;38: 815–20.
13. Candy B, Jones, Drake R, Leurent B, King M. Interventions for supporting informal caregivers of patients in the terminal phase of a disease. Cochrane Database Syst Rev. 2011;(6):CD007617.
14. Marcus DA, Bernstein CD, Constantin JM, Kunkel FA, Breuer P, Hanlon RB. Animal-assisted therapy at an outpatient pain management clinic. Pain Med. 2012; 13:45–57.
15. Spiegel D. Mind matters in cancer survival. JAMA. 2011;305:502–3.
16. Marcus DA. I have cancer: how can a dog help me? The power of wagging tails: a doctor's guide to dog therapy and healing. New York: Demos Health; 2011. p. 176.
17. Ussher J, Kirsten L, Butow P, Sandoval M. What do cancer support groups provide which other supportive relationships do not? The experience of peer support groups for people with cancer. Soc Sci Med. 2006; 62:2565–76.
18. Kvåle K. Do cancer patients always want to talk about difficult emotions? A qualitative study of cancer inpatients communication needs. Eur J Oncol Nurs. 2007; 11:320–7.
19. Gavriele-Gold J. The human-canine bond: new learning and a changing rationality from a psychoanalytic perspective. Psychoanal Rev. 2011;98:91–105.
20. Arora NK, Finney Rutten LJ, Gustafson DH, Moser R, Hawkins RP. Perceived helpfulness and impact of social support provided by family, friends, and health care providers to women newly diagnosed with breast cancer. Psycho Oncol. 2007;16:474–86.
21. Zilcha-Mano S, Mikulincer M, Shaver PR. Pets in the therapy room: an attachment perspective on animal-assisted therapy. Attach Hum Dev. 2011;13:541–61.

Incorporating Companion Dogs into Cancer Rehab: Benefits from Physical Exercise for Cancer Patients

7

Key Chapter Points

- The American Cancer Society recommends ≥150 minutes of moderate-intensity aerobic exercise per week.
- Recommended exercise targets are met by only one in three cancer survivors and half of young adult cancer survivors.
- Meeting exercise targets has been linked to reduced cancer risk, improved survival, and enhanced quality of life in cancer survivors.
- Walking is generally the preferred form of exercise for most people, and dog walking often improves compliance with a walking program.

Keywords

Fatigue • Lymphedema • Metabolic equivalent task-hours • Mortality • Quality of life • Survival • Walking

Healthy exercise can have a positive impact across cancer stages, with reduced cancer incidence and benefits for cancer patients, including symptomatic reduction and improved outcome (Fig. 7.1) [1, 2]. The American Cancer Society, World Cancer Research Fund/American Institute for Cancer Research, and the American College of Sports Medicine recommend an exercise target of ≥30 minutes of at least moderate-intensity aerobic exercise 5 days per week for most cancer patients and survivors (total weekly exercise target = 150 minutes; see Chap. 1) [3, 4]. Recommendations also note that individual patient programs may need to be modified based on patient health, treatment, and anticipated disease course. Exercise recommendations are based on data linking regular exercise with reduced cancer risk [5], with some evidence that physical activity may reduce cancer recurrence and extend survival [6–8]. In addition, engaging in routine physical activity and exercise improves aerobic capacity, physical functioning, psychosocial well-being, and quality of life in cancer survivors [9]. While achieving American Cancer Society exercise targets is ideal, data from studies (detailed below) show that even more modest levels of physical activity can be beneficial for cancer patients.

D.A. Marcus, *Therapy Dogs in Cancer Care: A Valuable Complementary Treatment*,
DOI 10.1007/978-1-4614-3378-1_7, © Springer Science+Business Media New York 2012

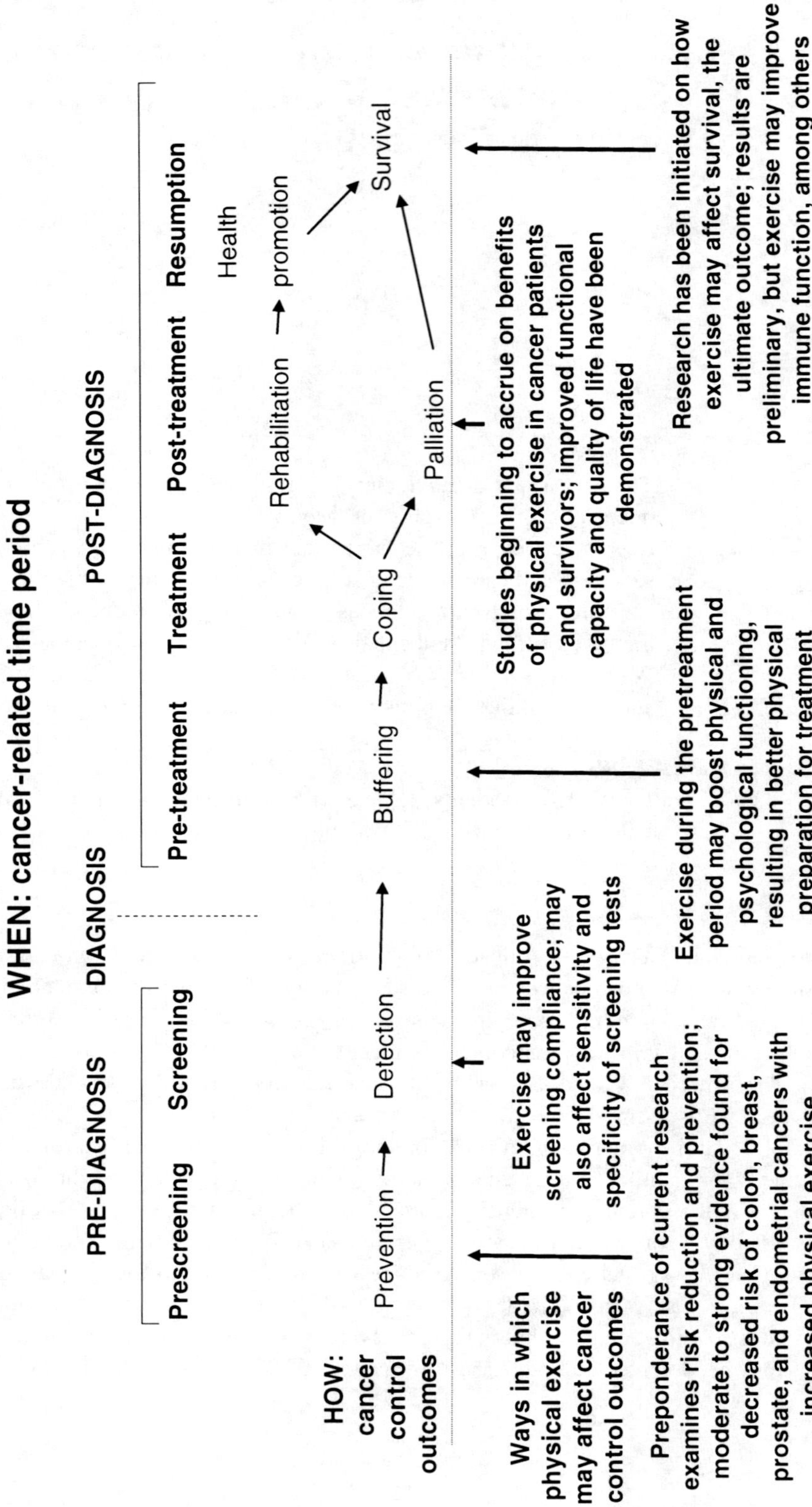

Fig. 7.1 Model describing when and how physical exercise may benefit patients with cancer (Reproduced with permission from [1])

Practical Pointer The American Cancer Society recommends cancer patients and survivors engage in ≥150 minutes of moderate-to-strenuous or ≥60 minutes of strenuous physical activity per week.

Experimental studies support a beneficial role of exercise for reducing factors associated with increased cancer risk. Several studies have shown that physical activity improves concentrations of biomarkers implicated in breast and colon cancer, as well as improving immune function in these patients [10]; these data support clinical studies linking physical activity with reduced cancer risk and improved survival. Animal data also link exercise with cancer incidence and progression. For example, running on an exercise wheel reduces both development and growth of prostate tumors in rodents [11, 12]. Some of the relationship between physical activity and cancer risk reduction may be related to links between obesity and increased cancer risk, potentially due to metabolic stresses and the proinflammatory nature of adipose cells [13, 14]. In addition, changes in the production of reactive oxygen species with exercise have also been postulated to influence the protective effect of exercise against cancer [5].

Unfortunately, many individuals, including those at higher risk for developing cancer, do not exercise sufficiently. Data from the 2009 Sister Study, evaluating sisters of women with breast cancer ($N=44{,}364$), reported that American Cancer Society exercise targets were met by only 26% of Caucasian and 18% of African–American sisters of women with breast cancer [15]. These data support findings from a previously published study showing that awareness of the relationship between physical activity and cancer risk was lower in African–Americans compared with Caucasians [16]. Focus group discussions with women with breast cancer who were undergoing or had completed treatment similarly reported lack of awareness by patients about the protective role exercise has against cancer, with this knowledge deficit acting as a major barrier to physical exercise engagement [17]. The authors of this study supported increased efforts for health-care providers to educate and counsel patients about the important impact from exercise for cancer patients.

Quantifying Exercise Level

A number of studies evaluating exercise effects detailed below used metabolic equivalent task-hours (MET-hours) to describe exercise intensity. Because walking is the most convenient exercise for most patients, studies typically convert MET-hours into equivalent hours of walking. In general, one hour of brisk walking is equivalent to 4–5 MET-hours. Brisk walking time is, therefore, used as the primary intensity marker throughout this chapter for ease of understanding, particularly when offering information to patients.

Practical Pointer

- 1 hour casual walking (2–2.5 miles/hour) = 3 MET-hours
- 1 hour brisk walking = 4–5 MET-hours
- 30 minutes of moderate-intensity bicycling = 2 MET-hours

Using MET-hours as an exercise measure, some studies have been able to determine exercise quantity that is important for achieving different targets for cancer patients. For example, an observational study of women with stage I–III colorectal cancer showed a significant reduction in overall mortality with exercise >9 MET-hours per week (the equivalent of 2.5 hours of brisk walking per week) and a significant reduction in cancer-related mortality when exercising 18 MET-hours per week (the equivalent of 5 hours of brisk walking per week; see Fig. 7.2) [18].

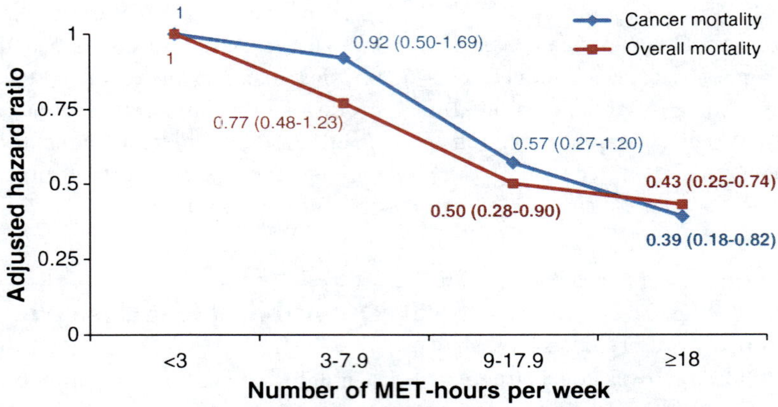

Fig. 7.2 Hazard ratios (95% confidence intervals) for mortality in patients with colorectal cancer, adjusted for cancer variables, age at diagnosis, treatment, obesity variables, and smoking. Values <1 signify lower mortality risk. Significant values are shown in bold (Based on [18])

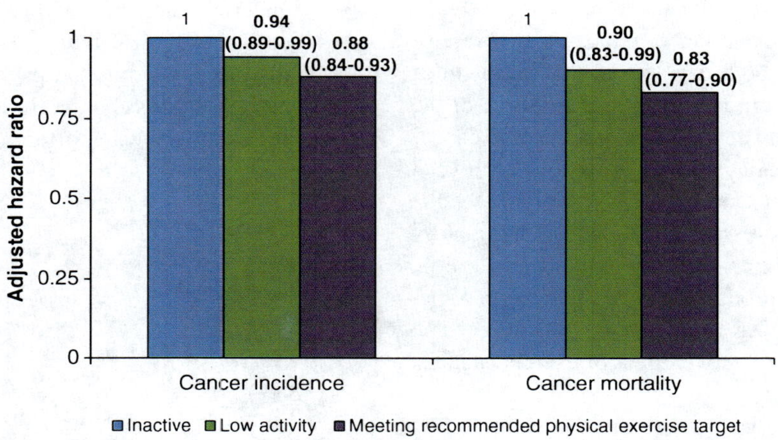

Fig. 7.3 Hazard ratios (95% confidence intervals) are adjusted for age, gender, education, work activity, and cardiovascular risk factors. Significantly reduced hazard ratios are marked with bold text. Risk was significantly reduced with increased exercise for both cancer incidence and mortality ($P<0.0001$ for each) (Based on [20])

Prevention Benefits from Exercise

American Cancer Society exercise recommendations are supported by data confirming a cancer protective effect from exercise. Epidemiological and experimental studies support an inverse relationship between regular exercise and risk for developing intestinal, colon, pancreatic, breast, lung, skin, endometrial, and prostate cancers [5]. For example, a case control study reported that past history of not exercising between ages 45 and 54 years old nearly tripled prostate cancer risk (adjusted odds ratio = 2.9, $P<0.05$) [19].

A large, prospective, cohort study evaluated the effects of exercise in over 416,000 adults ≥20 years old followed for 13 years [20]. As expected, exercise was linked with reduced mortality and cardiovascular deaths. Exercise was also linked with reduced cancer incidence and cancer deaths (Fig. 7.3). In addition, for every additional 15-minute increase in daily exercise beyond a minimum of 15 minutes, there was a further 1% reduction in cancer mortality.

Practical Pointer Increased physical activity and exercise significantly reduce cancer incidence and mortality.

Benefits of Physical Exercise After a Cancer Diagnosis

Physical activity can be an important aspect of cancer rehabilitation. For example, the American Cancer Guidelines note that clinical trials in cancer survivors show benefit with programs typically involving 45 minutes of moderate-to-vigorous physical activity at least 3 days per week, with improvements noted in mood and fatigue [3]. Physical exercise may also benefit patients with more advanced disease. A palliative care study randomized patients with a life expectancy ≤2 years ($N = 231$) to a physical exercise program 60 minutes twice weekly for 8 weeks or a nonexercise control [21]. Walking ($P=0.008$) and handgrip ($P=0.01$) were significantly better after 8 weeks with exercise, with improvements noted in both variables among exercising patients and losses seen in both among nonexercisers. This study supports that exercise can be useful to help maintain physical functioning in patients with advanced cancer.

In addition, research has shown improvement in cancer survival benefits with physical activity [1, 22]. Physical exercise may improve cancer survival through reduced cancer recurrence or progression (e.g., breast and colon cancer recurrence) and by reducing the development of other health problems, including other primary cancers.

Reduced Symptoms

Physical exercise has been linked to a wide range of physical and emotional benefits in cancer survivors (Table 7.1) [1]. Exercise may also offer therapeutic impact for reducing some cancer-related symptoms. For example, a review of 14 randomized, controlled trials evaluating exercise intervention in patients with breast cancer linked exercise with significant improvement in physical functioning and fitness, reduced fatigue, and enhanced quality of life [23]. Physical exercise has also been linked to improved health, functioning, and quality of life among pediatric cancer survivors [24].

Table 7.1 Benefits identified in research studies evaluating effects of physical activity in cancer survivors (Based on [1])

Physical benefits	Emotional benefits
• Improved strength • Increased flexibility • Better functional ability and physical well-being • Reduced fatigue • Less nausea and diarrhea • Decreased pain • Maintained body weight	• Reduced depression • Less anxiety • Decreased anger • Improved self-esteem • Increased life satisfaction

Practical Pointer The American Cancer Society recommends exercise, including daily walking, to improve physical fitness, reduce fatigue, improve digestion, and reduce mood problems and stress effects.

Fatigue

A systematic review of 44 randomized controlled trials supported that exercise interventions significantly reduced cancer-related fatigue ($P<0.001$) [25]. Significant reductions were shown in subgroup analyses for patients with breast and prostate cancer. Reductions failed to achieve significance for leukemia, lymphoma, and colorectal cancer survivors, although these analyses were based on a single study evaluated each for leukemia and colorectal cancer and 4 studies for lymphoma. In general, exercise was effective when it was of moderate intensity; low-intensity exercise was not effective.

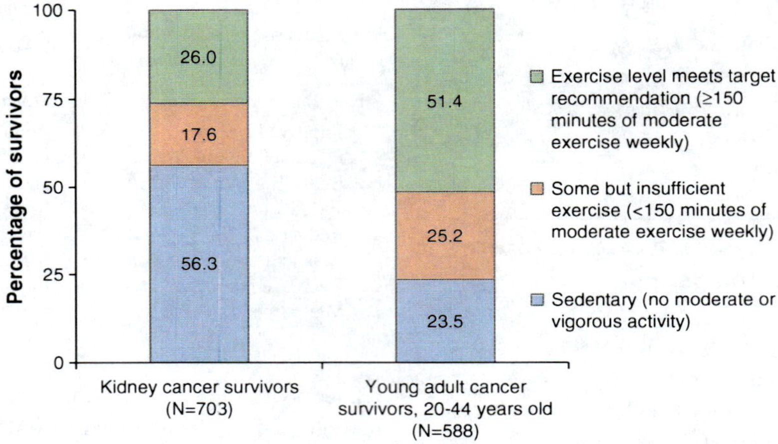

Fig. 7.4 Self-reported levels of physical activity (Based on [26, 27])

Improved Quality of Life

A dose–response relationship has been shown between physical exercise and quality of life among kidney cancer survivors (mean age = 65.0 ± 11.1 years) [26] and young adult cancer survivors (ages 20–44 years, mean age = 38.2 ± 5.6 years) [27] using data from a Canadian provincial registry. Standard physical activity guidelines were used to establish an exercise target, with adults recommended to participate in either 75 minutes of vigorous activity per week or 150 minutes of moderate activity per week. Recommended physical exercise targets were achieved by one in four kidney cancer survivors and half of young adult cancer survivors (Fig. 7.4). As exercise increased, both physical and emotional measures of quality of life likewise improved for cancer survivors (Fig. 7.5). These data support that patients may achieve quality-of-life benefits even when they have not achieved recommended exercise targets.

Quality of life was likewise linked with physical activity in a national cross-sectional survey of 9,105 cancer survivors (2,885 breast, 2,226 prostate, 1,918 colorectal, 586 bladder, 729 uterine, 761 melanoma) [28]. The American Cancer Society's recommendation of ≥150 minutes of moderate-to-strenuous or ≥60 minutes of strenuous physical activity per week was achieved by 38% of cancer survivors. Among those patients meeting recommended exercise targets, health-related quality-of-life scores were significantly better, even after adjusting for potentially confounding demographic and disease factors (Fig. 7.6).

Improved Survival

Observational studies in breast and colorectal cancer support that exercise may reduce cancer recurrence and prolong survival [29]. The amount of physical activity significantly linked with reduced cancer mortality has varied in studies between 9 and 27 MET-hours per week (Table 7.2) [30]. In one study, 4,826 women with breast cancer (stages I–III) within about 6 months of diagnosis were followed for about 60 months [31]. Women reporting regularly exercising at least twice weekly were considered to be exercisers, while others were labeled as nonexercisers. The most commonly reported exercise was walking. A significant inverse association was seen between exercise and total mortality in women with advanced disease (IIb–III), with reduced risk of recurrence/disease-specific mortality linked with exercise regardless of disease stage (Fig. 7.7). Benefits were also affected by estrogen/progesterone receptor status, with significant risk reduction only in women with estrogen/progesterone receptor-negative cancer. This study additionally identified benefits for patients participating in lower levels of exercise. While exercise

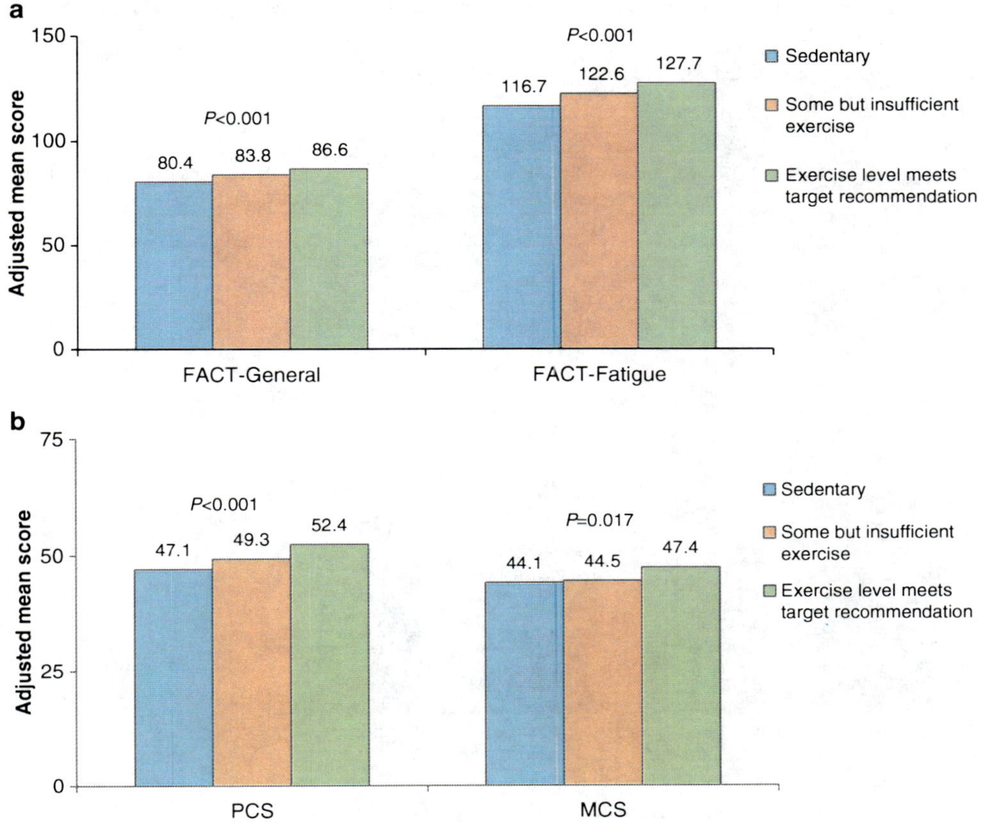

Fig. 7.5 Quality of life and exercise. With all quality-of-life measures used, higher scores indicate better quality of life. Scores were adjusted for age, gender, marital status, education, ethnicity, body mass index, months since diagnosis, drug treatment, current treatment status, recurrence, current disease status, drinking, and number of comorbidities. Trends for improved quality of life with increasing exercise were significant for all measures in both patient samples (Based on [26, 27]). (**a**) Kidney cancer survivors. Functional Assessment of Cancer Therapy (FACT) scale scores include a FACT-General score (including physical, functional, emotional, and social well-being; possible score range 0–108) and a FACT-Fatigue score (FACT-General plus fatigue; possible score range 0–160). (**b**) Young adult cancer survivors. Medical Outcomes Study 36-Item Short Form (SF-36) physical component scores (PCS) and mental component scores (MCS). PCS and MCS scores have possible score range from 0 to100, with a mean of 50 (SD 10) for a US normative population

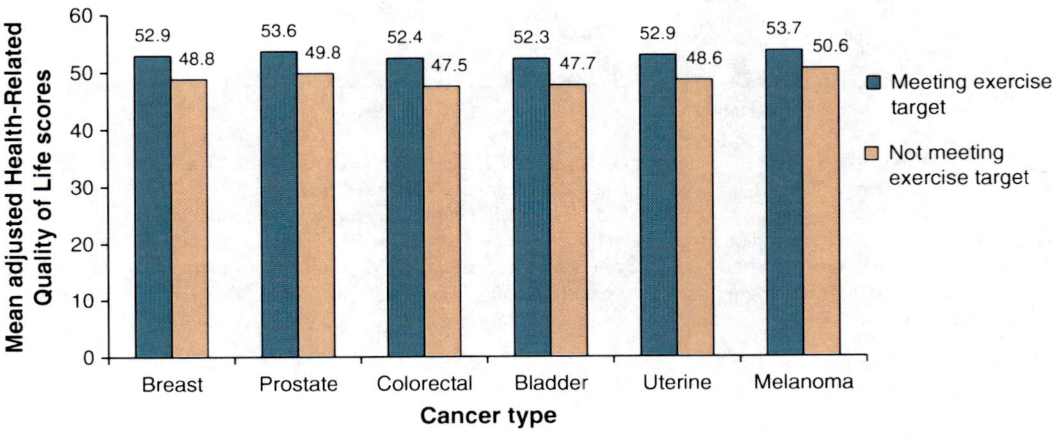

Fig. 7.6 Mean health-related quality-of-life scores, adjusted for age, race, cancer stage, marital status, education, number of comorbidities (possible range 0–100, with higher scores representing better quality of life). Quality-of-life scores were significantly higher in all cancer groups meeting exercise target (Based on [28])

Table 7.2 Exercise level associated with reduced cancer mortality (Based on [30])

Exercise level	Breast cancer	Colorectal cancer
MET-hours per week	9–21	18–27
Equivalent walking	30–75 minutes of brisk walking, 5 days per week	60–90 minutes of brisk walking, 5 days per week

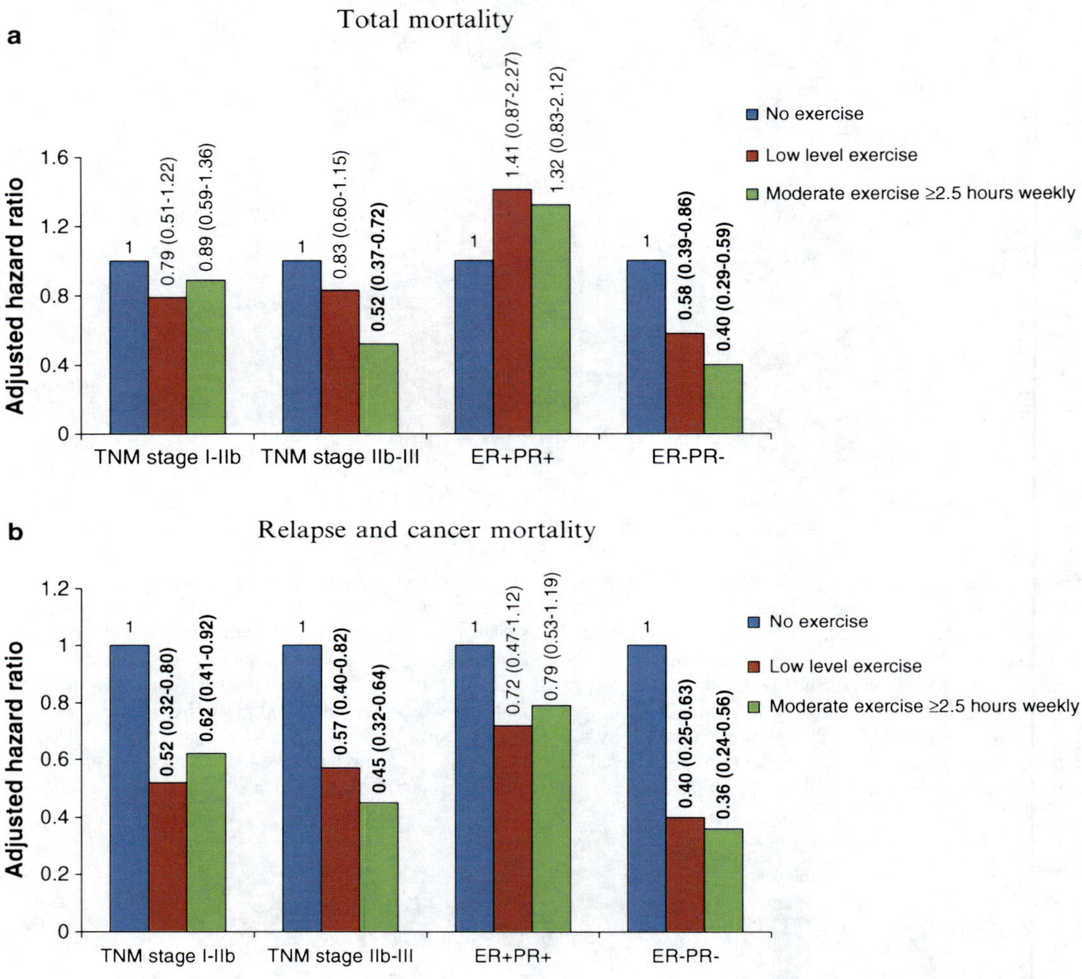

Fig. 7.7 Hazard ratios (95% confidence interval) over 36 months after breast cancer diagnosis, adjusted for age, baseline obesity, menopausal status, social factors, quality of life, treatment, and dietary intake. Hazard ratios based on stage were adjusted for estrogen/progesterone receptor status; ratios based on receptor status were adjusted for disease stage. Hazard ratio value <1 represents reduced risk. Significantly reduced hazard ratios are marked with bold text. Low exercise <8.3 MET-hours per week; moderate exercise ≥8.3 MET-hours per week. ER, estrogen receptor; PR, progesterone receptor; TNM, tumor-node-metastasis stage (Based on [31]). (**a**) Total mortality. (**b**) Relapse and cancer mortality

benefits for improved survival are likely to be multifactorial, a small study ($N=12$) evaluating DNA methylation linked increased physical activity after a breast cancer diagnosis with epigenetic regulation of tumor suppressor genes as an explanation for improved survival [32].

Practical Pointer Cancer mortality has been linked with briskly walking at least 150 minutes per week in patients with breast cancer and at least 300 minutes per week in patients with colorectal cancer.

Feasibility

Aerobic exercise is often feasible for cancer patients, although modifications are frequently needed for individual patients, based on physical limitations, treatment status, and general health condition. Tailoring exercise to meet individual patient conditions was used in a pilot study that evaluated aerobic exercise impact on 20 patients at least 30 days after surgery for non-small cell lung cancer (mean age 62 ± 11 years; 71% post-lobectomy; 42% with adjunctive chemotherapy; mean time from diagnosis = 30 ± 3 days) [33]. Exercise consisted of 20–30 minutes of bicycle training three times weekly for 14 weeks, with all sessions customized to the abilities of each individual patient. This study showed that aerobic exercise was safe and feasible for postsurgical patients, with significant improvements in quality of life and some cardiovascular measures. Significant quality-of-life changes included an 18% increase in functional well-being ($P=0.007$) and a 37% decrease in fatigue ($P=0.03$). Similarly, a randomized study showed that Pilates exercise was safe and effective in improving overall fitness in women who had been treated for breast cancer ($N=52$; mean age = 49 years old; mean time after diagnosis = 38 months) [34].

In addition to feasibility, cancer survivors are often interested in becoming more physically active. A Canadian survey of 588 young adult cancer survivors (20–44 years old) reported that 78% were interested in participating in a physical activity program and 88% believed they were capable of participating [35]. Walking was listed most commonly as the favorite activity or sport during summer (51% of patients) and winter (40% of patients). Patients reported interest in beginning a program at various stages during cancer treatment and recovery, although two in three patients were interested in physical activity starting after treatment completion (Fig. 7.8).

Lymphedema After Breast Cancer Surgery with Axillary Node Dissection

Concern about possible lymphedema development should not prevent patients from participating in exercise. Four randomized studies evaluated the effect of early exercise on the development of lymphedema in patients treated for breast cancer with axillary lymph node dissection [36]. These studies either showed a reduction in lymphedema or no increase in lymphedema with exercise, including supervised resistance and weight training. A more recent study, the Physical Activity and Lymphedema trial, randomized women at risk for breast cancer-related lymphedema ($N=154$) to a slowly progressive weight lifting program twice weekly supervised for 13 weeks and then without supervision for 9 months or a 1-year no exercise control [37]. Women were required to have a diagnosis of unilateral, nonmetastatic breast cancer, have had at least 2 lymph nodes previously resected, and be currently cancer-free. Average age of participants was 55 years (range 36–75 years old), with an average time since cancer diagnosis of 3 years. Onset of lymphedema during the 1-year study was not increased among women engaged in exercise (Fig. 7.9). Indeed, overall incidence of lymphedema in all women and those who had had more extensive lymph node dissection was significantly less among women engaged in twice weekly weight lifting.

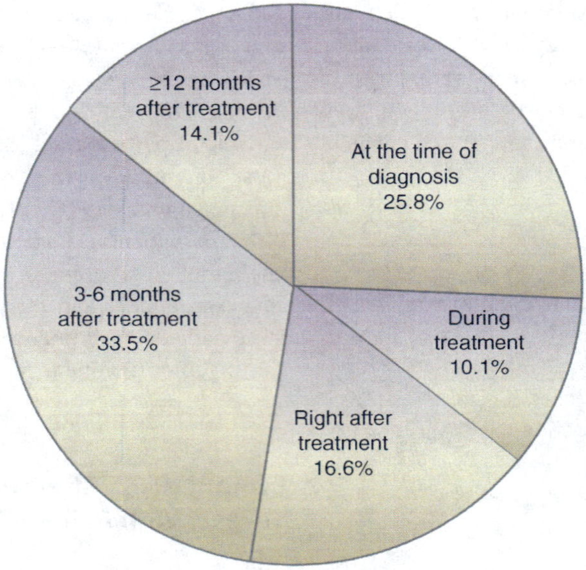

Fig. 7.8 Time during cancer care when patients are interested in starting a physical activity program (Based on [35])

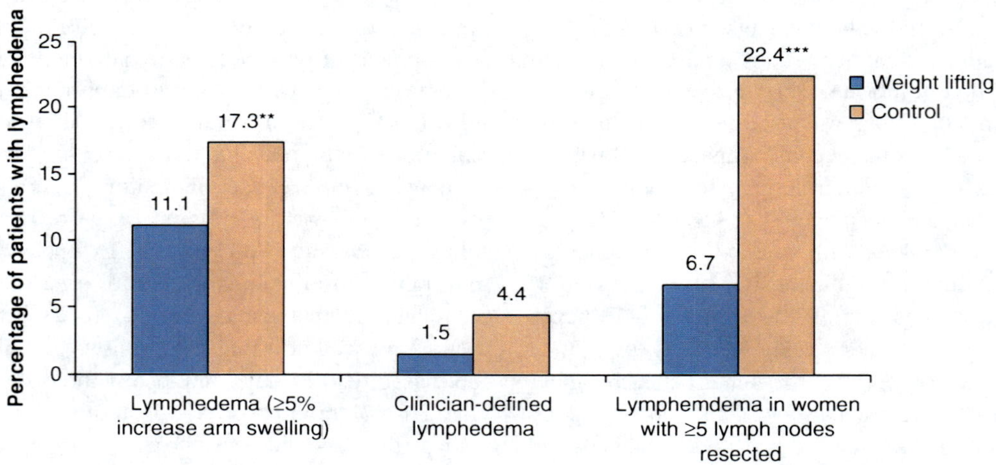

Fig. 7.9 Incident lymphedema in women treated for breast cancer. Clinician-defined lymphedema required 12 months of follow-up. Significant differences favored weight lifting: $^{**}P=0.003$, $^{***}P=0.001$ (Based on [37])

These data support considering the addition of supervised exercise with weight lifting after breast cancer surgery.

> **Practical Pointer** Breast cancer patients undergoing axillary node dissection should not expect increased risk for lymphedema from participating in supervised exercise.

Walking for Cancer Patients

Walking is the often listed as a preferred exercise for adults. According to data from the 2005 National Health Interview Survey, 42% of adults in the United States walk for a leisure activity [38]. The National Population Health Survey and Canadian Community Health Survey reported 30% of Canadian adults walk regularly, while

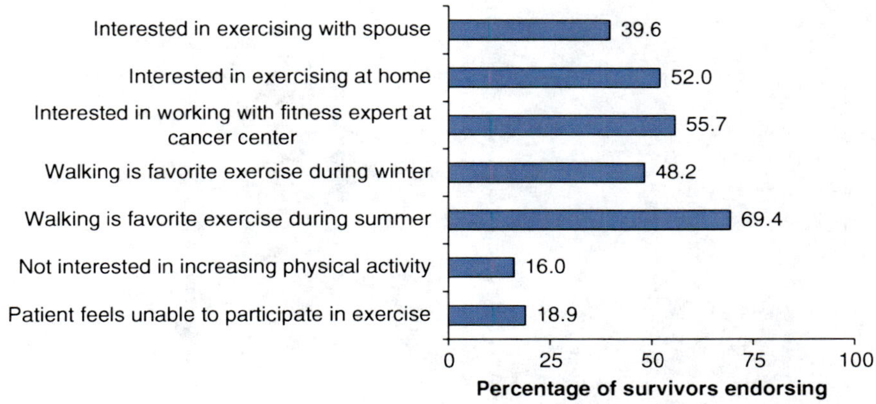

Fig. 7.10 Exercise perceptions and preferences in kidney cancer survivors (Based on [40])

70% had walked for exercise at least once during the previous 3 months [39].

Walking is also usually the preferred exercise for many cancer patients. The survey of 703 kidney cancer survivors reported above additionally queried survivors about their interest in participating in exercise [40]. Most patients endorsed a perceived ability and interest in participating in exercise, with walking often selected as a preferred exercise (Fig. 7.10). In addition, cancer survivors who were currently sedentary were most likely to prefer exercising at home (57%); this group, in particular, may be an ideal group to target with a home walking program. Similarly, a survey of 91 cancer patients undergoing chemotherapy in Taiwan (mean age = 53.3 ± 12.6 years; most common cancer diagnoses colorectal [35%], breast [33%], and lung [21%]) identified that two in five patients were successfully achieving World Health Organization exercise recommendation standards (i.e., 150 minutes of moderate activity or 60 minutes of vigorous activity weekly) [41]. The most commonly used exercise was walking. The average time patients spent walking was 163 minutes weekly compared with 16 minutes weekly doing any other moderate or vigorous exercise.

> **Practical Pointer** Walking is generally selected as the preferred form of exercise.

Walking Exercise Reduces Symptoms

Exercise improves both physical and emotional health in cancer patients. Researchers in Germany randomized 58 women with metastatic breast cancer who had completed chemotherapy/radiation therapy at least 4 weeks earlier to a 10-week exercise and walking program or a waiting control [42]. Participants in the walking group met twice weekly for 90 minutes. After 10 weeks, those women participating in the walking group experienced significantly improved fitness, as well as decreases in anxiety and depression scores (Fig. 7.11).

Researchers at Johns Hopkins University likewise showed significant improvements from a home-based walking program in cancer patients [43]. In this study, 126 patients (mean age 60.2 ± 10.6) were randomized to a walking program (20–30 minutes of brisk walking followed by a 5-minute cool down 5 times per week) throughout their cancer treatment or a usual care control group. The most common diagnoses were prostate (56%) and breast (35%) cancer, and most patients had stage II disease (70%). Half of the patients were being treated with radiation (52%) and 35% with chemotherapy. Measures were obtained before starting and after completion of cancer treatment. In general, patients in the walking program maintained or improved cardiorespiratory fitness and physical function and

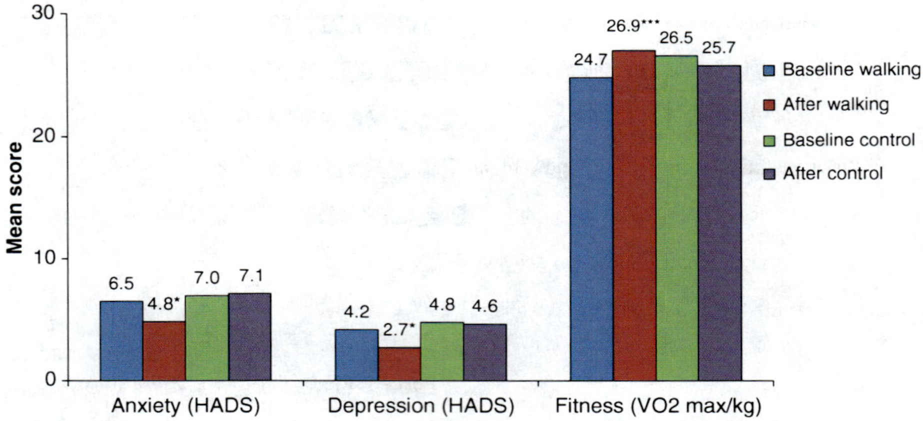

Fig. 7.11 Pre- and post-treatment hospital anxiety and depression scale (HADS) and maximal oxygen uptake (VO_2 max/kg) scores. Significant improvement occurred after 10 weeks of walking exercise (*$P \leq 0.05$; ***$P < 0.001$) (Based on [42])

experienced less pain during cancer treatment compared with those who were sedentary. Improvements were most notable in patients with prostate cancer. Furthermore, walking was helpful in reducing losses in capabilities among patients undergoing chemotherapy. A secondary analysis of this study additionally reported 10% less fatigue ($P < 0.001$), 13% more vigor ($P < 0.01$), and 3% less emotional distress ($P = 0.021$) among those exercising during cancer treatment [44].

Walking Exercise Improves Survival

Higher levels of physical activity have also been linked with improve survival in postmenopausal women with breast cancer, even among women who reported low physical activity prior to their diagnosis. A longitudinal study conducted by Yale School of Public Health evaluated the relationship between walking and other recreational activities and survival in 4,643 postmenopausal women with breast cancer participating in the Women's Health Initiative [45]. Mortality information was gathered every 2 years for 6 years. After a diagnosis of breast cancer, 40% of these women increased their physical activity level, while 25% decreased exercise and 35% remained unchanged. Compared with women who remained sedentary, mortality from all causes and from breast cancer was significantly reduced in those women walking briskly about 3 hours per week (9 MET-hours per week; Fig. 7.12). Overall mortality reduction benefits were realized by women exercising post-diagnosis, even if their exercise level had been low pre-diagnosis. Compared with women with breast cancer who were inactive before and after their diagnosis, those increasing physical activity after their diagnosis had a 45% lower mortality risk [46]. Furthermore, women reducing activity level after breast cancer diagnosis had a 4 times greater risk of death.

Brisk walking has also been linked to reduced prostate cancer progression in men with localized disease [47]. Risk of cancer progression was shown to be 57% lower among men walking briskly for at least 3 hours per week.

Prescribing a Walking Program During Cancer Recovery

Health-care providers should discuss exercise targets with patients throughout cancer care. A survey of patients with early stage (localized or in situ) breast ($N = 531$) or prostate cancer ($N = 447$) at Duke University reported that 58% of patients routinely exercised for an average of 43 minutes four times weekly, achieving exercise guidelines [48]. Conversely, the National Health

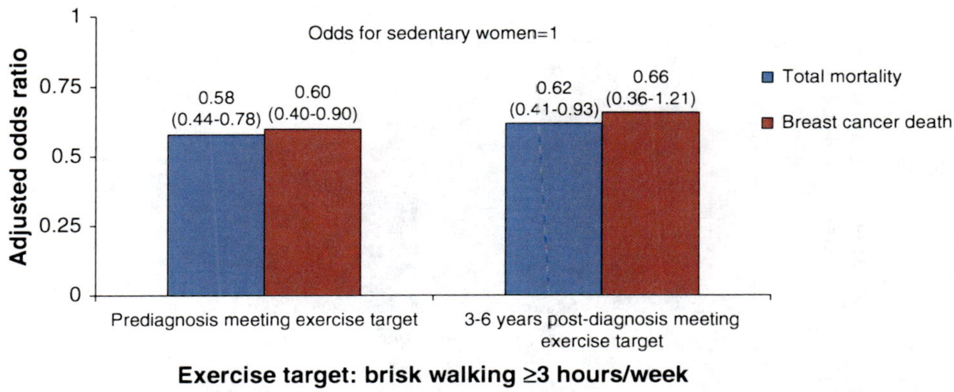

Fig. 7.12 Odds ratios (95% confidence intervals) for mortality risk among women exercising ≥9 MET-hours per week (about 3 hours per week of brisk walking) compared with sedentary women, adjusted for age, ethnicity, treatment, body mass index, diabetes, alcohol, smoking, dietary factors, and vigorous intensity exercise (Based on [45])

Interview Survey evaluating behaviors in 7,384 cancer survivors (adults stating they had ever been diagnosed with cancer) and 121,347 non-cancer controls identified through a population-based survey in the United States reported 30% of cancer survivors and 37% of controls participated in 150 minutes of moderate-intensity exercise weekly [49]. These data support an important role for health-care providers in encouraging patients to continue exercise into their cancer survivor period.

Dog Walking Improves Exercise Adherence

Incorporating companion dogs into an exercise routine can improve patients' motivation and compliance for maintaining healthy exercise. Research consistently shows that dog owners walk more than those without dogs. A recent survey of Canadians living in the Calgary metropolitan area reported that adults owning dogs were more likely to consistently exercise through recreational neighborhood walking (83% of dog owners were consistent walkers vs. 59% of those without a dog, $P=0.001$) [50]. Average recreational walking time was significantly higher among dog owners, with mean walking times exceeding the World Health Organization [51], the US Department of Health and Human Services [52], and Centers for Disease Control [53] recommendation for 150 minutes of exercise weekly (Fig. 7.13). Chapter 8 describes specific exercise routines that can incorporate a companion dog and provides practical resources that can be adapted for individual cancer patients.

Healthy Hydration

Proper hydration is essential to good health and successful exercise. Fluid deficits may be a particular concern in cancer patients due to a propensity for volume deficits from a variety of mechanisms, including decreased fluid intake, central mechanisms, renal effects, etc. [54]. While dehydration is well known to occur during the terminal stages of end-of-life care [55], therapy-induced nausea frequently leads to dehydration in early treatment, too. For example, a survey of 104 patients undergoing radiation therapy for head and neck cancer identified severe dehydration or malnutrition in 26% of patients [56]. Chemotherapy was also linked to a greater than threefold risk of developing severe dehydration in patients with breast cancer compared with patients not receiving chemotherapy [57]. Anorexia and early satiety in cancer patients may also contribute to dehydration [58]. Cancer patients should, therefore, be counseled about hydration prior to beginning a new exercise program.

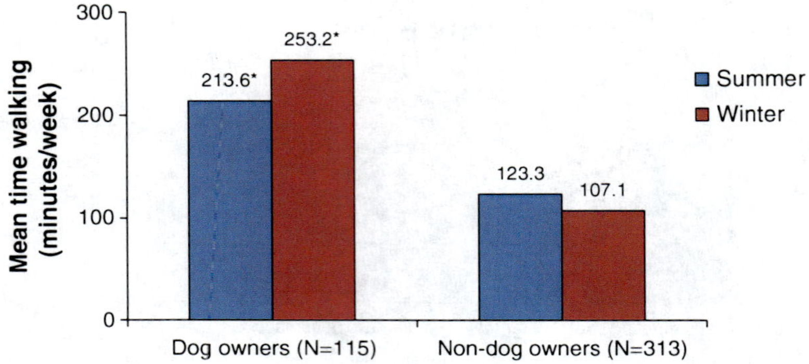

Fig. 7.13 Recreational walking in adult dog owners vs. adults without dogs. Differences in mean walking times between dog owners and nonowners were significant: $*P<0.05$ (Based on [50])

Adequate hydration improves exercise performance [59, 60]. In addition, inadequate hydration may reduce persistence with exercise. Researchers from the University of Bath noted generally poor water replacement among 52 healthy adults during exercise [61]. Average observed fluid intake during exercise was 390 ± 298 mL, while estimated sweat loss was 794 ± 391 mL. Poor fluid replacement is particularly important as hypohydration (defined as random urine osmolality >900 mOsmol/kg) was already identified in 37% of participants prior to exercising. Furthermore, hypohydrated patients experienced a more negative psychological affect to exercise. These data suggest that pre-exercise hydration may be important to facilitate a more positive perception of exercise that will motivate patients for better exercise adherence.

In general, urine color, particularly with first morning urine, can be used as a reasonable measure of hydration status when laboratory indices are not readily available [62]. Light, clear urine represents good hydration, while darker yellow or brown urine represents inadequate hydration [63]. In addition, patients should be encouraged to drink on average about 500 mL of water before exercise, with additional water taken during and after exercise.

> **Practical Pointer** Urine identified as "pale yellow" or "straw colored" suggests adequate hydration for exercise [63].

Summary

- Numerous studies support exercise as an independent predictor for cancer risk, recurrence, survival, and well-being in cancer survivors.
- Exercise helps reduce fatigue and mood disturbances and improve quality of life and physical fitness in cancer patients.
- While cancer mortality reduction has been linked to meeting or exceeding American Cancer Society exercise targets, important benefits in symptom reduction, quality-of-life improvement, and reduced overall mortality have been seen with lower levels of physical activity.
- Walking is the most commonly preferred exercise for cancer patients.
- Walking has been linked with reduced symptoms (including fatigue and emotional distress) and improved survival among cancer patients.

References

1. Rajarajeswaran P, Vishnupriya R. Exercise in cancer. Indian J Med Paediatr Oncol. 2009;30:61–70.
2. Courneya KS. Physical activity in cancer survivors: a field in motion. Psychooncology. 2009;18:337–42.
3. Doyle C, Kushi LH, Byers T, et al. Nutrition and physical activity during and after cancer treatment: an American Cancer Society guide for informed choices. CA Cancer J Clin. 2006;56:323–53.

4. Pekmezi DW, Demark-Wahnefried W. Updated evidence in support of diet and exercise interventions in cancer survivors. Acta Oncol. 2001;50:167–78.
5. Na HK, Oliynyk S. Effects of physical activity on cancer prevention. Ann N Y Acad Sci. 2011;1229: 176–83.
6. Courneya KS, Friedenriech CM. Physical activity and cancer: an introduction. Recent Results Cancer Res. 2011;186:1–10.
7. Schmitz K. Physical activity and breast cancer survivorship. Recent Results Cancer Res. 2011;186: 189–215.
8. Denlinger CS, Engstrom PF. Colorectal cancer survivorship: movement matters. Cancer Prev Res. 2011; 4:502–11.
9. Wiggins MS, Simonavice EM. Cancer prevention, aerobic capacity, and physical functioning in survivors related to physical activity: a recent review. Cancer Manag Res. 2010;2:157–64.
10. Winzer BM, Whiteman DC, Reeves MM, Paratz JD. Physical activity and cancer prevention: a systematic review of clinical trials. Cancer Causes Control. 2011;22:811–26.
11. Zheng X, Cui XX, Huang MT, et al. Inhibitory effect of voluntary running wheel exercise on the growth of human pancreatic Panc-1 and prostate PC-3 xenograft tumors in immunodeficient mice. Oncol Rep. 2008; 19:1583–8.
12. Zheng X, Cui XX, Gao Z, et al. Inhibitory effect of dietary atorvastatin and celecoxib together with voluntary running wheel exercise on the progression of androgen-dependent LNCaP prostate tumors to androgen independence. Exp Ther Med. 2010;2:221–8.
13. Harvey AE, Lashinger LM, Hursting SD. The growing challenge of obesity and cancer: an inflammatory issue. Ann N Y Acad Sci. 2011;1229:45–52.
14. Sung M, Yeon J, Park S, Park JY, Choi M. Obesity-induced metabolic stresses in breast and colon cancer. Ann N Y Acad Sci. 2011;1229:61–8.
15. Spector D, Deroo LA, Sandler DP. Lifestyle behaviors in black and white women with a family history of breast cancer. Prev Med. 2011;52:394–7.
16. Oh A, Shaikh A, Waters E, et al. Health disparities in awareness of physical activity and cancer prevention: findings from the National Cancer Institute's 2007 Health Information National Trends Survey (HINTS). J Health Commun. 2010;15 suppl 3:60–77.
17. Loh SY, Chew SL, Lee SY. Physical activity and women with breast cancer: insights from expert patients. Asian Pac J Cancer Prev. 2011;12:87–94.
18. Meyerhardt JA, Giovannucci EL, Holmes MD, et al. Physical activity and survival after colorectal cancer diagnosis. J Clin Oncol. 2006;24:3527–34.
19. Shahar S, Shafurah S, Hasan Shaari NS, et al. Roles of diet, lifetime physical activity and oxidative DNA damage in the occurrence of prostate cancer among men in Klang Calley, Malaysia. Asian Pac J Cancer Prev. 2011;12:605–11.
20. Wen CP, Wai JP, Tsai MK, et al. Minimum amount of physical activity for reduced mortality and extended life expectancy: a prospective cohort study. Lancet. 2011;378:1244–53.
21. Oldervoll LM, Loge JH, Lydersen S, et al. Physical exercise for cancer patients with advanced disease: a randomized controlled trial. Oncologist. 2011;16: 1649.
22. Barbaric M, Brooks E, Moore L, Cheifetz O. Effects of physical activity on cancer survival: a systematic review. Physiother Can. 2010;62:25–34.
23. McNeely ML, Campbell KL, Rowe BH, et al. Effects of exercise on breast cancer patients and survivors: a systematic review and meta analysis. CMAJ. 2006;175:34–41.
24. San Juan AF, Wolin K, Lucia A. Physical activity and pediatric cancer survivorship. Recent Results Cancer Res. 2011;186:319–47.
25. Brown JC, Huedo-Medina TB, Pescatello LS, et al. Efficacy of exercise interventions in modulating cancer-related fatigue among adult cancer survivors: a meta-analysis. Cancer Epidemiol Biomarkers Prev. 2011;20:123–33.
26. Trinh L, Plotnikoff RC, Rhodes RE, North S, Courneya KS. Association between physical activity and quality of life in a population-based sample of kidney cancer survivors. Cancer Epidemiol Biomarkers Prev. 2011;20:859–68.
27. Bélanger LJ, Plotnikoff RC, Clark A, Courneya KS. Physical activity and health-related quality of life in young adult cancer survivors: a Canadian provincial survey. J Cancer Surviv. 2011;5:44–53.
28. Blanchard CM, Courneya KS, Stein K. Cancer survivors' adherence to lifestyle behavior recommendations and associations with health-related quality of life: results from the American Cancer Society's SCS-II. J Clin Oncol. 2008;26:2198–204.
29. Speed-Andrews AE, Courneya KS. Effects of exercise on quality of life and prognosis in cancer survivors. Curr Sports Med Rep. 2009;8:176–81.
30. Jones LW, Peppercorn J, Scott JM, Battaglini C. Erratum to: exercise therapy in the management of solid tumors. Curr Treat Opt Oncol. 2010;11:73–86.
31. Chen X, Lu W, Zheng W, et al. Exercise after diagnosis of breast cancer in association with survival. Cancer Prev Res. 2011;4:1409–18.
32. Zeng H, Irwin ML, Lu L, et al. Physical activity and breast cancer survival: an epigenetic link through reduced methylation of a tumor suppressor gene L3MBTL1. Breast Cancer Res Treat, in press.
33. Jones LW, Eves ND, Peterson BL, et al. Safety and feasibility of aerobic training on cardiopulmonary function and quality of life in postsurgical nonsmall cell lung cancer patients. A pilot study. Cancer. 2008;113:3430–9.
34. Eyigor S, Karapolat H, Yesil H, Uslu R, Durmaz B. Effects of pilates exercise on functional capacity, flexibility, fatigue, depression and quality of life in female breast cancer patients: a randomized study. Eur J Phys Rehabil Med. 2010;46:481–7.
35. Bélanger LJ, Plotnikoff RC, Clark A, Courneya KS. A survey of physical activity programming and counseling

preferences in young-adult cancer survivors. Cancer Nurs. 2012;35:48–54.

36. Cavanaugh KM. Effects of early exercise on the development of lymphedema in patients with breast cancer treated with axillary lymph node dissection. J Oncol Pract. 2011;7:89–93.
37. Schmitz KH, Ahmed RL, Troxel AB, et al. Weight lifting for women at risk for breast cancer-related lymphedema: a randomized trial. JAMA. 2010;304: 2699–705.
38. Kruger J, Ham SA, Berrigan D, Ballard-Barbask R. Prevalence of transportation and leisure walking among U.S. adults. Prev Med. 2008;47:329–34.
39. Bryan SN, Katzmarzyk PT. Patterns and trends in walking behaviour among Canadian adults. Can J Public Health. 2009;100:294–8.
40. Trinh L, Plotnikoff RC, Rhodes RE, North S, Courneya KS. Physical activity preferences in a population-based sample of kidney cancer survivors. Support Care Cancer, in press.
41. Liou YM, Lee HL, Chien LY, et al. Daily-life physical activity and related factors among patients with cancer receiving chemotherapy in Taiwan. Cancer Nurs. 2011;34:443–52.
42. Mehnert A, Veers S, Howaldt D, et al. Effects of a physical exercise rehabilitation group program on anxiety, depression, body image, and health-related quality of life among breast cancer patients. Onkologie. 2011;34:248–53.
43. Griffith K, Wenzel J, Shange J, et al. Impact of a walking intervention on cardiorespiratory fitness, self-reported physical function, and pain in patients undergoing treatment for solid tumors. Cancer. 2009; 115:4874–84.
44. Wenzel J, Griffith K, Shange J, et al. Results of a home-based walking intervention for patients undergoing cancer treatment. Presented at the 16th international conference of cancer nursing. Atlanta, 7–11 March 2010.
45. Irwin ML, Tiernan A, Manson JE, et al. Physical activity and survival in postmenopausal women with breast cancer: results from the Women's Health Initiative. Cancer Prev Res. 2011;4:522–9.
46. Irwin ML, Smith AW, McTiernan A, et al. Influence of pre- and postdiagnosis physical activity on mortality in breast cancer survivors: the health, eating, activity, and lifestyle study. J Clin Oncol. 2008;26: 3958–64.
47. Richman EL, Kenfield SA, Stampfer MJ, et al. Physical activity after diagnosis and risk of prostate cancer progression: data from the cancer of the prostate strategic urologic research endeavor. Cancer Res. 2011;71:3889–95.
48. Demark-Wahnefried W, Peterson B, McBride C, et al. Current health behaviors and readiness to pursue life-style changes among men and women diagnosed with early stage prostate and breast carcinoma. Cancer. 2000;88:674–84.
49. Bellizzi KM, Rowland JH, Jeffrey DD, McNeel T. Health behaviors of cancer survivors: examining opportunities for cancer control intervention. J Clin Oncol. 2005;23:8884–93.
50. Lail P, McCormack GR, Rock M. Does dog-ownership influence seasonal patterns of neighbourhood-based walking among adults? A longitudinal study. BMC Public Health. 2011;11:148.
51. World Health Organization website. Available at http://www.who.int/dietphysicalactivity/factsheet_adults/en/index.html. Accessed May 2011.
52. US Department of Health and Human Services physical activity guidelines for Americans. Available at http://www.health.gov/PAGuidelines/guidelines/. Accessed May 2011.
53. Centers for Disease Control and Prevention website. Available at http://www.cdc.gov/physicalactivity/everyone/guidelines/adults.html. Accessed May 2011.
54. Srhill N, Walsh D, Nelson K, Davis M. Evaluation and treatment of cancer-related fluid deficits: volume depletion and dehydration. Support Care Cancer. 2001;9:408–19.
55. Dalal S, Bruera E. Dehydration in cancer patients to treat or not to treat. J Support Oncol. 2004;2:467–86.
56. Givens DJ, Karnell LH, Gupta AK, et al. Adverse events associated with concurrent chemoradiation therapy in patients with head and neck cancer. Arch Otolaryngol Head Neck Surg. 2009;135:1209–17.
57. Hassett MJ, O'Malley AJ, Pakes JR, Newhouse JP, Earle CC. Frequency and cost of chemotherapy-related serious adverse effects in a population sample of women with breast cancer. J Natl Cancer Inst. 2006;98:1108–17.
58. Davis MP, Walsh D, Lagman R, Yavuzsen T. Early satiety in cancer patients: a common and important but underrecognized symptom. Support Care Cancer. 2006;14:693–8.
59. Kavouras SA, Arnaoutis G, Makrillos M, et al. Educational intervention on water intake improves hydration status and enhances exercise performance in athletic youth. Scand J Med Sic Sports, in press.
60. Von Duvillard SP, Braun WA, Markofski M, Beneke R, Leithäuser R. Fluids and hydration in prolonged endurance performance. Nutrition. 2004;20:651–6.
61. Peacock OJ, Stokes K, Thompson D. Initial hydration status, fluid balance, and psychological affect during recreational exercise in adults. J Sports Sci. 2011; 29:897–904.
62. Kavouras SA. Assessing hydration status. Curr Opin Clin Nutr Metab Care. 2002;5:519–24.
63. Armstrong LE, Maresh CM, Catellani JW, et al. Urinary indices of hydration status. Int J Sport Nutr. 1994;4:265–79.

8 Incorporating Companion Dogs into Cancer Rehab: Dog-Themed Exercise Program for Cancer Patients

Key Chapter Points

- Exercise should be modified for individual patient capabilities, with additional adjustments on treatment days and when symptoms are more severe.
- This chapter provides dog-themed stretching and strength exercises for cancer patients, along with patient educational handouts including exercise tips and an exercise log.
- Walking, including dog walking, can be an ideal aerobic exercise that is easy to modify, based on symptoms, physical limitations, and treatment.
- Exercising should be performed with well-behaved dogs to avoid accidental injuries from disobedient dogs pulling or jumping.

Keywords

Aerobic • Diary • Isometric • Lymphedema • Stretching • Walking

Exercise is an important component of managing cancer patients as they undergo treatment and rehabilitation as cancer survivors [1] (see Chap. 7 for details). A variety of resources are available describing specific exercise recommendations for cancer patients (see Chap. 10). In general, exercise duration and intensity need to be adjusted based on an individual's physical capabilities. In addition, periodic adjustments within a program are generally needed to incorporate reduced intensity for treatment days and days when symptoms are more severe. All patients should begin any new exercise at a low-intensity level and very gradually increase as tolerated.

Exercise Prescription for Cancer Patients

The American Cancer Society recommends 30–60 min of moderate to vigorous physical activity at least 5 days per week in healthy adults to reduce cancer risk and in cancer survivors, as tolerated [2]. In 2010, the American College of Sports Medicine published exercise guidelines for cancer survivors that endorse stretching, strength training, and aerobic activity (Box 1) [3]. Reduced exercise intensity and impact (e.g., avoiding running and jumping exercises) are needed in patients with metastatic disease or

D.A. Marcus, *Therapy Dogs in Cancer Care: A Valuable Complementary Treatment*,
DOI 10.1007/978-1-4614-3378-1_8, © Springer Science+Business Media New York 2012

treatments likely to result in osteoporosis (e.g., hormonal therapies for breast cancer). In addition, exercise level will likely need to be adjusted as patients undergo treatments.

> **Practical Pearl** Cancer patients starting exercise should start low and go slow, starting with short sessions of low-intensity exercise.
>
> Gradual progression as tolerated should focus on increasing exercise frequency and duration before adding more intensity.

Patients should begin their exercise program slowly, about 5–10 min daily, with gradual increases to 20–30 min daily (Table 8.1, Box 2). Sessions should include a 5- to 10-min warm-up and cool-down before and after exercise sessions. Aerobic exercise should be performed 3–5 times weekly, as tolerated. Patients should also be sure to drink water before and after walking to maintain hydration.

> **Box 1 American College of Sports Medicine Exercise Guidelines for Cancer Survivors (Based on [3])**
>
> - Inactivity should be avoided.
> - A general exercise target is 150 min of moderate-intensity exercise weekly.
> - Flexibility stretching exercises should be included with exercise.
> - Strength training should occur about 2–3 times weekly.

Why Include a Companion Dog in an Exercise Program?

As described in Chap. 1, dog owners are more likely to adhere to regular exercise programs [4]. Research shows that having an exercise partner is a major contributor to successfully maintaining an exercise program, [5, 6] and a companion dog can be a reliable exercise partner. For example, a 4-year longitudinal study among patients with diabetes identified dog walking as a major factor in successful exercise maintenance [7]. Including dogs in exercise may also make exercise sessions more enjoyable as attention can be shifted onto the dog as a form of positive distraction and patients may appreciate both the emotional support and tactile benefits from dog companionship (see Chap. 6).

When dogs are incorporated into exercise or walking, the dog must be well behaved, obedient, and able to consistently walk well on a loose leash without pulling. Dogs that are prone to pulling on leashes, bolting for other dogs, squirrels, or birds, or jumping on humans might put the patient at risk for falls or other injuries. Patients with a less reliable dog may need to include a human companion during walks and exercise sessions that can assist with managing the dog when necessary.

Dog-Themed Exercise Program Designed for Cancer Patients and Survivors

Paula Breuer is a physical therapist working at the University of Pittsburgh and herself a breast cancer survivor. She has developed an exercise

Table 8.1 Exercise prescription for cancer patients (based on the Foundation for Cancer Research & Wellness [8])

Patients who fatigue with mild exertion	Patients undergoing chemotherapy or radiation	Patients after cancer treatment or in remission
Range of motion Gentle resistive exercise Progress to 3–5 min of walking several times daily, as tolerated	Moderate-intensity aerobic exercise to maintain physical and emotional reserves and to reduce fatigue and nausea Strength training to prevent weakness	Moderate-intensity aerobic exercise to improve fitness, progressing to more intense exercise, as tolerated

Box 2 Contraindications and Cautions to Exercise (Based on [2, 3] and [9])

- Contraindications:
  - Acute nausea with exercise or vomiting within 24 h
  - Severe fatigue, weakness, faintness, disorientation, or blurred vision
  - Cardiovascular insufficiency
  - Acute infection
  - Severe metabolic disease
  - Severe anemia
  - Neutrophil count $<0.5 \times 10^9$ μL
  - Platelet count $<50 \times 10^9$ μL
  - Recent cancer treatment:
    - ≤2 h after radiation
    - Intravenous chemotherapy within 24 h
- Limit use of public gyms:
  - If immunosuppressed until white blood cell count $>500/mm^3$
  - For one year after bone marrow transplant
  - Patients undergoing radiation therapy should avoid exposing irradiated skin to chlorinated pools
- Patients with indwelling catheters should avoid resistance exercises that might dislodge catheter
- Resistance exercise should be limited after bowel surgery
- Caution may be needed in patients with neuropathy with sensory or motor loss that may make area prone to injury
- Patients with severe fatigue should be encouraged to begin gentle stretching exercises
- Resistance exercises may need to be limited in patients with breast cancer if lymphedema develops

program to incorporate an individual's companion dog to make the exercise sessions more enjoyable. Incorporating a dog into exercise can also be a powerful tool to motivate patients to maintain an exercise program [10]. In general, exercise programs should include stretching and strengthening of large muscles and aerobics. The following program can be modified to meet the needs and abilities of typical cancer patients.

In order to maintain physical gains, patients should try to perform some exercise each day. On treatment days or days when fatigue or pain is more problematic, patients should be encouraged to complete those exercises that are the most easy and comfortable for them to do. This helps maintain physical fitness and provides a psychological boost of having success with exercise even on more difficult days.

Before starting a new exercise program, patients should review proposed exercises with their treating doctor. Patients should plan to exercise each day, although exercise intensity may vary (Box 3). These exercises can be performed indoors, outdoors in a yard or park, or during a dog walk with a well-behaved, obedient dog.

Stretching Exercises

Stretches should be performed so that a gentle stretch is felt without pain. Humans should stretch like their dogs instinctively do—leisurely and slowly. If a stretch causes pain, the extent of the stretch should be reduced. Each stretch may be increased as comfortable as patients become more familiar with each exercise. Initially, each stretch should be held for about 5 s, followed by 5–10 s of relaxation. Over time, stretch duration may be increased as tolerated to 15–20 s per stretch, with relaxation between stretches. Each exercise may be repeated about three times initially, with more repetitions added as patients become more comfortable to a maximum of 5–8 repetitions. Patients would ideally perform some stretching exercises for about 10–15 min per session and a stretching session twice daily.

Upper Body Leash Exercises

These exercises can be performed using a standard dog leash. The leash used in the photos is a 4-ft leash; however, a 6-ft leash might also be

Box 3 ***Patient Instruction Sheet*****: Starting a New Exercise Program**

- Review the exercise program with your doctor before you get started.
- Plan to pace your activities throughout the day rather than trying to complete a full exercise program in one session to "get it out of the way." It is important to allow adequate recovery time between exercises rather than trying to do all exercises in a row. Many people will perform some exercises in the morning, several in the afternoon, and some in the evening.
- Start at a low intensity where you feel comfortable and increase gradually.
- Expect that some days you will feel more fatigued than others. On treatment days or days when you feel more fatigued, you should still do some exercise but only a few exercises. Choose those exercises that you are most comfortable doing and that you find the most soothing.

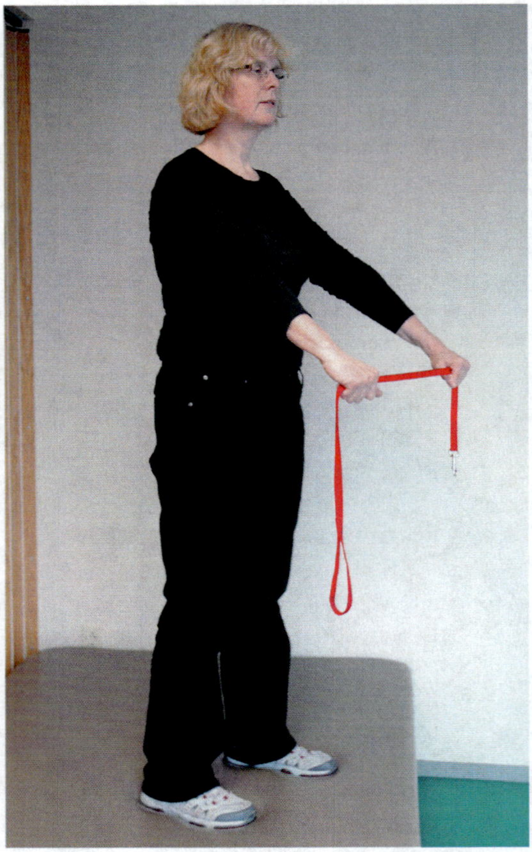

Fig. 8.1 Leash lift. Start position

used. Cloth or leather nonretractable leashes are acceptable. Leash exercises can be completed before going for a walk or when in a fenced area or an off-leash dog park where the dog's leash is available to use. An extra leash can alternatively be used for exercising, while keeping the dog on leash for dog control. When a few exercises are being performed, the dog can be asked to sit and stay.

Photographs show full movements for each exercise. Patients will often need to begin with partial movements, as comfortable, slowly advancing toward more complete movements as tolerated:

1. Leash lift. This exercise stretches the trunk and arms:
   A. Starting position: stand on a firm, level surface with the feet about shoulder width apart. Hold leash in front of the body, with arms shoulder width apart (Fig. 8.1).
   B. Keeping elbows extended, lift arms in front of the chest and then overhead (Fig. 8.2).
   C. With arms overhead, move hands toward the end of the leash, using a slow motion that allows the leash to slip through the hands (Fig. 8.3). The distance the hands reach apart from each other can vary, based on patient comfort. Hold stretch with arms apart. Relax and then return to the starting position to repeat. This stretch can be enhanced by breathing in deeply while the arms are in the overhead position.
2. Bow and arrow stretch. This exercise stretches the upper back and trunk:
   A. Starting position: stand on a firm, level surface with the feet about shoulder width apart. Turn toward the side and hold the leash as shown, with the left hand on top of the right (Fig. 8.4).
   B. Push left hand away from your body and pull the right hand toward your chin (Fig. 8.5).
   C. Pull your right hand backward, as though you are pulling back on a bow (Fig. 8.6).

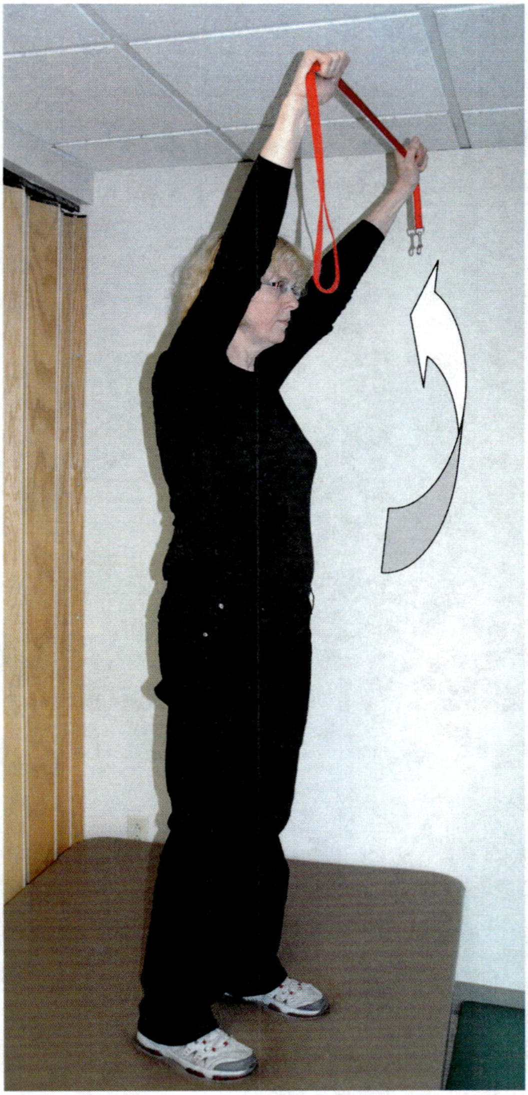

Fig. 8.2 Leash lift. Raise arms in an arc to overhead

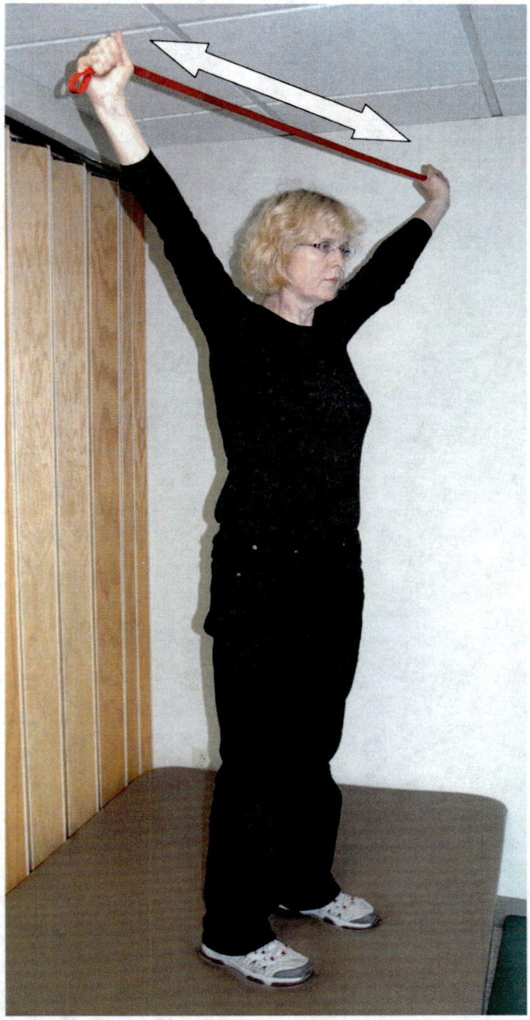

Fig. 8.3 Leash lift. Reach hands apart

Hold position, relax, and repeat. Then switch sides so your right hand starts on top, your right hand moves forward away from your chest, and your left hand pulls back on the bow.

3. Shoulder blade reach. This exercises stretches the shoulder:
   A. Starting position: stand on a firm, level surface with the feet about shoulder width apart. Turn toward the right. Loop one end of the leash around your left hand. Relax the left hand in the loop of the leash. Place the leash over your right shoulder and hold the clip end with your right hand (Fig. 8.7).
   B. Push your right hand away from your chest and slightly upward (Fig. 8.8). This will pull your left hand up toward your right shoulder blade.
   C. Pull with your right hand until the left hand is as close to the shoulder blade as is comfortable (Fig. 8.9). Hold, then relax, repeat, and switch sides.

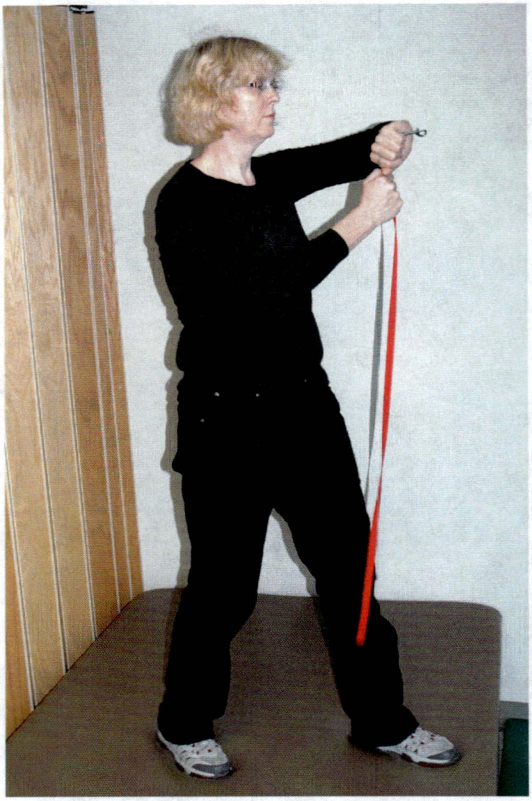

Fig. 8.4 Bow and arrow stretch. Start position

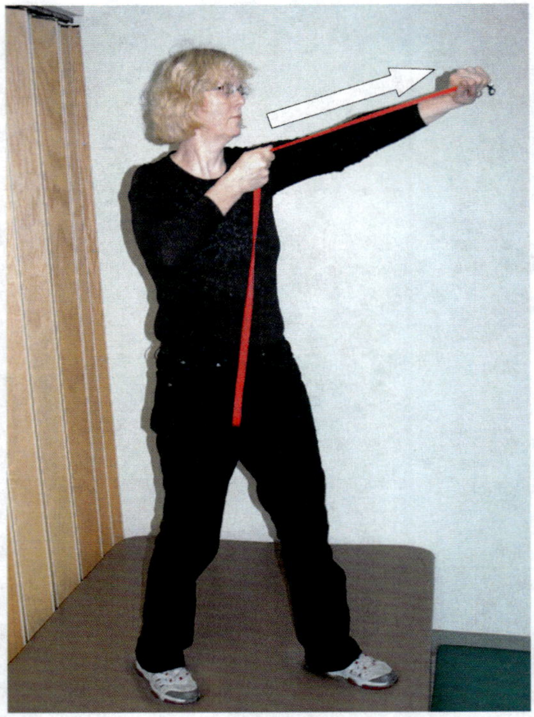

Fig. 8.5 Bow and arrow stretch. Push top hand away

4. Side stretch. This exercise stretches the shoulder blade muscles that form the back of the armpit (e.g., latissimus dorsi and teres major muscles). Restrictions in these muscles can often inhibit scapular movement in breast cancer patients following lymph node removal [11]:
   A. Starting position: stand on a firm, level surface with the feet about shoulder width apart. Hold the leash in both hands in front of your body. Separate your hands on the leash between a little more than shoulder width and about twice shoulder width, as is most comfortable (Fig. 8.10).
   B. Turn to your right. Keep your right hand low while elevating your left hand (Fig. 8.11). Hold.
   C. Return to the start position, facing forward with both hands holding the leash in front of your body (Fig. 8.12).

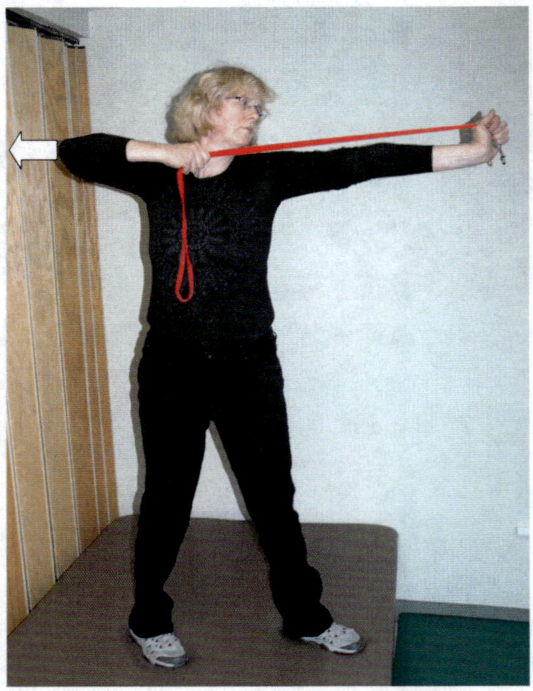

Fig. 8.6 Bow and arrow stretch. Pull back on the bow

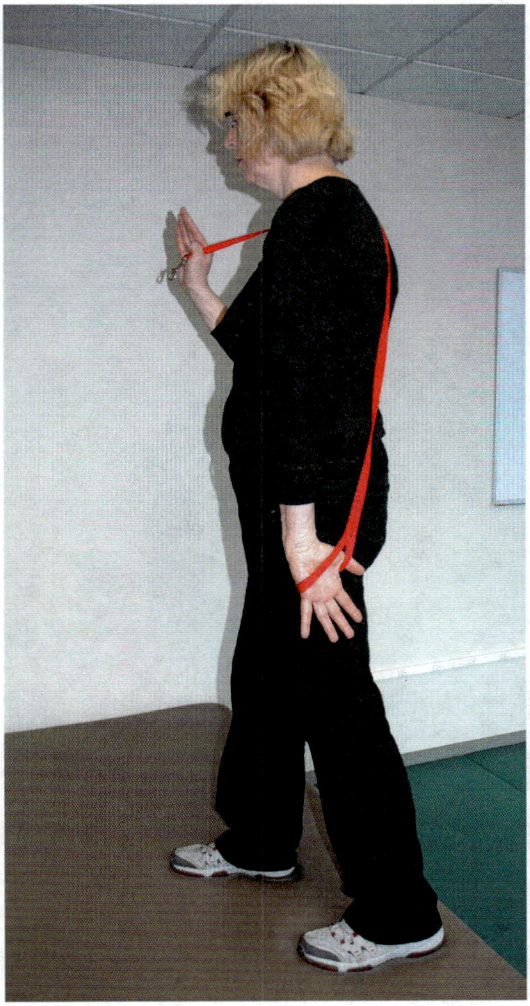

Fig. 8.7 Shoulder blade reach. Start position

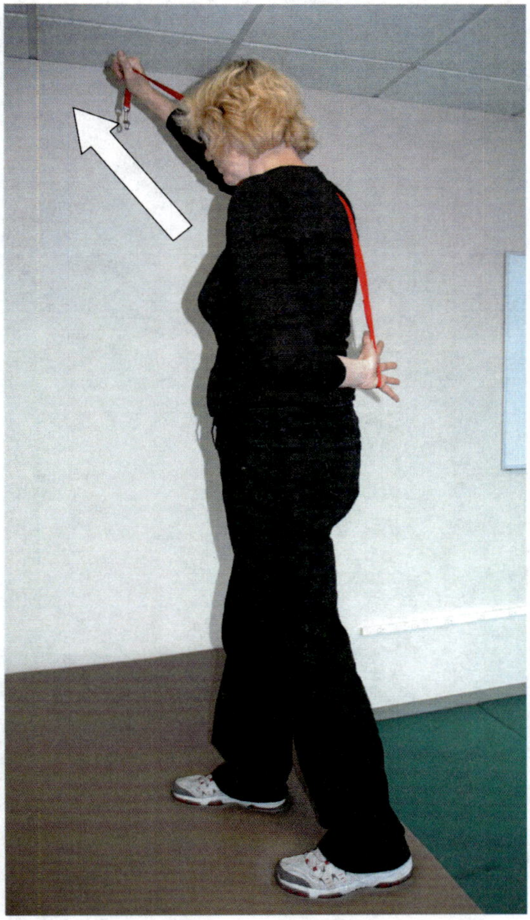

Fig. 8.8 Shoulder blade reach. Push hand away from your chest

D. Turn to your left. Keep your left hand low while elevating your right hand (Fig. 8.13). Hold. This exercise can be enhanced by shifting your weight to the left leg and turning the lower trunk slightly backward. Repeat sequence.

5. Leash circles. This exercise stretches the muscles in the upper back:

A. Starting position: stand on a firm, level surface with the feet about shoulder width apart. Hold leash in front of your body, hands slightly more than to twice shoulder width apart (Fig. 8.14).

B. Turn to your right while raising both arms to the side to start making your circle (Fig. 8.15).

C. Continue making a circle by moving your arms overhead, making sure your body is again facing forward (Fig. 8.16).

D. Continue the circle by turning toward your left and lowering your arms to your side (Fig. 8.17). Finish the circle by returning to the starting position. Relax and repeat. Then make circles by starting to move to the left, overhead, to the right, and back to the start position.

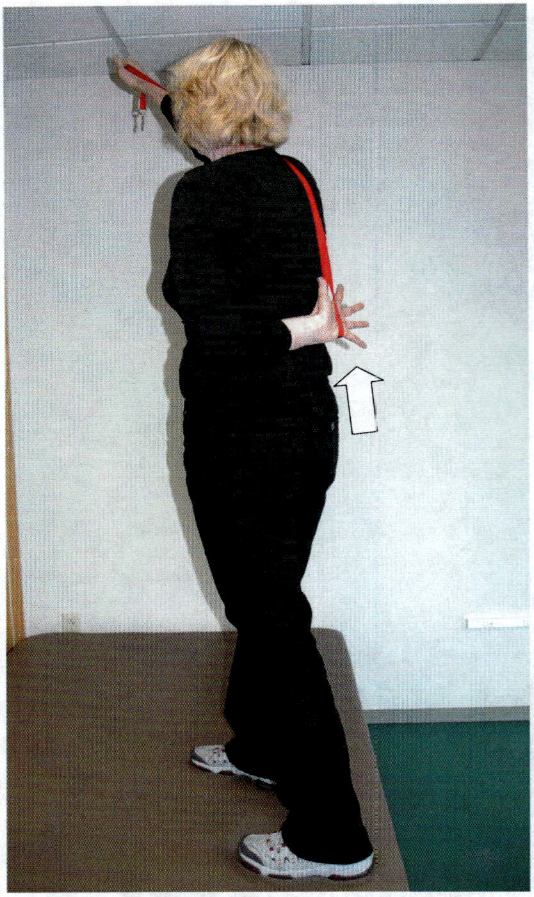

Fig. 8.9 Shoulder blade reach. Pull hand toward your shoulder blade

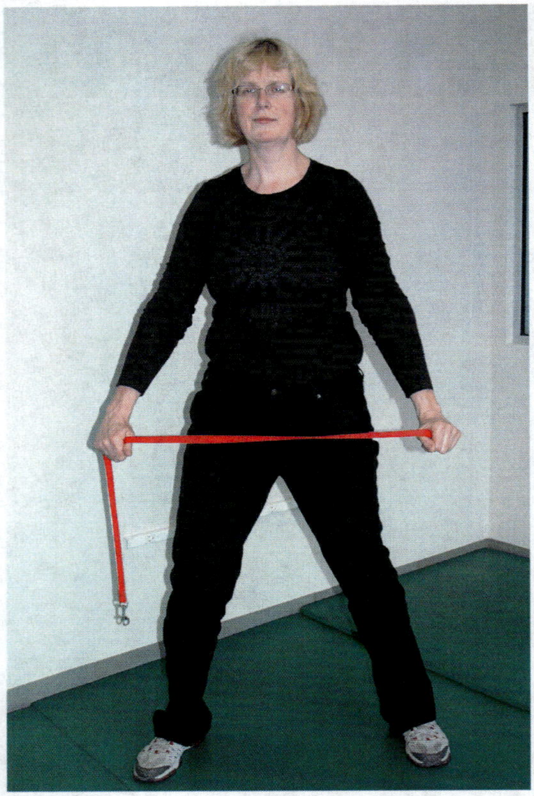

Fig. 8.10 Side stretch. Start position

6. Horizontal side shift. This exercise stretches the muscles in the upper back and shoulder:
   A. Starting position: stand on a firm, level surface with the feet about shoulder width apart. Hold leash in front of your body, hands about twice shoulder width apart (Fig. 8.18).
   B. Keeping your feet facing forward, turn your body to the right, reaching your arms out at your side away from your body (Fig. 8.19). Hold.
   C. Return to the start position. Then, keeping your feet facing forward, turn your body to the left, reaching your arms out at your side away from your body (Fig. 8.20). Hold. Relax. Repeat. Then perform this same exercise starting first to the left and then to the right.

Lower Body Leash Exercises

1. Calf and hamstring stretch. This exercise stretches the back of the leg:
   A. Starting position: sit on a firm surface (e.g., chair or park bench). Hook the middle of the leash under your right foot while holding both ends of the leash in your hands (Fig. 8.21).
   B. Keeping your back straight and heel on the ground, pull up on the leash to tip up your toes (Fig. 8.22). You will feel a stretch in your calf. Hold.

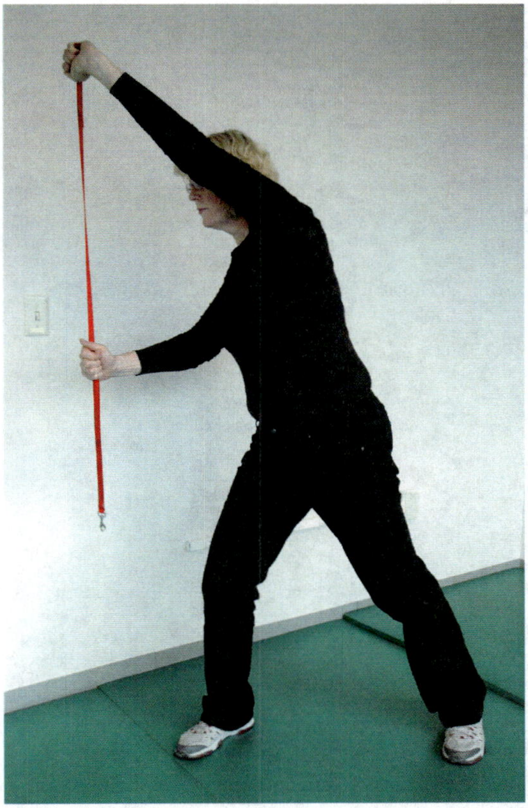

Fig. 8.11 Side stretch. Right turn

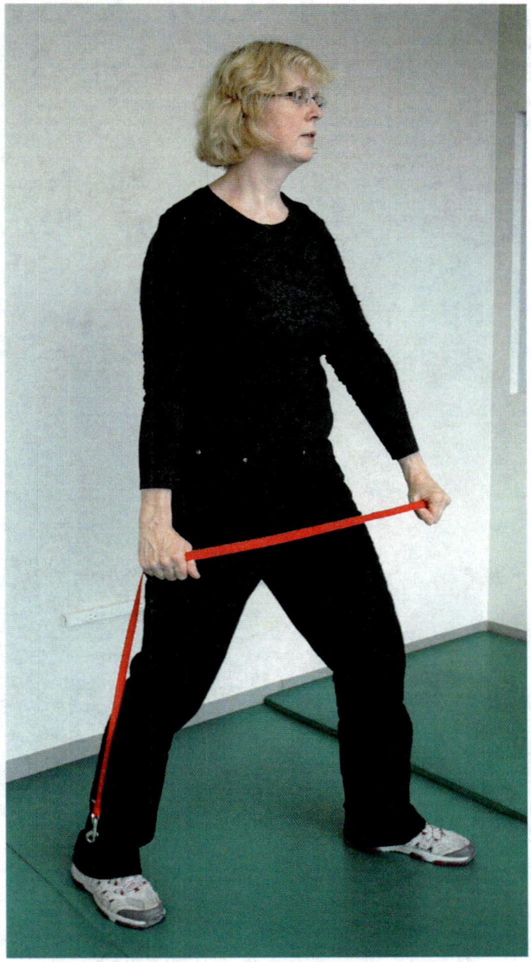

Fig. 8.12 Side stretch. Return to start position

C. While still sitting up straight and pulling back on your toes, straighten your knee to extend the leg while keeping your heel on the floor (Fig. 8.23). Hold.

D. While pulling back on your toe, lift your leg up off the floor and hold (Fig. 8.24).

E. Keeping your back straight, try leaning forward slightly to increase your stretch (Fig. 8.25). Be sure to lean forward from the hip. Hold. Relax. Repeat. Then repeat with the left leg.

2. Quad stretch. This exercise stretches the quadriceps, iliopsoas, and rectus muscles:
   A. Starting position: sit on the edge of a firm surface (e.g., chair or park bench). Hook the end loop of the leash around your right foot and drop your right knee toward the ground. Hold the other end of the leash in both hands in front of your body (Fig. 8.26).
   B. Pull up on the leash, lifting your right foot off the ground (Fig. 8.27). Pull up as high as is comfortable. Hold. Relax. Repeat. Repeat with left leg.

Neck Stretching

1. Range of motion:
   A. Starting position: sit tall on a firm surface with your hands resting in your lap and your back straight. Keep your head forward (Fig. 8.28). Relax.
   B. Slowly turn your head to the right (Fig. 8.29). Hold 3–5 s.

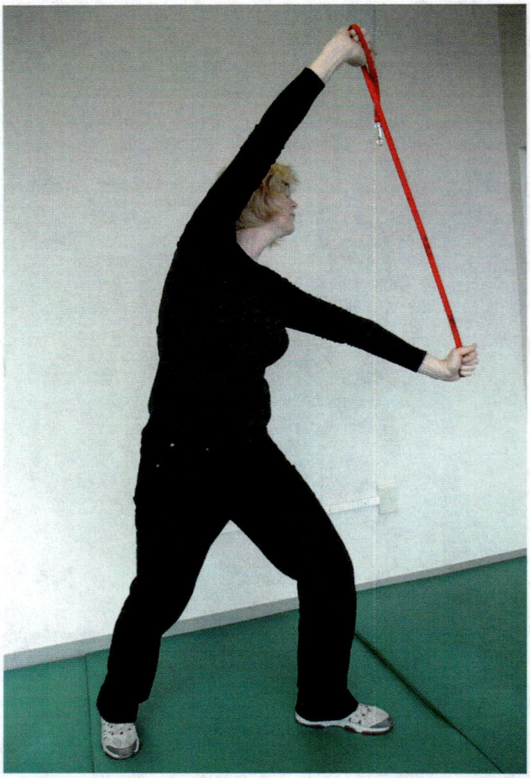

Fig. 8.13 Side stretch. Left turn

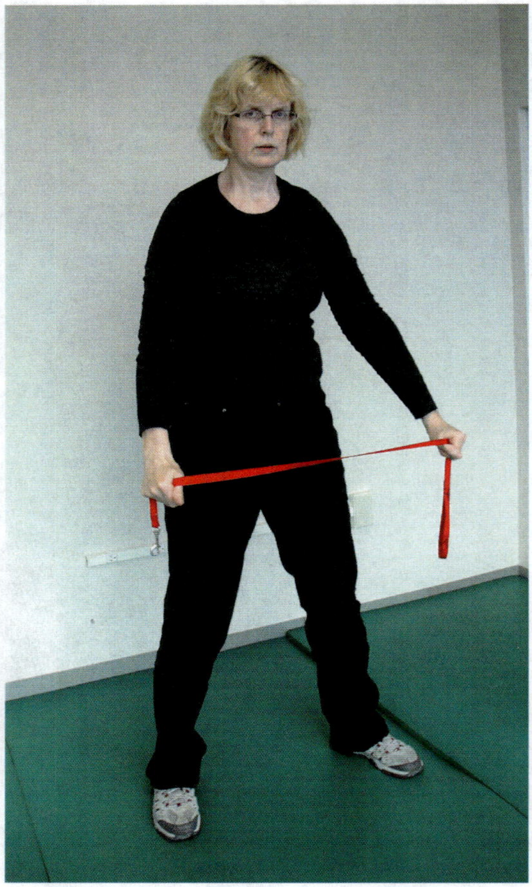

Fig. 8.14 Leash circles. Start position

C. Slowly turn your head to the left (Fig. 8.30). Hold 3–5 s.

D. Return to the start position and then tip your right ear toward your right shoulder (Fig. 8.31). Hold 3–5 s.

E. Tip your left ear toward your left shoulder (Fig. 8.32). Hold 3–5 s.

F. Return to the start position. Bend your head forward (Fig. 8.33). Hold 3–5 s. Relax. Repeat.

2. Chin tuck. A chin tuck is a safer exercise than tipping your head backward when performing range of motion exercises:

   A. Starting position: sit tall on a firm surface with your hands resting in your lap and your back straight. Look straight ahead (Fig. 8.34).

   B. Pull your chin backward as though trying to pull your chin toward the back of your head (Fig. 8.35).

Back Stretches

1. Flex and massage. This exercise stretches the back and arms:

   A. Starting position: sit on a firm surface (e.g., chair or park bench) and place your dog in front of you. Slowly lean forward from the hips, massaging your dog as your hands reach forward. Hold and massage the dog's head or shoulders (Fig. 8.36).

   B. Slowly start moving back, lifting your body but keeping your arms forward as you

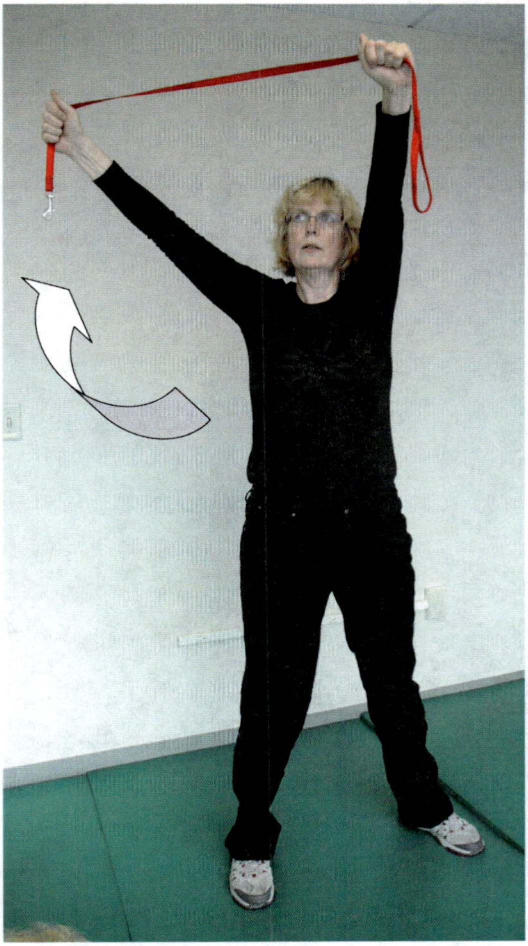

Fig. 8.15 Leash circles. Circle right

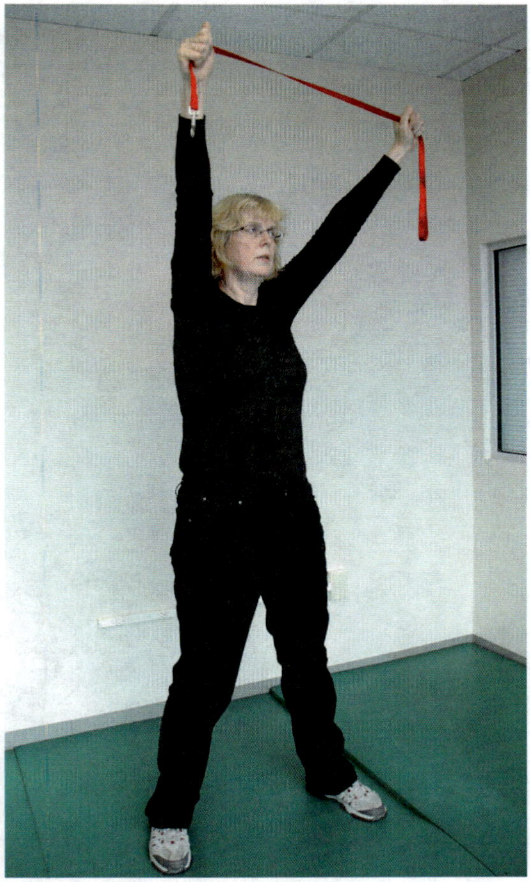

Fig. 8.16 Leash circles. Circle overhead

stroke and massage your dog (Fig. 8.37). Do not worry if your dog moves backward as you do.

C. Finish when you return to sitting upright with a straight back (Fig. 8.38). Relax. Repeat.

2. Long stroke dog pets. This exercise stretches your back and arms and can also help reduce lymphedema:

   A. Starting position: sit on a firm surface (e.g., chair or park bench) with your dog in front of you. Reach forward and stroke your dog along his sides, massaging your fingers into his fur (Fig. 8.39).

   B. Cross your right arm over to the left side of the dog and left arm to the right side of the dog to increase your stretch (Fig. 8.40).

3. Forward tilt:

   A. Starting position: sit on a firm surface (e.g., chair or park bench) with your feet together.

   B. Slowly bend forward. Drop your head and arms forward (Fig. 8.41).

4. Long stretch. This exercise stretches your back, arms, and legs:

   A. Starting position: stand on a firm, level surface about three feet away from a firm structure you can hold onto, like a wall, piece of furniture, or tree. Bend forward at the hips and reach forward with your hands

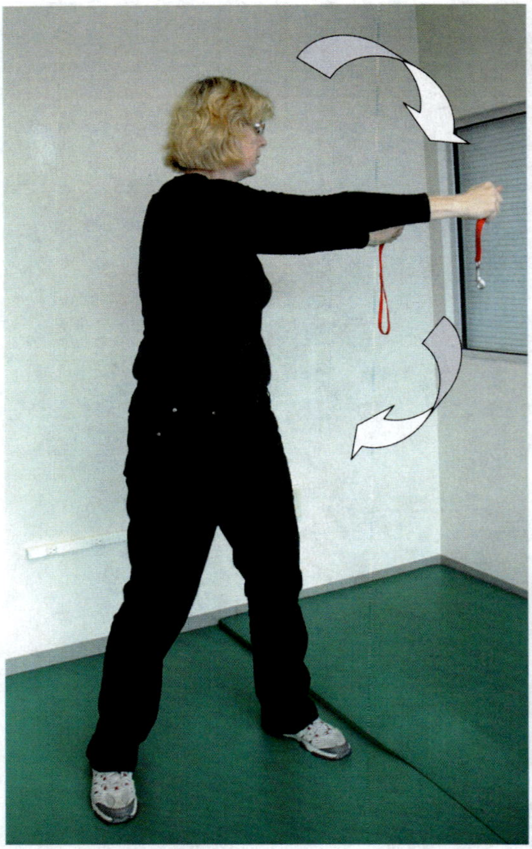

Fig. 8.17 Leash circles. Continue circle to left

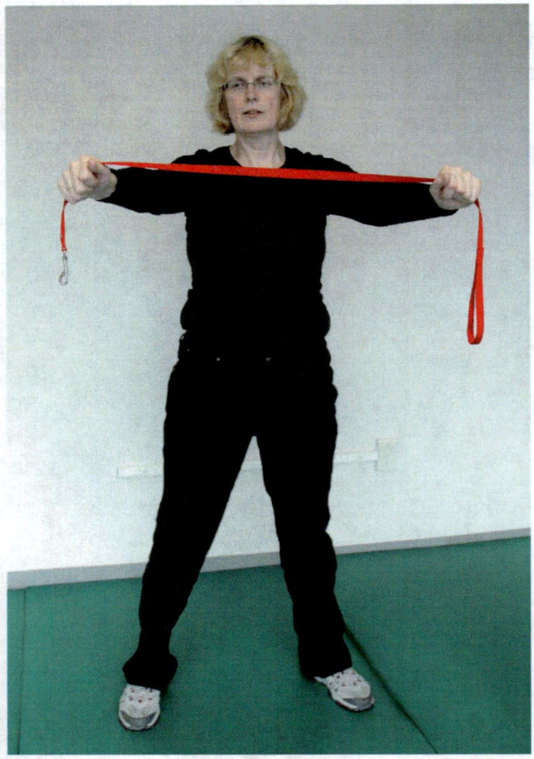

Fig. 8.18 Horizontal side shift. Start position

to hold onto the firm structure for support. Move away from the support as needed while holding onto it until you are in a forward-bending position and your body has made a 90° angle (Fig. 8.42). If needed, you may bend your knees slightly. Stretch by leaning away from the support (e.g., wall or tree). Hold. Relax. Repeat.

5. Lateral stretch. This exercise stretches the muscles on the sides of your trunk. Adjust the level of stretching as is comfortable for you:
   A. Starting position: stand on a firm, level surface with your right side toward a firm surface, like a wall or tree trunk. Stand about one foot from the wall, with your feet about shoulder width apart. Place your right hand on the wall (Fig. 8.43).
   B. Slowly push your right hand up the wall (Fig. 8.44).
   C. Continue reaching up the wall as high as is comfortable. Once you can comfortably reach all the way up, try leaning in toward the wall for a final stretch (Fig. 8.45).

Exercise with Dog Toys

1. Ball toss. This exercise stretches your upper back and arms and adds strengthening to the leg with lunges. Relax while your dog fetches the ball and brings it back to you. Repeat. Then try tossing with your other hand:
   A. Starting position: hold the ball at your side (Fig. 8.46).
   B. If you throw with your left hand, step forward with your right foot (Fig. 8.47). If you throw with your right hand, step forward with your left foot. Step forward a distance that is comfortable for you.

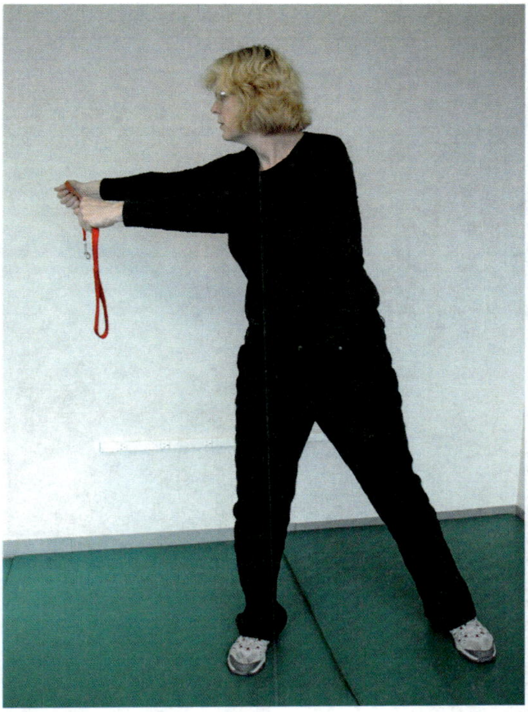

Fig. 8.19 Horizontal side shift. Turn and reach to right

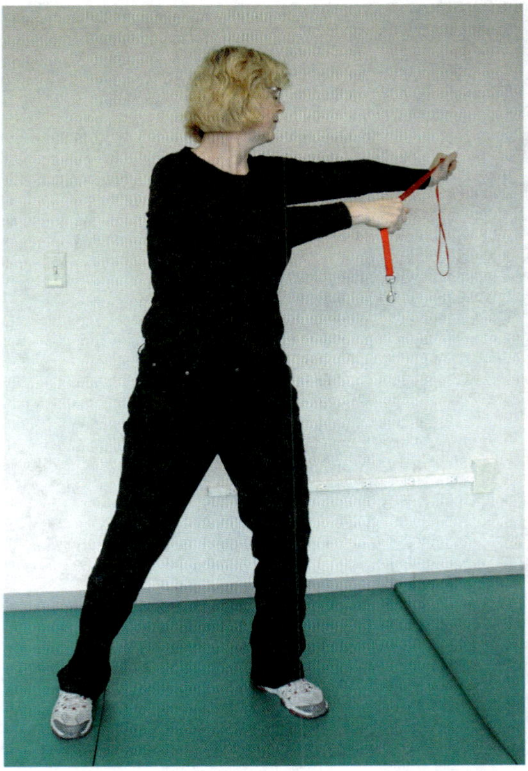

Fig. 8.20 Horizontal side shift. Turn and reach to left

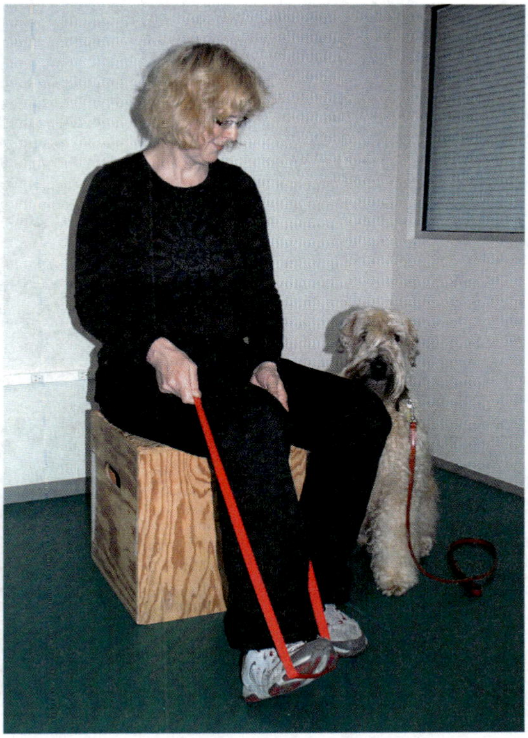

Fig. 8.21 Calf and hamstring stretch. Start position

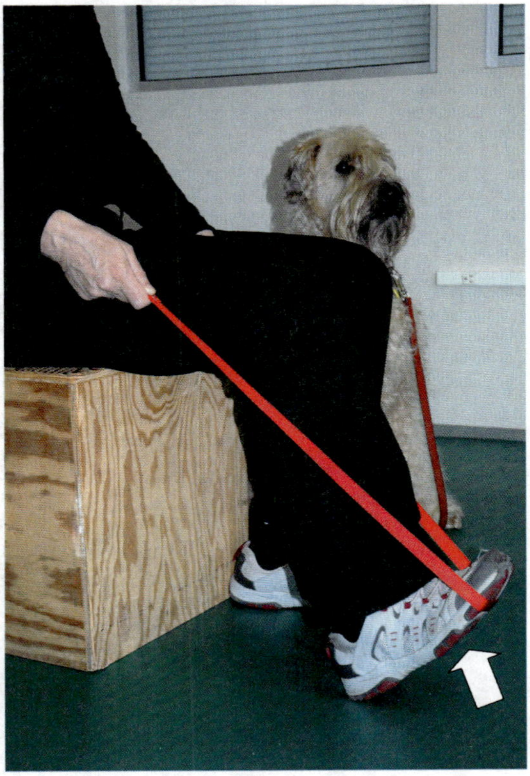

Fig. 8.22 Calf and hamstring stretch. Pull leash to raise toes

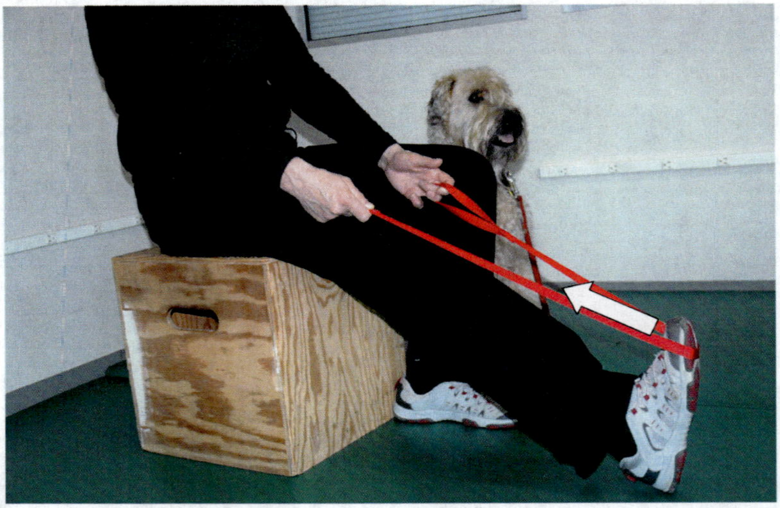

Fig. 8.23 Calf and hamstring stretch. Straighten knee

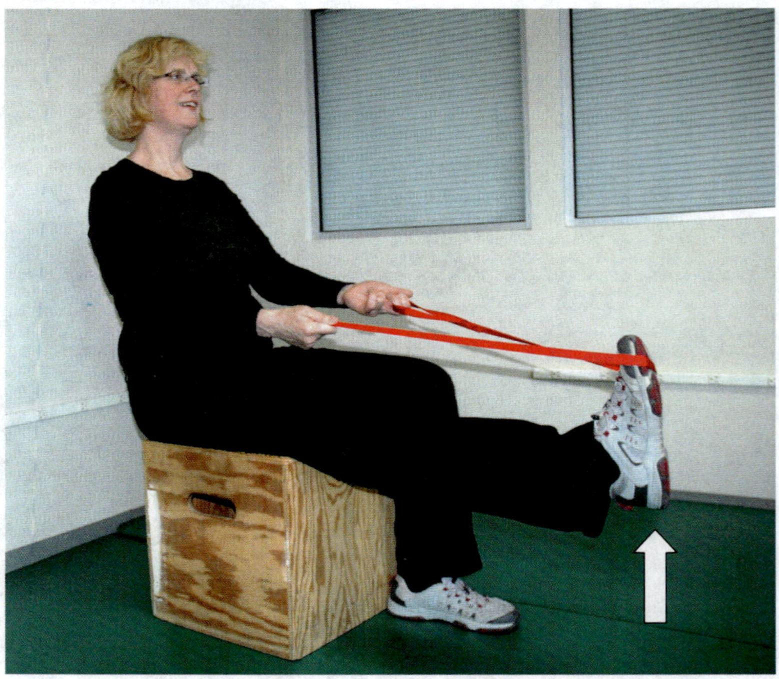

Fig. 8.24 Calf and hamstring stretch. Lift leg

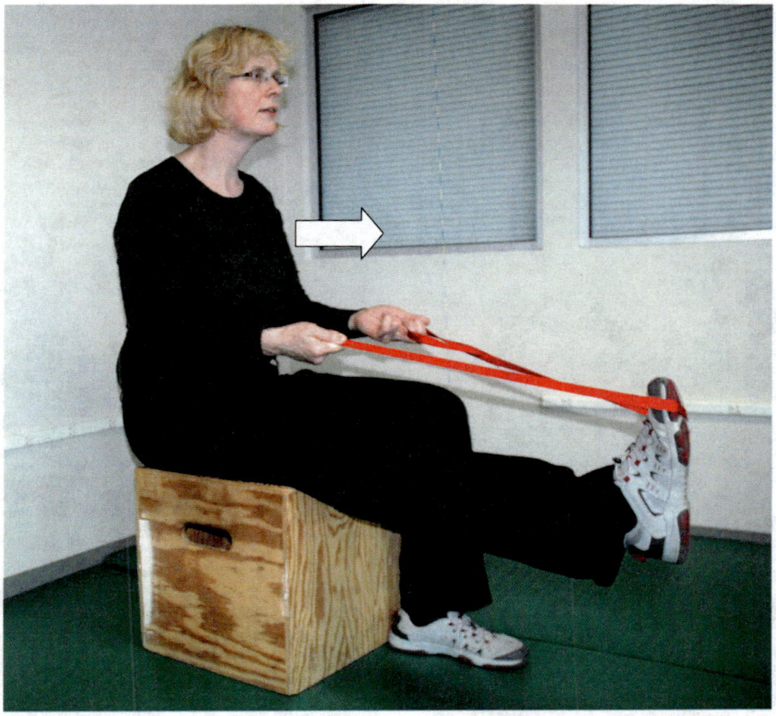

Fig. 8.25 Calf and hamstring stretch. Lean forward to increase stretch

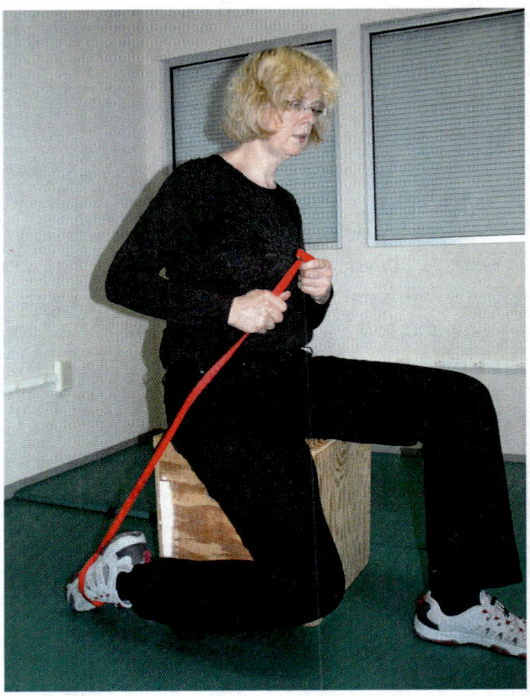

Fig. 8.26 Quad stretch. Start position

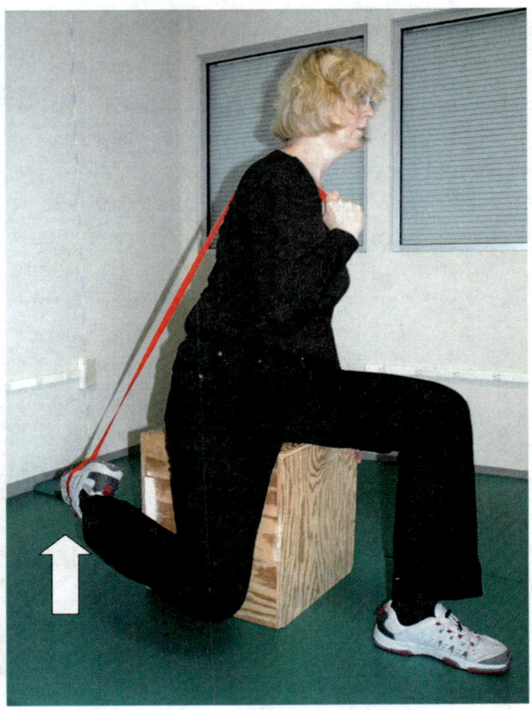

Fig. 8.27 Quad stretch. Pull foot up

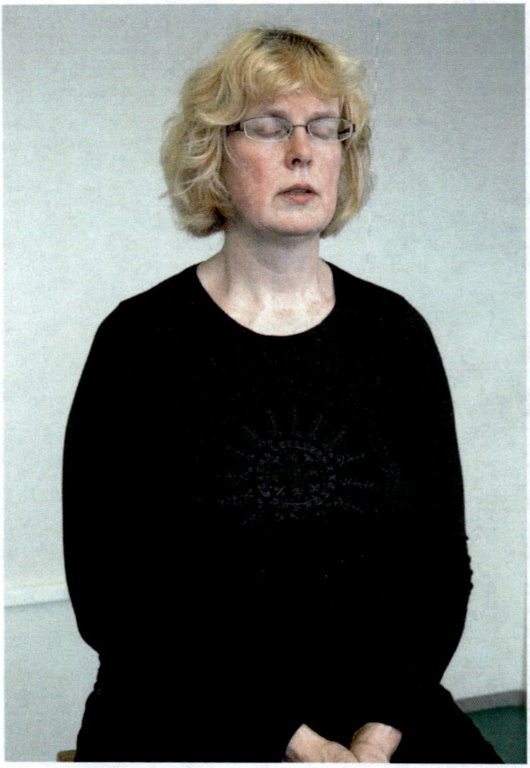

Fig. 8.28 Neck range of motion. Start position

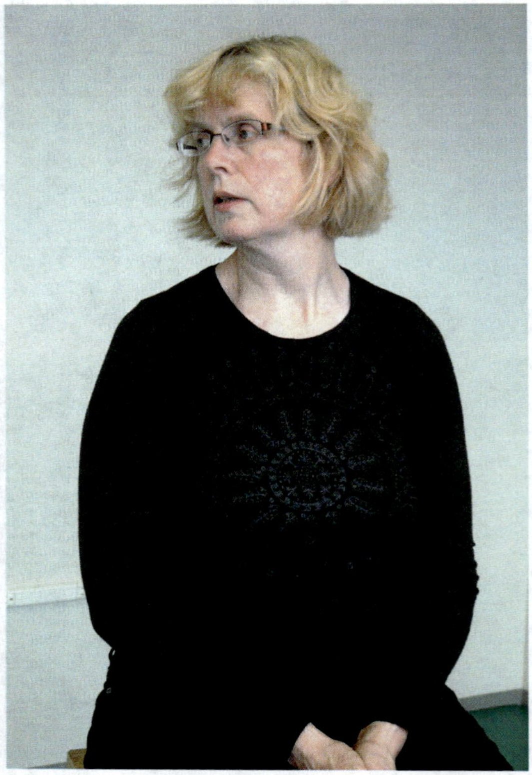

Fig. 8.29 Neck range of motion. Turn right

   C. As you throw the ball, bend the knee of your forward leg to make a lunge (Fig. 8.48). You can increase the lunge by widening your stride or bending your knee more. Do not bend your front knee more than 90°. If you have balance problems, support yourself by placing the hand that is not holding the ball on your forward leg before starting to bend your knee. You can alternatively hold onto a nearby tree or park bench for support if needed. You may also want to take a smaller forward step if you have balance problems.
2. Seated ball toss. This modified ball toss can be used for people with balance problems:
   A. Starting position: sit on the edge of a firm surface (e.g., chair or park bench). If you throw with your left hand, step forward with your right foot (Fig. 8.49). Hold or lean onto your right leg with your right arm for added support. If you throw with your right hand, reverse the position with your left foot forward and lean or hold onto your left leg.
   B. Reach forward with your left arm for a good stretch as you toss the ball (Fig. 8.50).
3. Ball pass. This is a shoulder range of motion exercise. If you have a gentle dog that will not jump, this can also be a fun game of hide-and-show the ball for your dog. As long as you are comfortable and do not move too quickly, you can add ball tosses for your dog after completing this exercise:
   A. Starting position: while standing, place the ball in your right hand (Fig. 8.51).
   B. Move the ball in front of your body and grab with your left hand (Fig. 8.52).
   C. Move the ball to your back and grab it with your right hand (Fig. 8.53).
   D. Return the ball to the front and continue (Fig. 8.54). Relax. Repeat with the ball moving in the other direction.

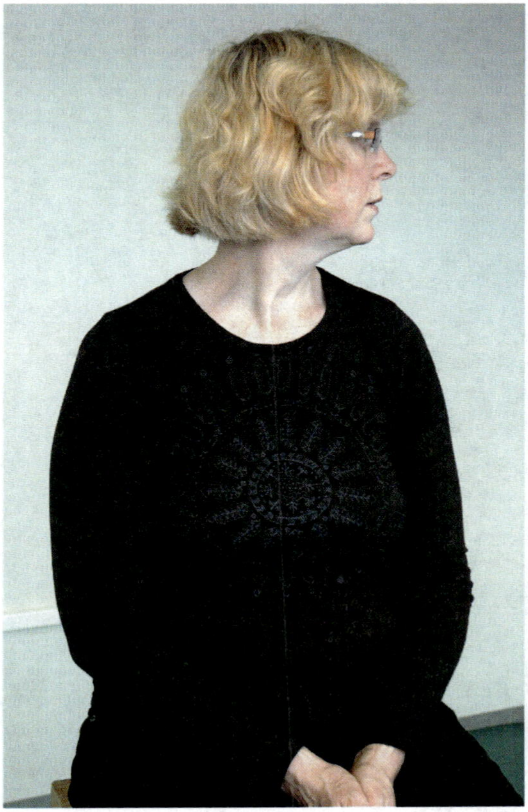

Fig. 8.30 Neck range of motion. Turn left

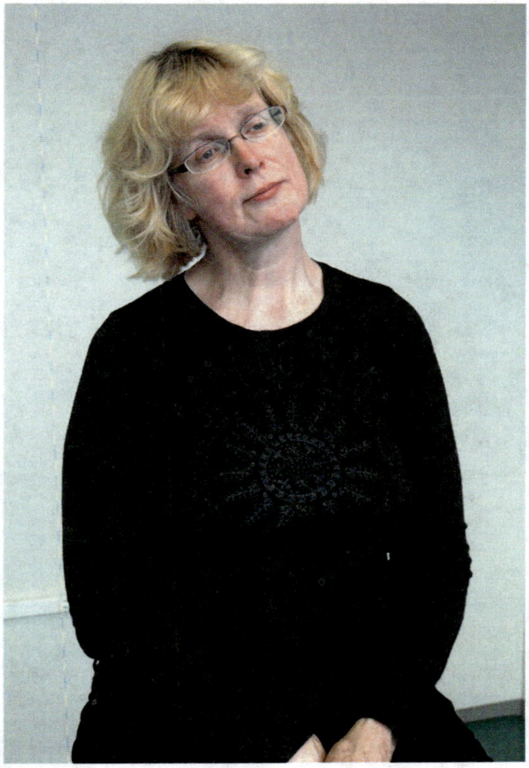

Fig. 8.31 Neck range of motion. Tip ear right

4. Two-handed ball toss. This exercise stretches the shoulder and arm:
   A. Starting position: stand on a firm, level surface with your feet about shoulder width apart. Hold the ball in both hands in front of you (Fig. 8.55).
   B. Slowly lift the ball in an arc in front of your body and overhead (Fig. 8.56).
   C. Step forward with one foot as you prepare to gently toss the ball forward (Fig. 8.57).
   D. After tossing the ball, hold hand overhead and stretch out fingers for an extra stretch (Fig. 8.58). Hold. Then relax as your dog retrieves the ball. Repeat.
5. Flying disk toss. This exercise stretches the shoulder and arm:
   A. Starting position: stand on a firm, level surface with your feet about shoulder width apart. Place your left foot forward and hold the disk in your left hand (Fig. 8.59).
   B. Toss the disk with a soft throw to achieve a gentle stretch (Fig. 8.60). Do not whip the disk. Relax while your dog retrieves the disk. Repeat. Switch sides by placing your right foot forward and try tossing with your right hand.

Balance Exercises

1. Side stepping:
   A. Starting position: stand on a firm, level surface with your feet about shoulder width apart. Place your hands on your hips (Fig. 8.61).
   B. Optional starting position for added balance support: stand on a firm, level surface with your feet about shoulder width apart. Hold your arms at your sides (Fig. 8.62). You might also hold onto the back of a park bench or railing for support.
   C. With arms on your hips or out at your sides, take a small step to the right (Fig. 8.63).

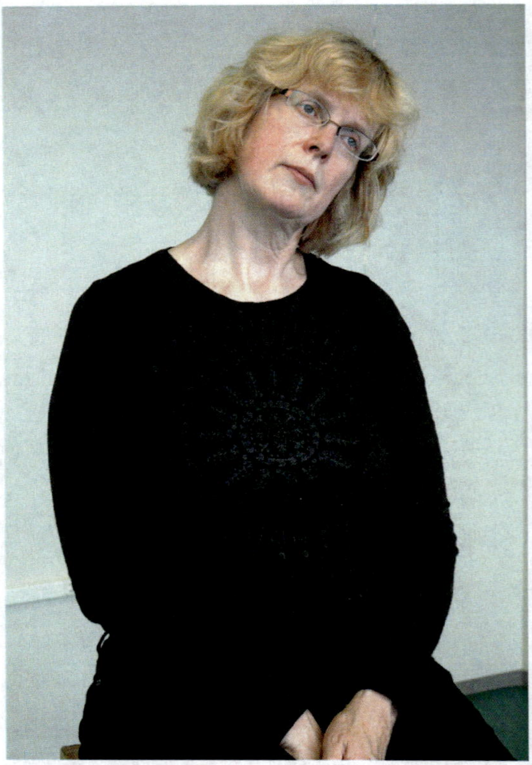

Fig. 8.32 Neck range of motion. Tip ear left

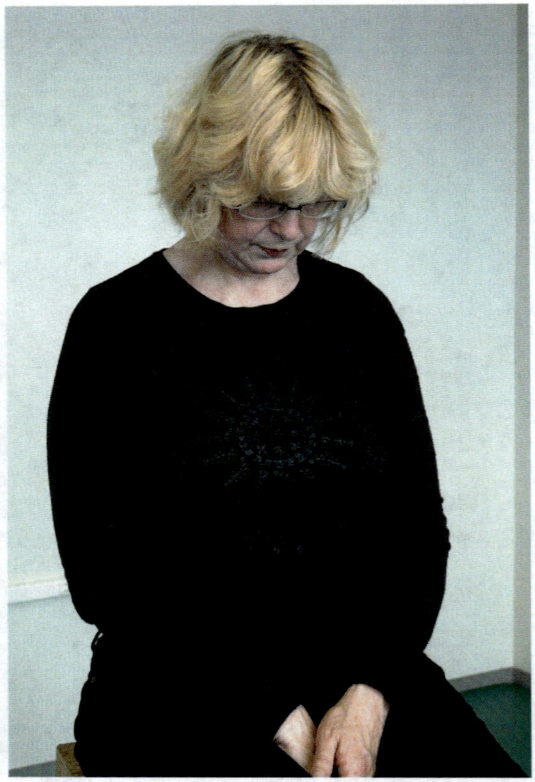

Fig. 8.33 Neck range of motion. Bend head forward

Make sure you lift your foot up as you step to the side. When you become more comfortable with this exercise, you might try increasing your step size.

D. Bring your left foot in to meet your right foot (Fig. 8.64) and repeat by taking another step to the right. Continue this pattern for several steps. Relax. Then repeat taking steps to the left.

2. March walk:
   A. Starting position: stand on a firm, level surface. Place your dog on your side (Fig. 8.65).
   B. Begin walking forward slowing, keeping your dog at your side or in a heel position. If your dog tends to want to walk in front of you, hold a treat in your hand in front of his nose to entice him to stay at your side (Fig. 8.66).
   C. While your dog is walking nicely at your side, start making slow, high steps as though you were marching slowly (Fig. 8.67). Adjust the height of your step as is comfortable for you. Return to walking after several march steps. Repeat.
3. Heel walking:
   A. Starting position: stand on a firm, level surface. Place your dog on your side.
   B. Start walking slowly on your heels, keeping your toes pointed up off the floor (Fig. 8.68). After several steps, walk normally. Repeat.

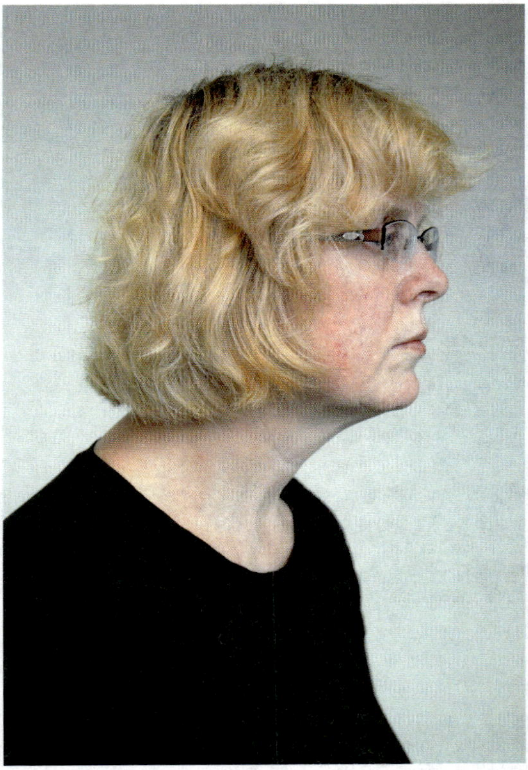

Fig. 8.34 Chin tuck. Start position

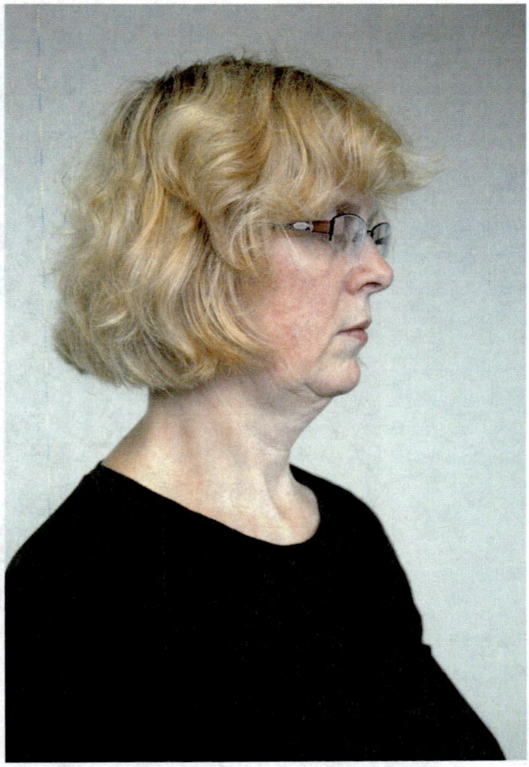

Fig. 8.35 Chin tuck. Pull chin backward

4. Toe walking:
   A. Starting position: stand on a firm, level surface. Place your dog on your side.
   B. Start walking slowly on your tip toes, keeping your heels off of the floor. After several steps, walk normally. Repeat.
5. Backward walk and recall. This exercise should only be performed on a very level surface if your feel comfortable walking backward:
   A. Starting position: stand on a firm, level surface. Place your dog in front of you and slowly back away from your dog while asking him to stay (Fig. 8.69).
   B. If your dog tends to follow you when in a standing position, you may first ask him to sit and then stay (Fig. 8.70). Walk back to the end of the leash. If your dog was standing, ask him to sit. Rest.
   C. Recall your dog, asking him to slowly walk toward you while you slowly and carefully take several steps backward (Fig. 8.71). Rest. Repeat.
6. Tandem stance:
   A. Starting position: stand tall on a firm, level surface. Place your dog at your side. Take a step with one foot in front of you so that one foot is placed about 6–12 in. in front of the other (Fig. 8.72). Hold and count to 5 s. Then move your feet together and relax. If you feel comfortable and secure in this position, you can add a balance strengthening component to this exercise by slowly looking over your right shoulder and then your left shoulder. Repeat. As you get more comfortable with this exercise, work on increasing the time you are able to stand in this tandem stance. Slowly increase to 10 s and eventually to 30 s.

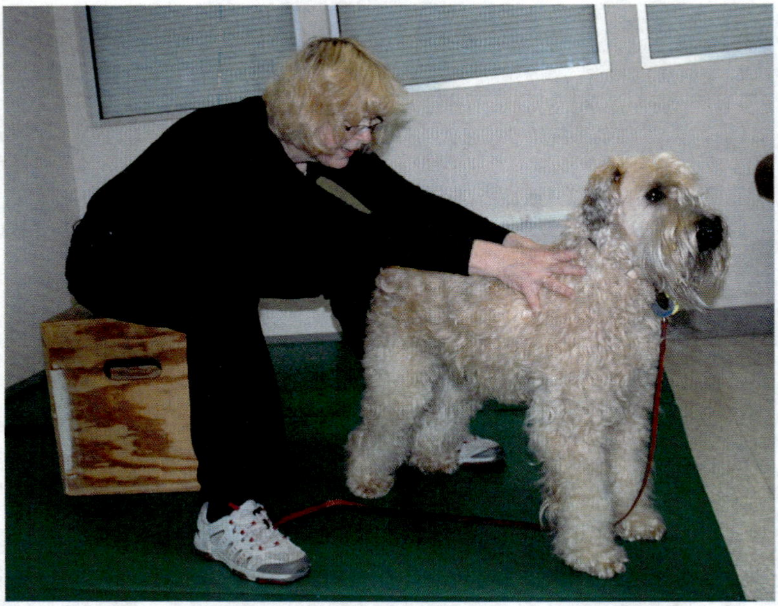

Fig. 8.36 Flex and massage. Start position

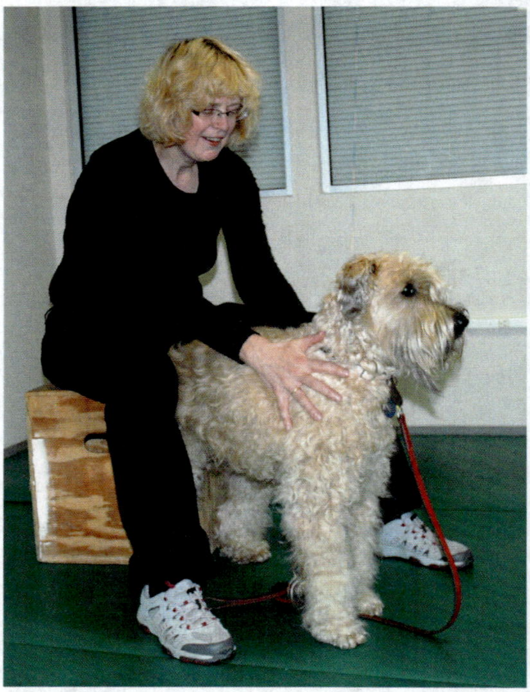

Fig. 8.37 Flex and massage. Begin to sit up, keeping hands forward on dog

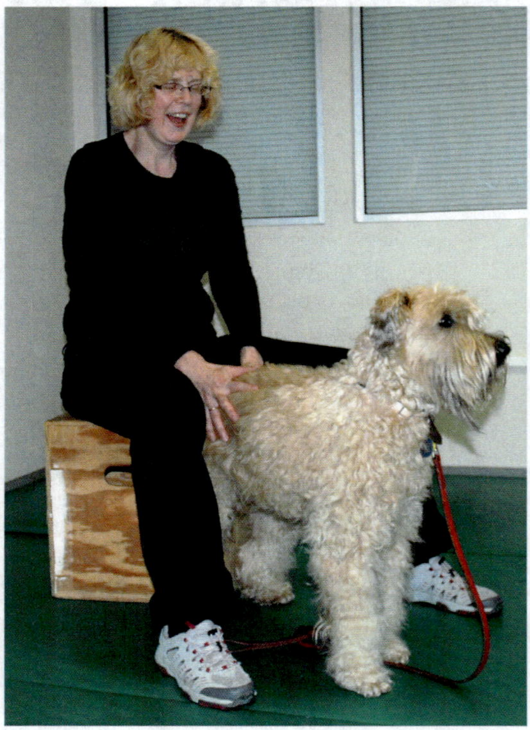

Fig. 8.38 Flex and massage. Pull hands toward you and sit upright

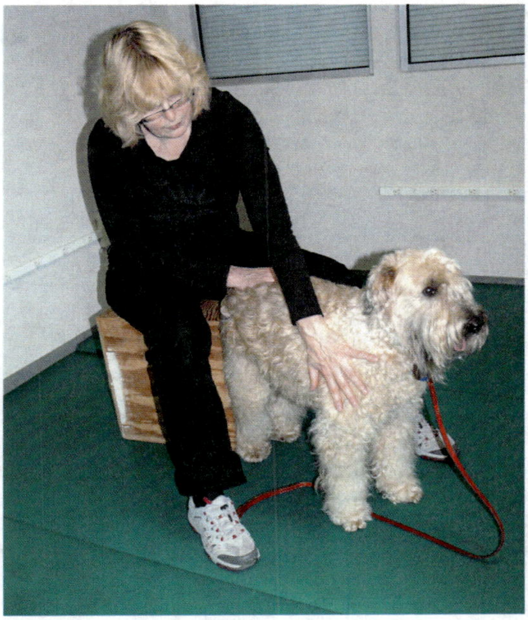

Fig. 8.39 Long stroke dog pets. Reach forward and massage your dog's sides

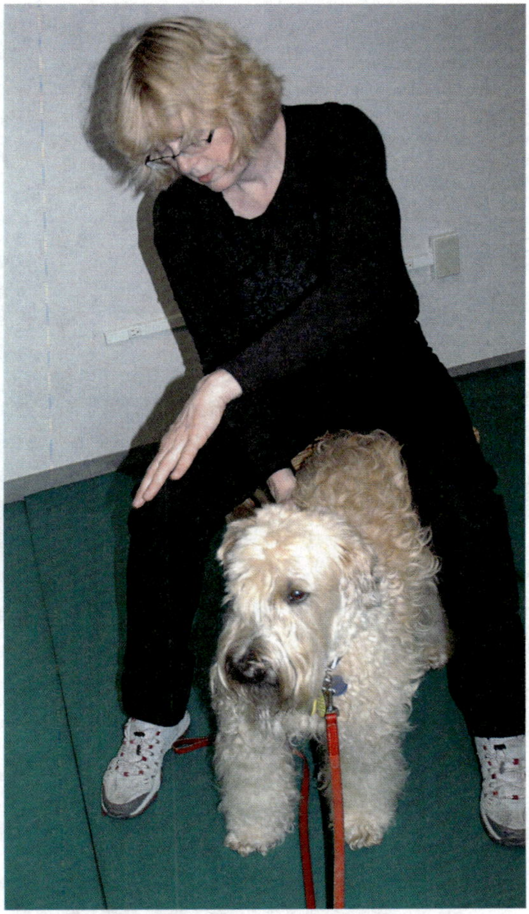

Fig. 8.40 Long stroke dog pets. Cross arms to increase your stretch

Strengthening Exercises

Strengthening exercises should be performed about three times a week on nonconsecutive days. Patients should complete 1–3 sets of each exercise, as is comfortable, during each session. Each set should include several repetitions of each exercise, building over time as tolerated to a maximum of 8–10 repetitions of each exercise. The number of repetitions performed during a set should not be increased more often than once each week. Each exercise should be held for about 5 s before relaxing. Patients should watch for signs of fatigue and limit these exercises to avoid excessive fatigue.

1. Bear hug. This isometric exercise strengthens the interscapular muscles:
   A. Starting position: stand on a firm, level surface with the feet about shoulder width apart (Fig. 8.73). Hold your head high. Hold leash in front of your body, thumbs up and elbows out.
   B. While holding leash in front, squeeze the shoulder blades together as shown in the drawing (Figs. 8.74 and 8.75). Try not to move your elbows back so that you maintain the hug position.
2. Isometric push. This exercise strengthens the arm and back muscles:
   A. Starting position: sit on a firm surface (e.g., chair or park bench) with your feet firmly on the ground. Place your hands against the front of your seat. Press backward firmly (Fig. 8.76). Count to 5 s. Relax. Repeat.
   B. Move your hands to the back of your seat and push toward you (Fig. 8.77). Count to 5 s. Relax. Repeat.
   C. Move your hands to the sides of your seat and push in toward your sides, as though you were trying to squeeze the seat together (Fig. 8.78). Count to 5 s. Relax. Repeat.

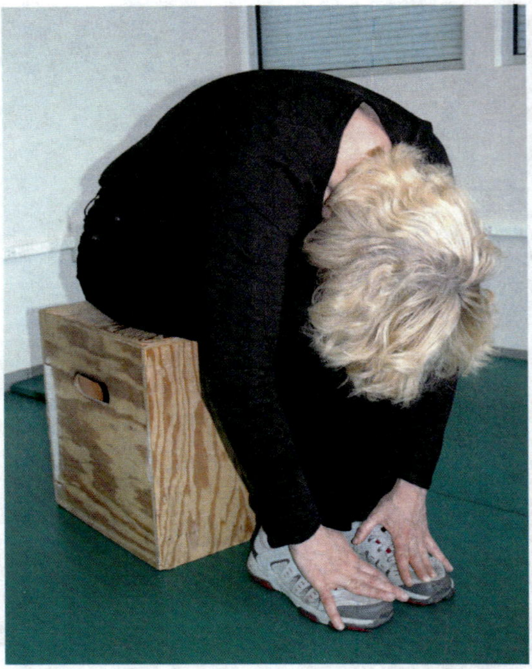

Fig. 8.41 Forward tilt. Bend forward over your knees

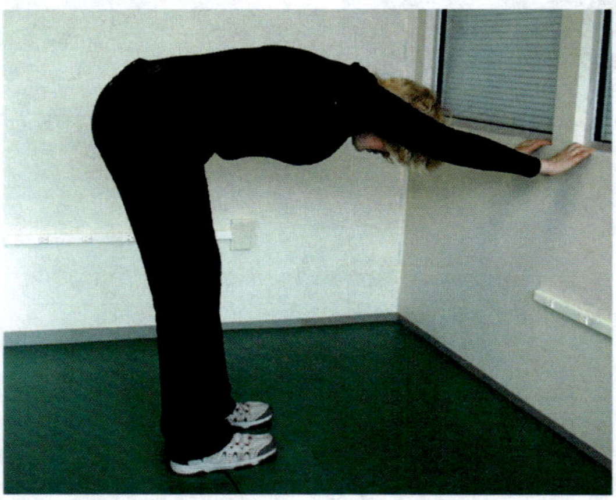

Fig. 8.42 Long stretch. Hold onto a firm object and bend forward to make a 90 degree angle

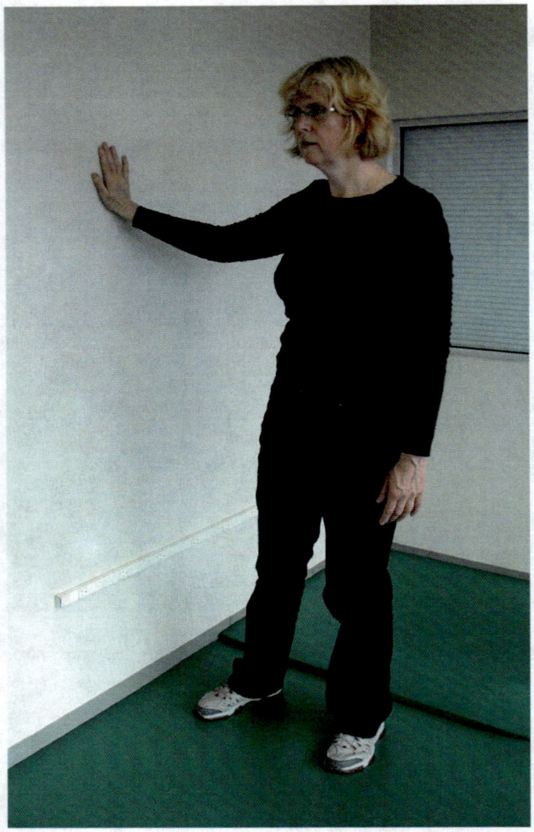

Fig. 8.43 Lateral stretch. Start position

3. Seated march. This exercise strengthens the abdominal and core muscles:
   A. Starting position: sit tall on a firm surface with your back straight. Place your hands on the sides of your seat for added support (Fig. 8.79).
   B. Tighten your abdominal muscles and begin marching by first lifting your right leg off of the floor (Fig. 8.80), then putting your right foot back on the floor, and then lifting your left leg off the floor. Repeat. Your abdominal muscles should be tight while you are lifting a leg. Then you can relax your abdominal muscles when you have both feet on the floor.
   C. Try placing one hand over the abdomen while marching to feel that the muscles are tight (Fig. 8.81).
4. Ball squeeze. This isometric exercise strengthens the leg adductors:
   A. Starting position: sit tall on a firm surface with your back straight. Place a ball between your knees (Fig. 8.82).

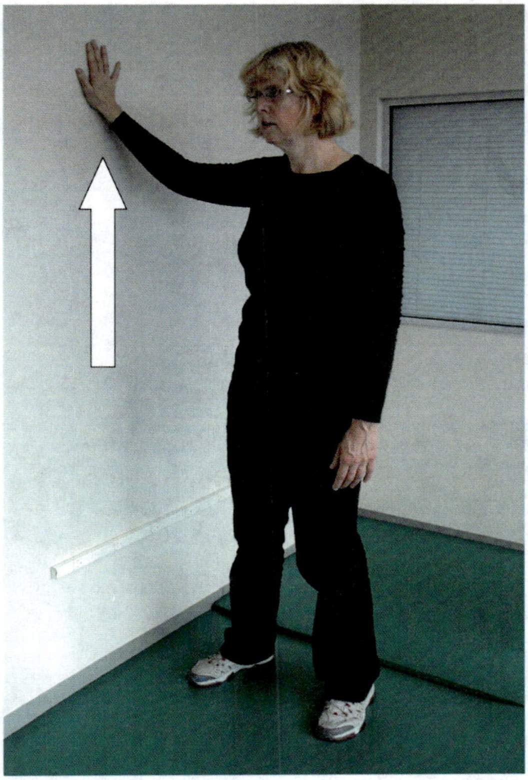

Fig. 8.44 Lateral stretch. Slowly push hand up the wall

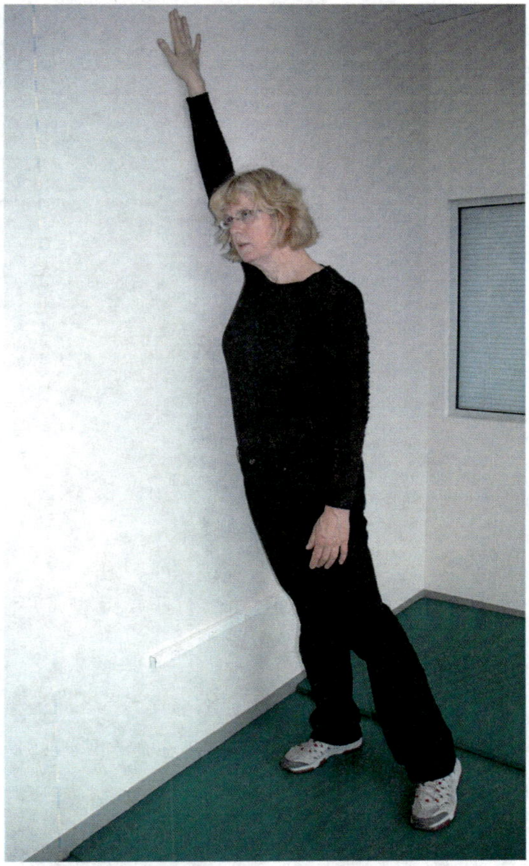

Fig. 8.45 Lateral stretch. Lean toward the wall after reaching maximum reach to increase the stretch

B. Push your knees together (Fig. 8.83). Hold for 5 s.

C. Relax your legs, allowing your knees to move apart from each other while still holding the ball (Fig. 8.84). Repeat.

5. Unleash the legs. This isometric exercise strengthens the leg abductors:

   A. Starting position: sit tall on a firm surface with your back straight and your feet flat on the ground. Loop the leash around both legs and hold the ends in your hands (Fig. 8.85).

   B. While holding the leash tightly to try to hold your legs together, push your knees apart (Fig. 8.86).

   C. Maintain pressure on the leash so that your legs open slowly (Fig. 8.87).

   D. Tighten the leash as you relax and return your knees together (Fig. 8.88). Repeat.

Exercises for Lymphedema

1. Pet the dog:

   A. Starting position: sit on a firm surface and invite your dog to sit in front of you (Fig. 8.89).

   B. Enjoy working your hands as you pet and stroke through your dog's fur (Fig. 8.90).

2. Grip a clean dog toy. This exercise should be done with a new soft dog toy or a soft toy that was laundered to avoid germs:

   A. Starting position: hold the toy in both hands (Fig. 8.91).

   B. Squeeze the toy and twist the toy while squeezing it (Fig. 8.92).

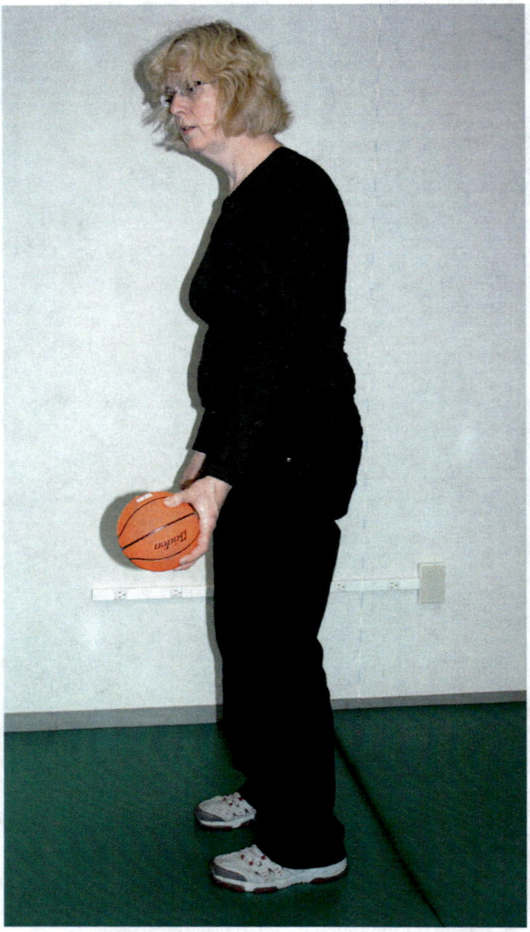

Fig. 8.46 Ball toss. Start position

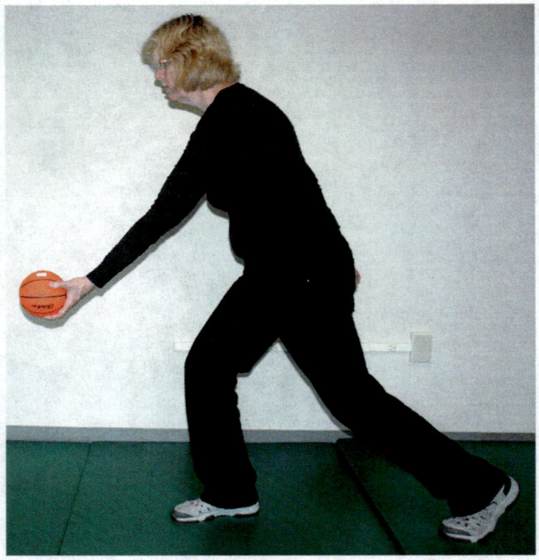

Fig. 8.47 Ball toss. Step forward as you prepare to toss the ball

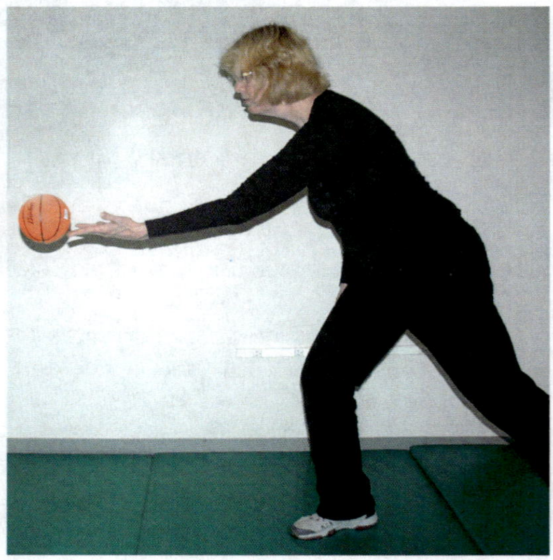

Fig. 8.48 Ball toss. Bend your forward knee to lunge as you toss the ball

C. Bend the toy into an arch in front of your body and straighten again (Fig. 8.93). This also exercises your shoulders. Relax. Repeat.

3. Bonus home exercise—rice squeeze. This exercise helps with grasping and decreasing sensitivity (or desensitization). Empty a fresh bag of rice into a clean container. After completing the exercise, place a lid on the container to keep the rice clean for the next time you want to exercise with it. Do not use this rice for cooking:

A. Starting position: place your hand into the container of rice (Fig. 8.94).

B. Make a fist while grabbing the rice (Fig. 8.95). Release your grip and press your hand back under the rice. Repeat.

Aerobic Exercise

Walking, cycling, and swimming are all aerobic exercises that utilize large muscle groups that promote benefits in cancer patients. Walking may be an ideal exercise, as it allows for adjustments in intensity level based on an individual's tolerance

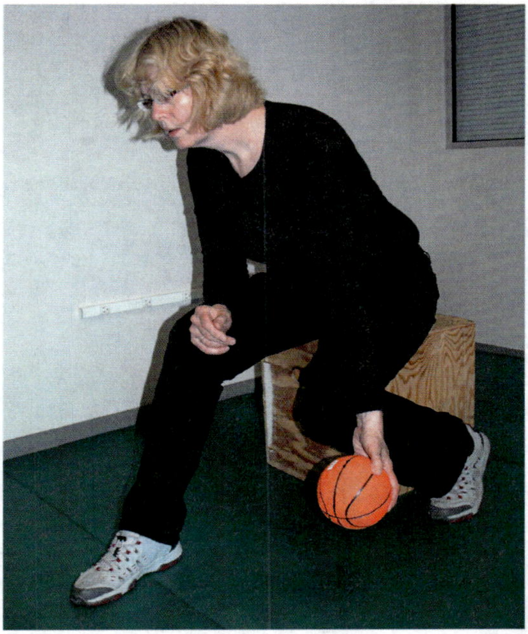

Fig. 8.49 Seated ball toss. This modified position for the ball toss exercise should be used if you have balance problems

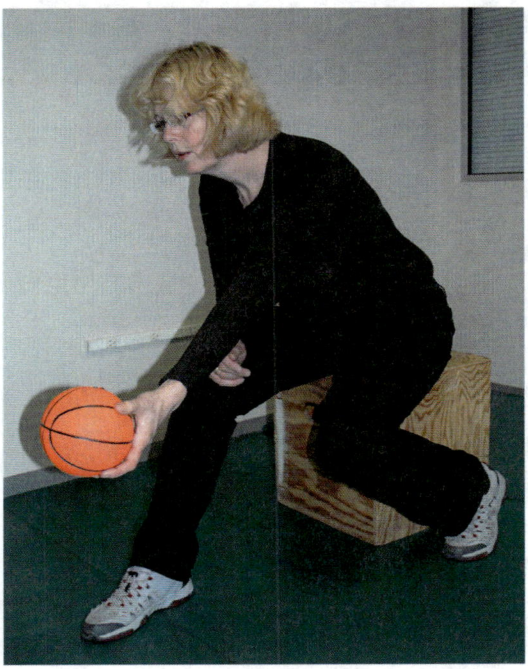

Fig. 8.50 Seated ball toss. Reach forward for a good stretch as you toss the ball

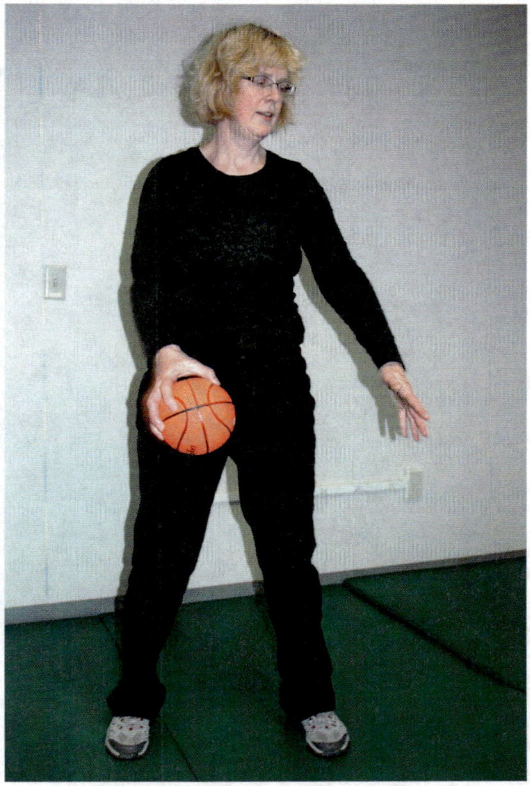

Fig. 8.51 Ball pass. Start position

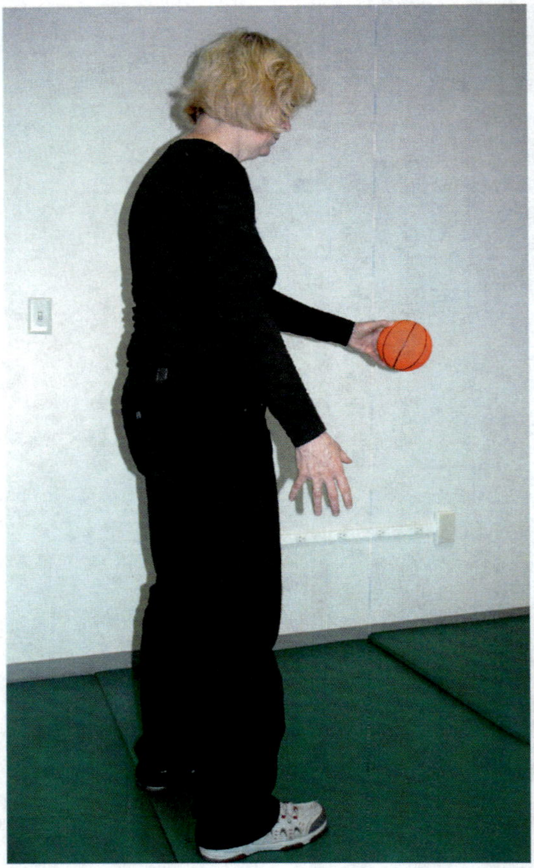

Fig. 8.52 Ball pass. Bring the ball to the front of your body

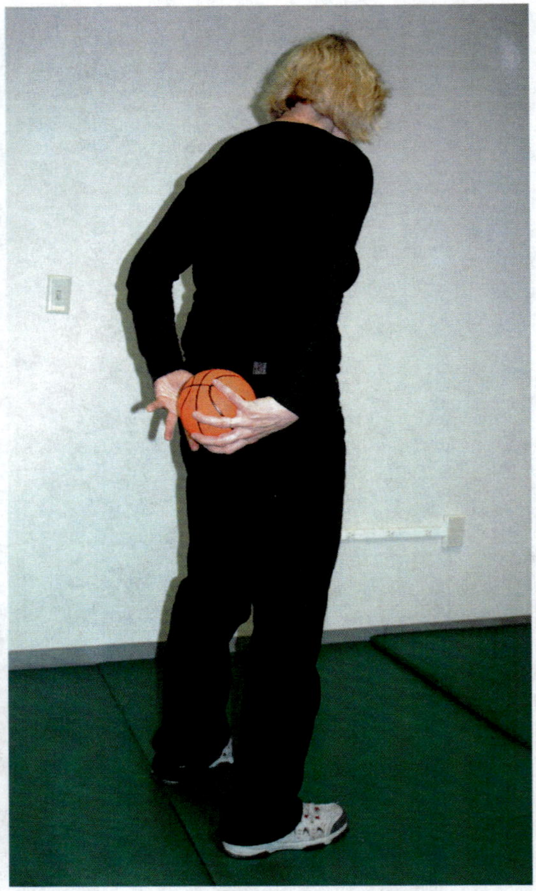

Fig. 8.53 Ball pass. Move the ball around to your back

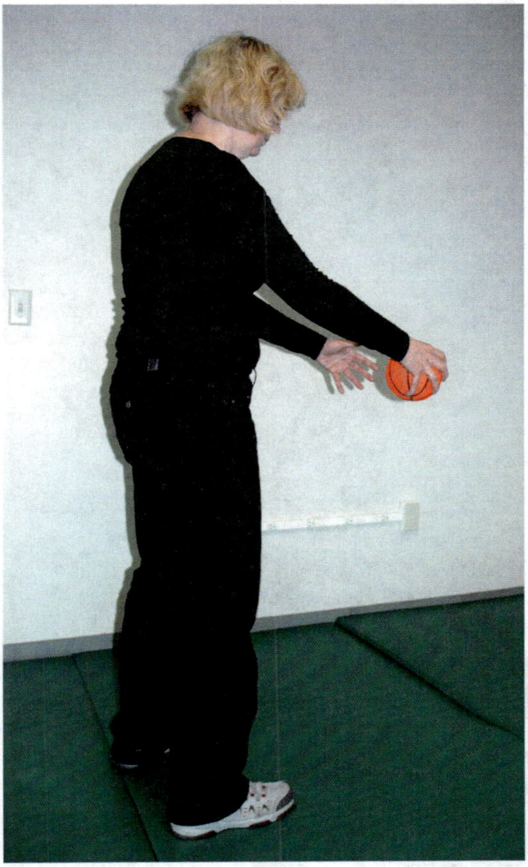

Fig. 8.54 Ball pass. Continue moving the ball around your body to your front again

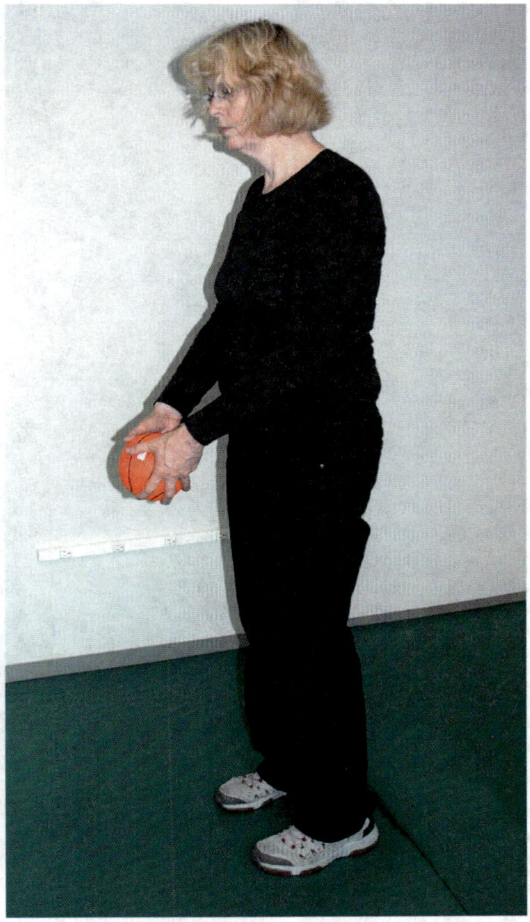

Fig. 8.55 Two-handed ball toss. Start position

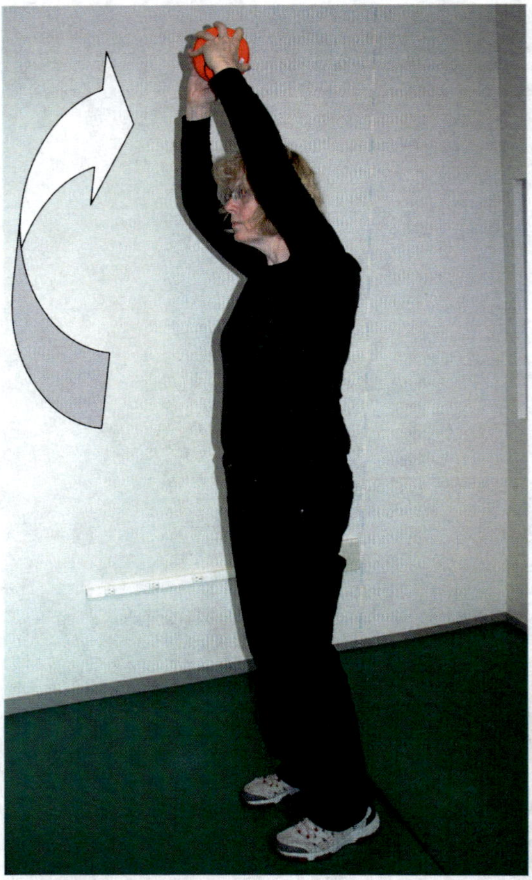

Fig. 8.56 Two-handed ball toss. Lift ball in front of the body in an arc to overhead

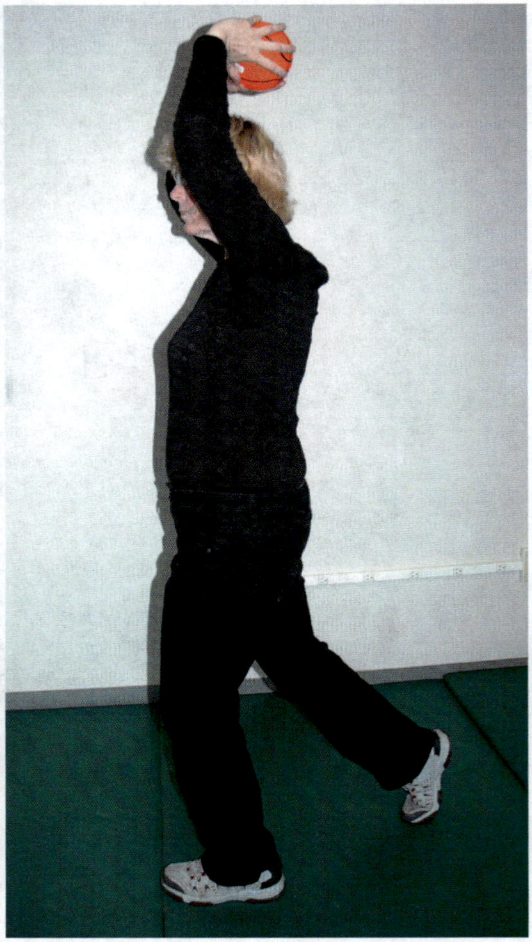

Fig. 8.57 Two-handed ball toss. Step forward as you prepare your toss

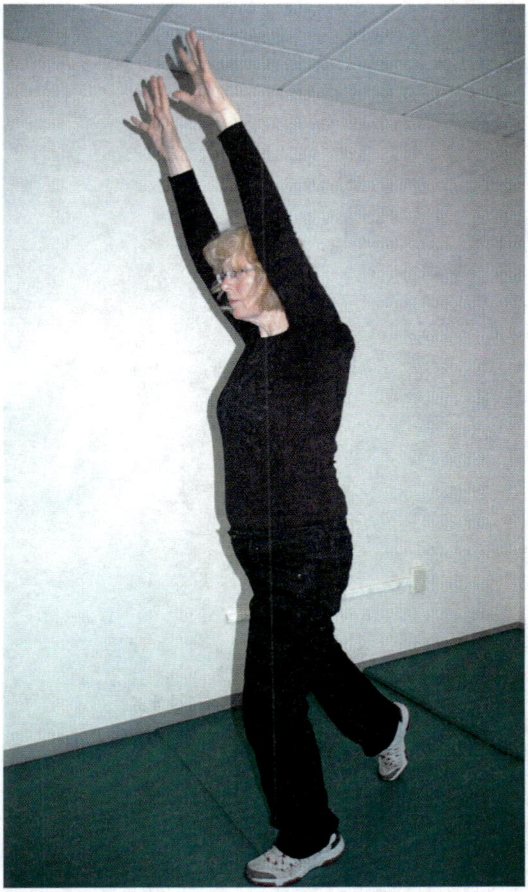

Fig. 8.58 Two-handed ball toss. Toss the ball, keeping hands overhead for a final stretch

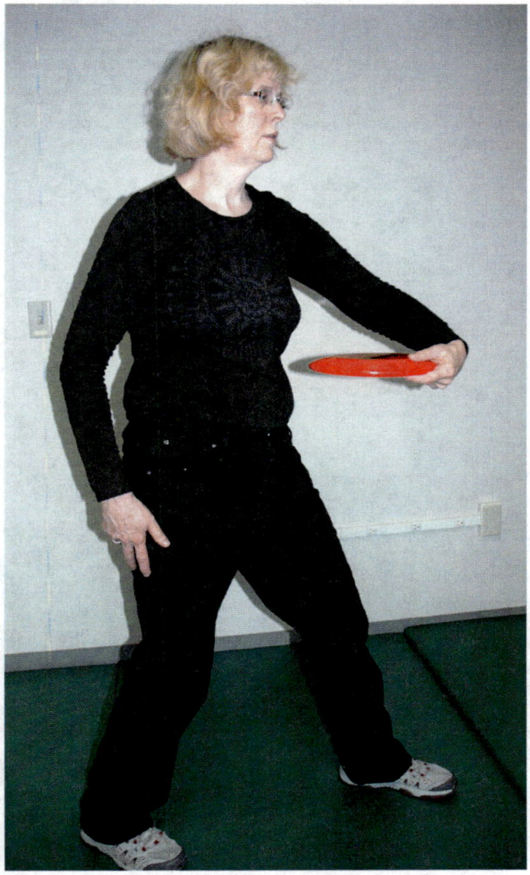

Fig. 8.59 Flying disk toss. Start position

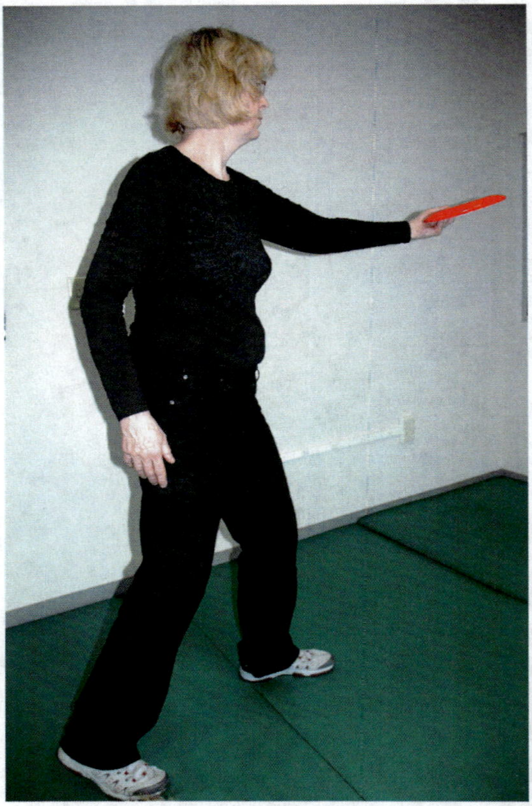

Fig. 8.60 Flying disk toss. Gently toss disk

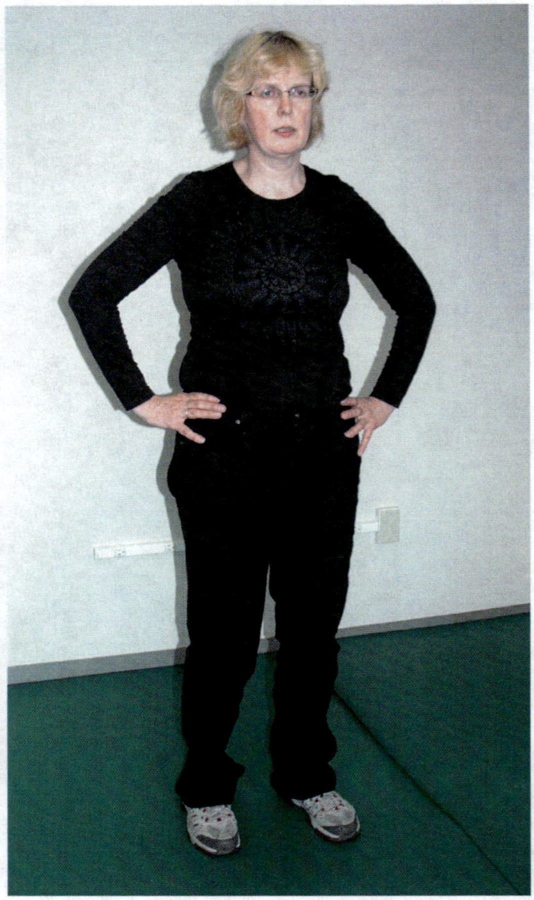

Fig. 8.61 Side stepping. Start position

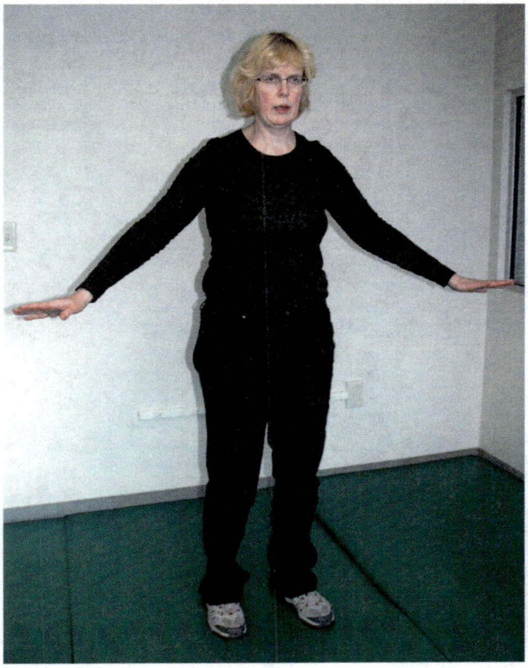

Fig. 8.62 Side stepping. Modified start position to increase balance

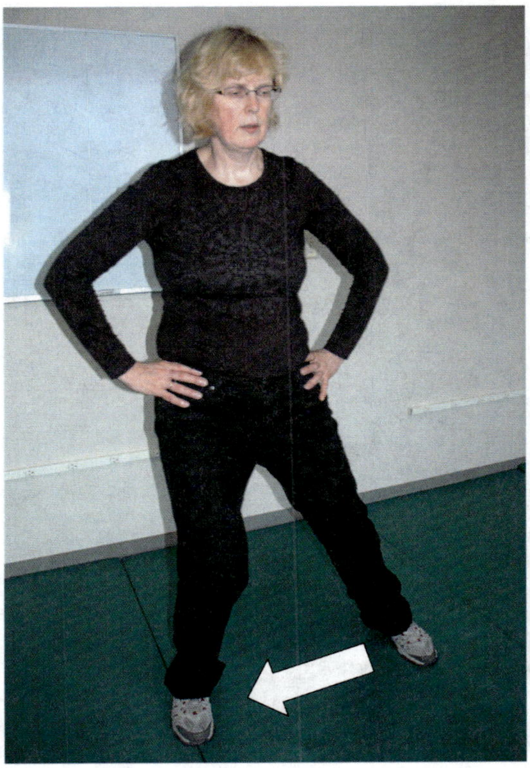

Fig. 8.63 Side stepping. Lift foot and make a small step to the side

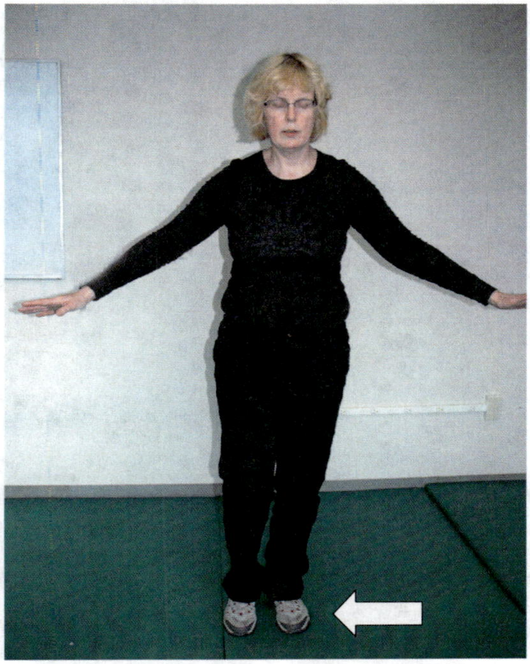

Fig. 8.64 Side stepping. Bring your other foot over to meet the foot that stepped to the side

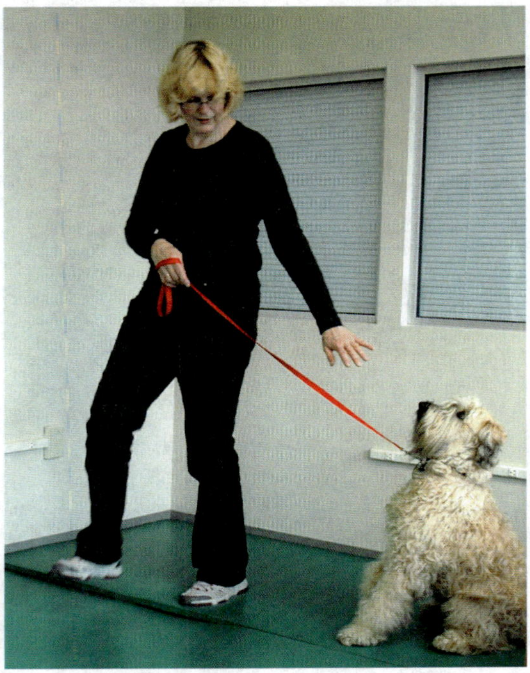

Fig. 8.65 March walk. Start position

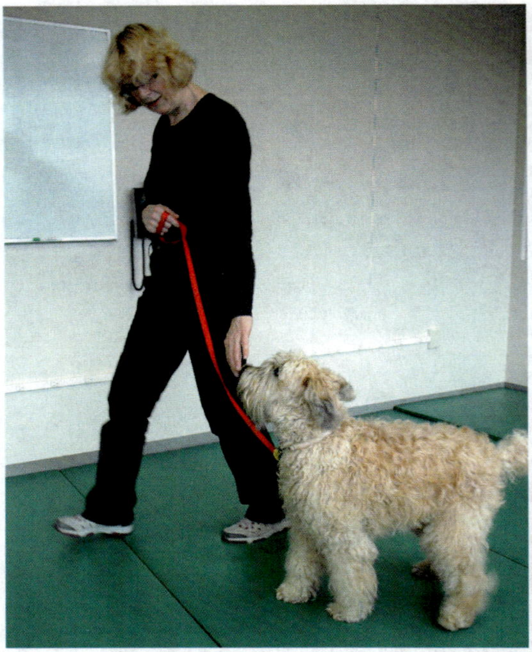

Fig. 8.66 March walk. Walk forward slowly with your dog at your side

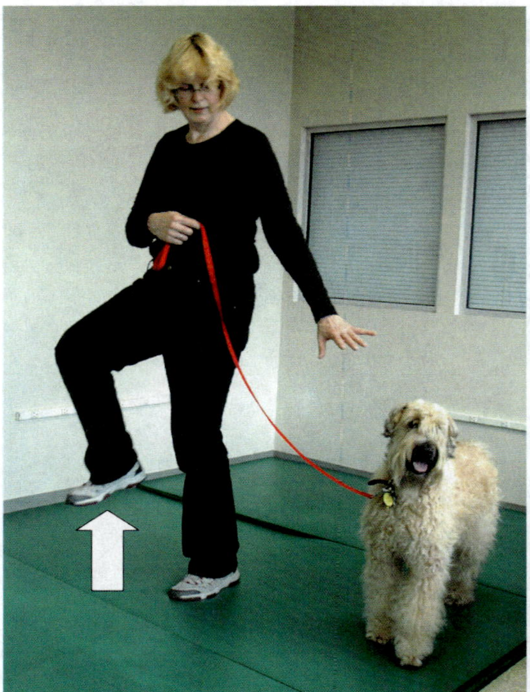

Fig. 8.67 March walk. Make high steps as you walk, as you find comfortable

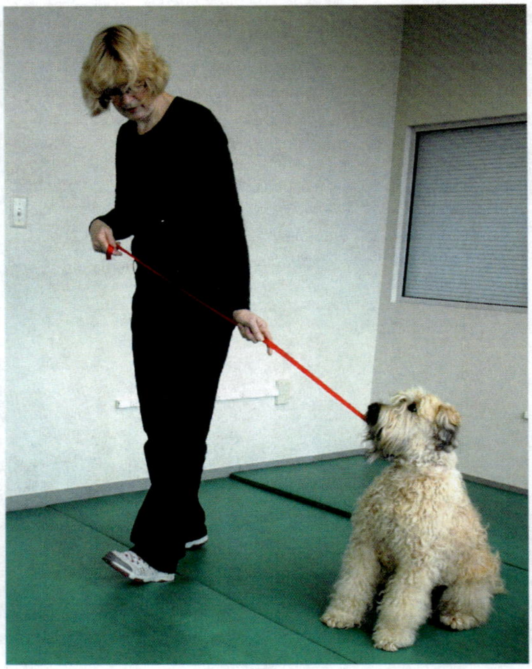

Fig. 8.68 Heel walking. With your dog walking slowly at your side, walk forward on your heels

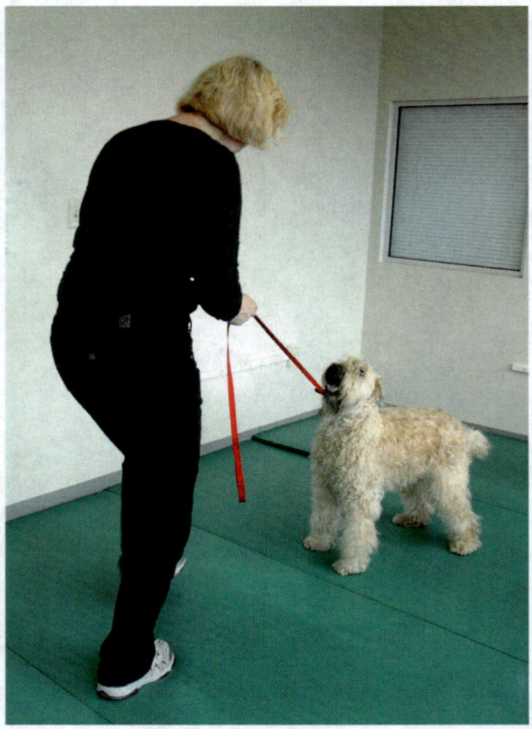

Fig. 8.69 Backward walk and recall. Start position

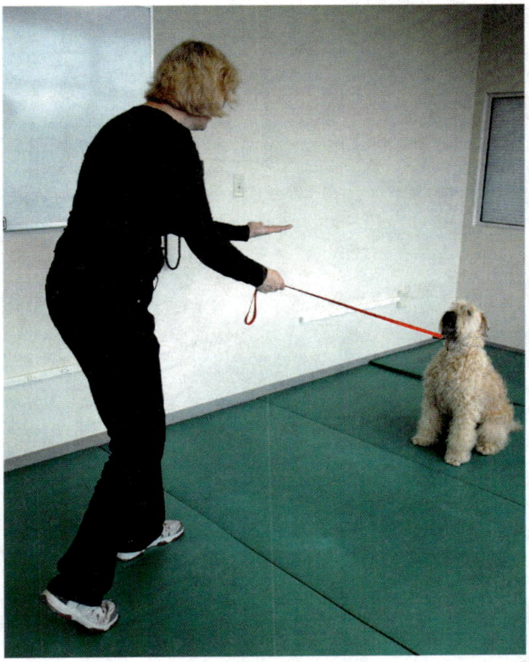

Fig. 8.70 Backward walk and recall. You may opt to ask your dog to sit as you move away from the dog

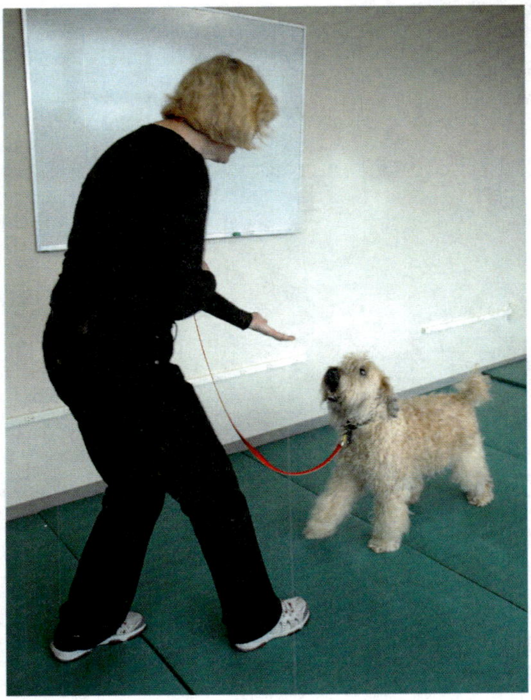

Fig. 8.71 Backward walk and recall. Call your dog to come to you

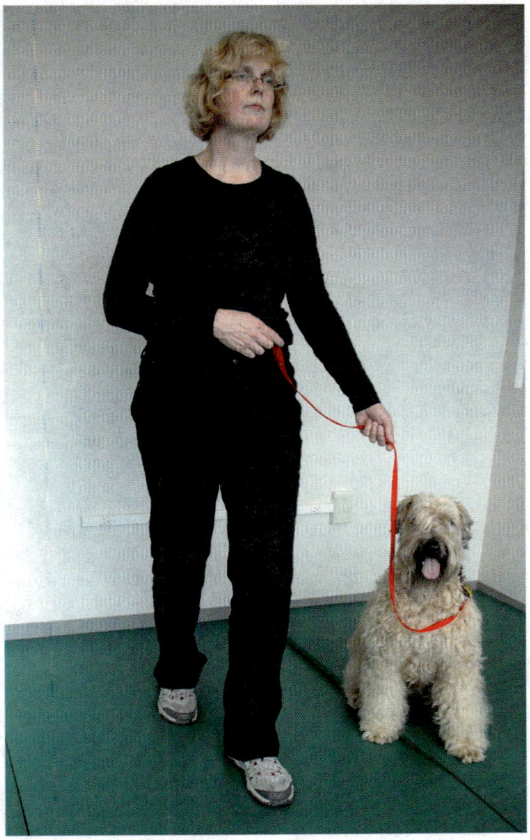

Fig. 8.72 Tandem stance. Start position

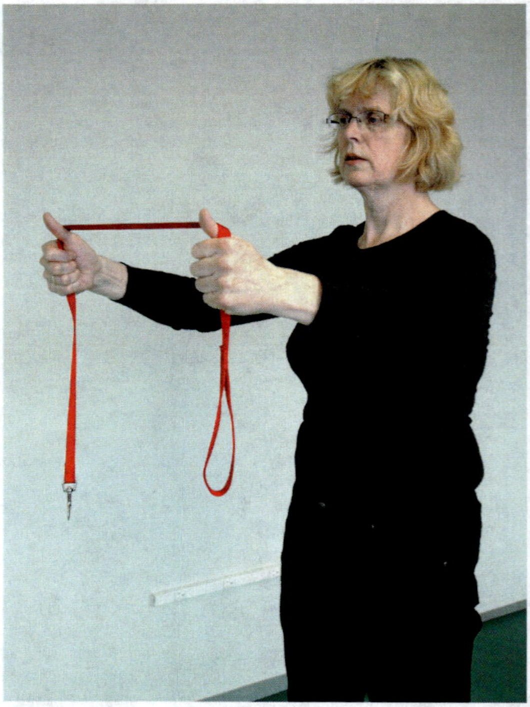

Fig. 8.73 Bear hug. Start position

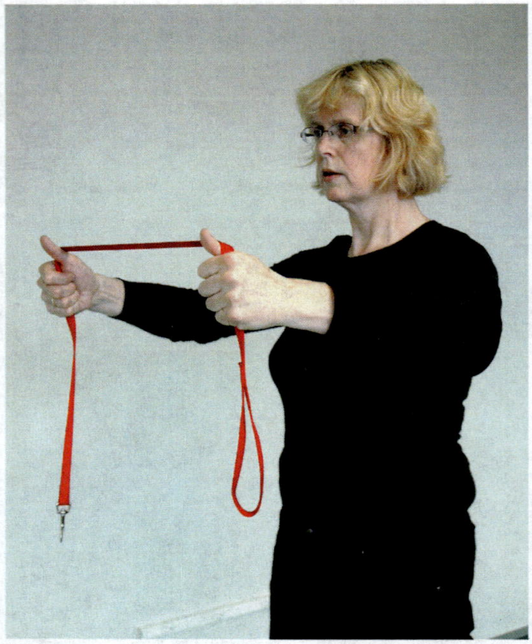

Fig. 8.74 Bear hug. Squeeze shoulder blades together while keeping your arms and leash raised in front of your chest

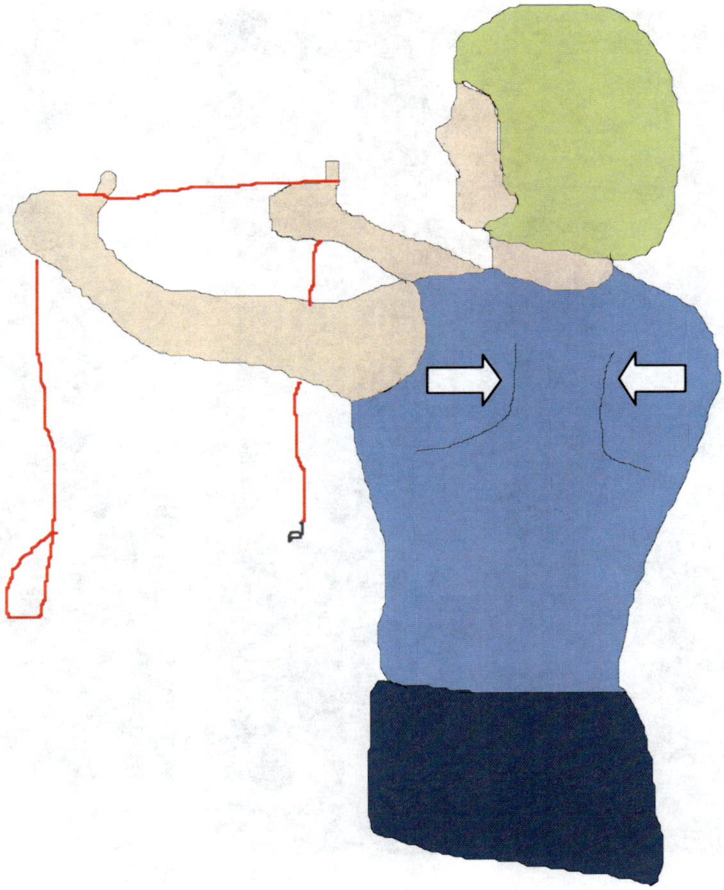

Fig. 8.75 Bear hug. As you squeeze your shoulder blades together, picture them moving together toward the middle of your back. The movement should be felt in your shoulders and upper back and you should not move your elbows backward

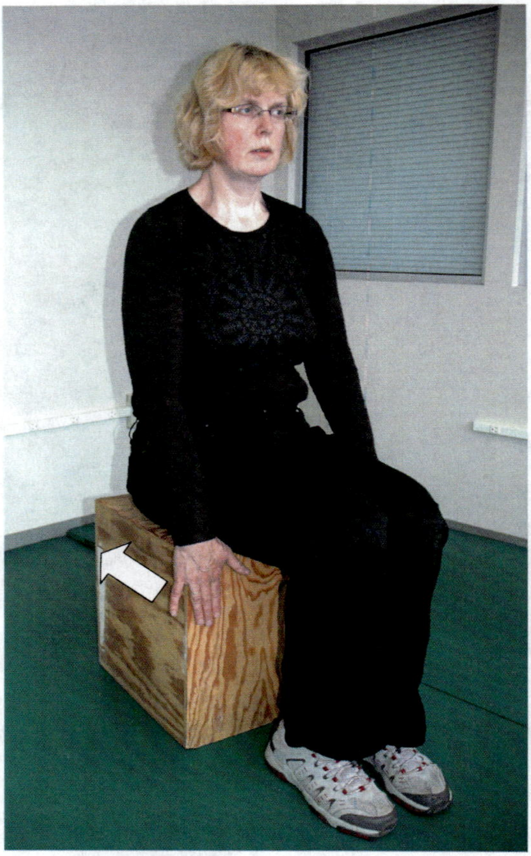

Fig. 8.76 Isometric push. Place your hands on the front of your seat and press the seat backward. Neither you nor the seat should move

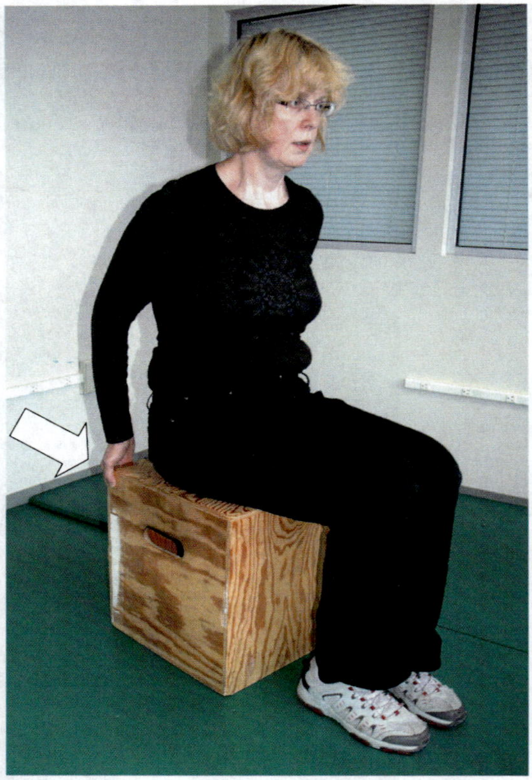

Fig. 8.77 Isometric push. Put your hands on the back of your seat and press forward against your seat. Neither you nor the seat should move

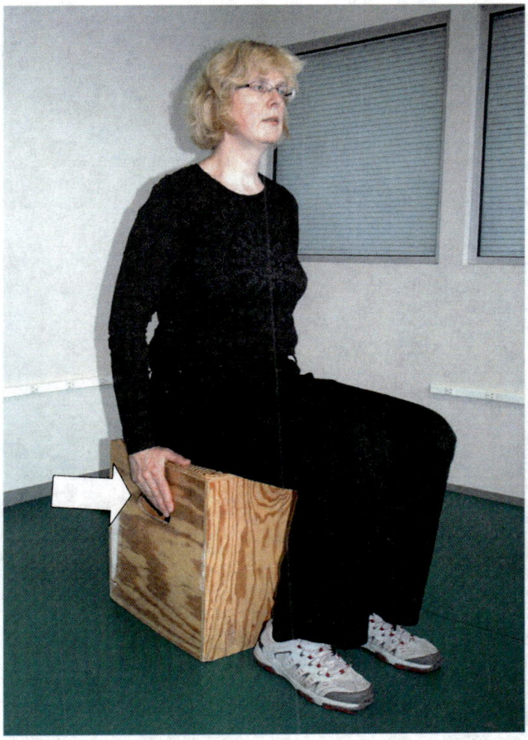

Fig. 8.78 Isometric push. Put your hands on the sides of your seat and press your hands toward each other, like you are trying to squeeze the seat. Neither you nor the seat should move

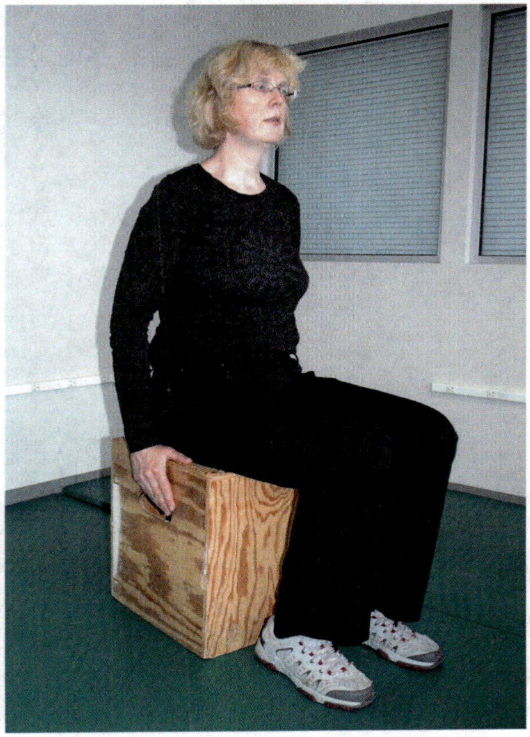

Fig. 8.79 Seated march. Start position

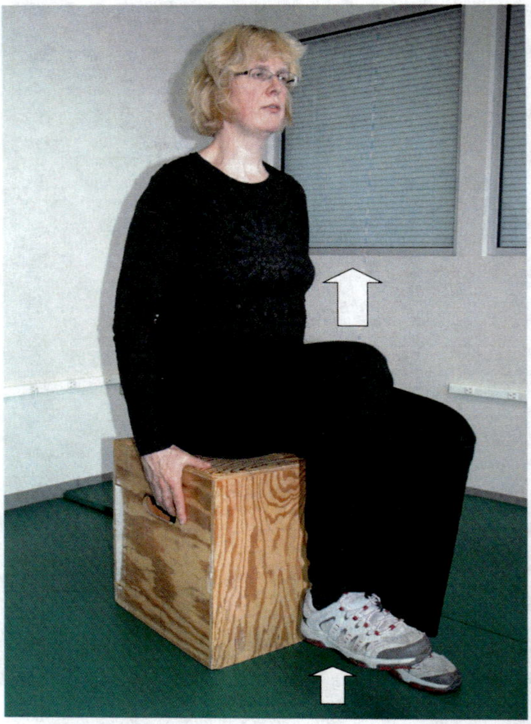

Fig. 8.80 Seated march. Lift one leg at a time off the floor

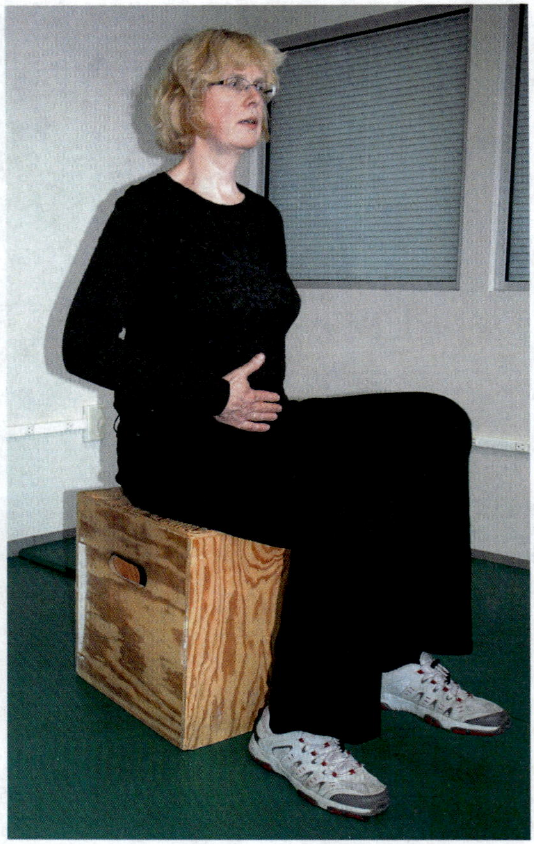

Fig. 8.81 Seated march. Press your abdomen to feel your abdominal muscles tightening as you lift each leg

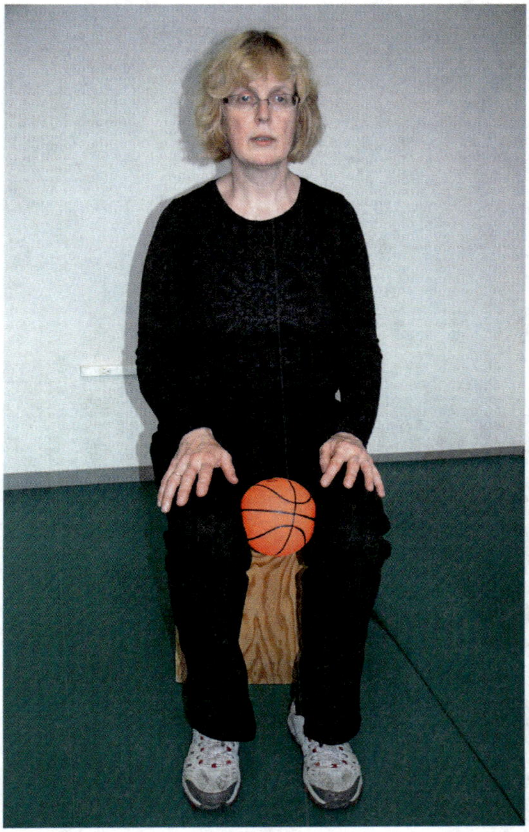

Fig. 8.82 Ball squeeze. Start position. Place a ball between your knees

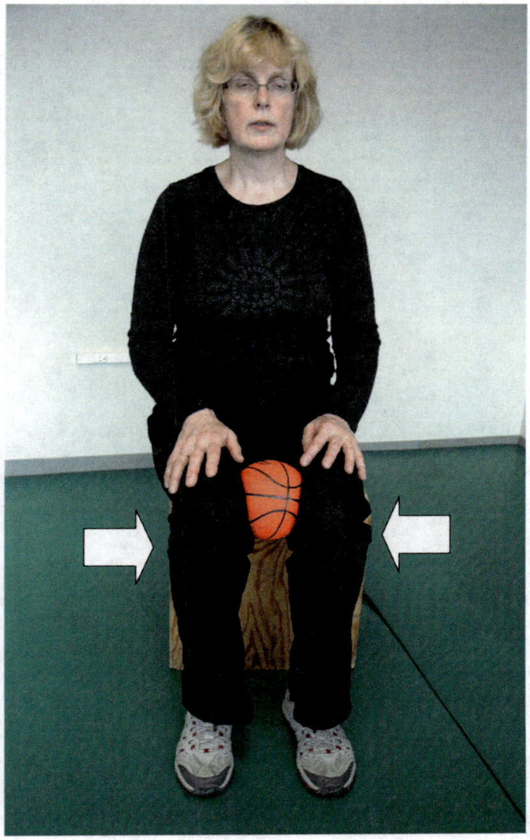

Fig. 8.83 Ball squeeze. Squeeze the ball by pressing your knees together

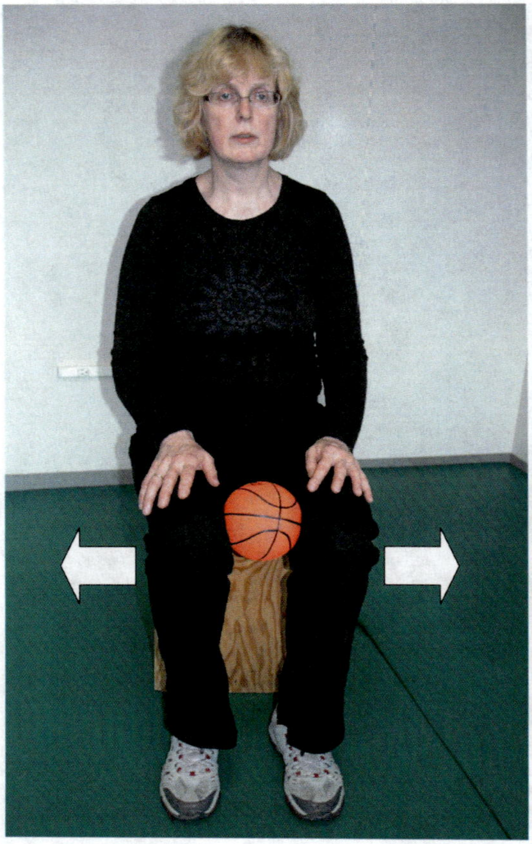

Fig. 8.84 Ball squeeze. Relax by stopping squeezing. Then repeat

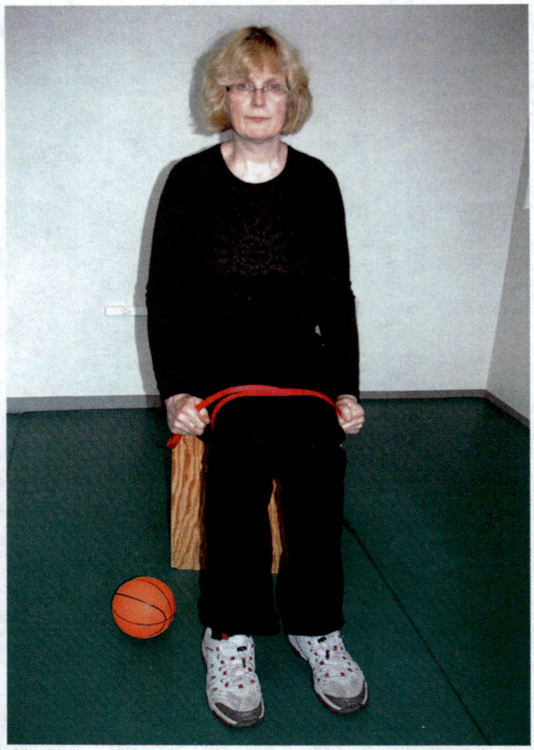

Fig. 8.85 Unleash the legs. Start position. Wrap a leash around your thighs and hold the ends

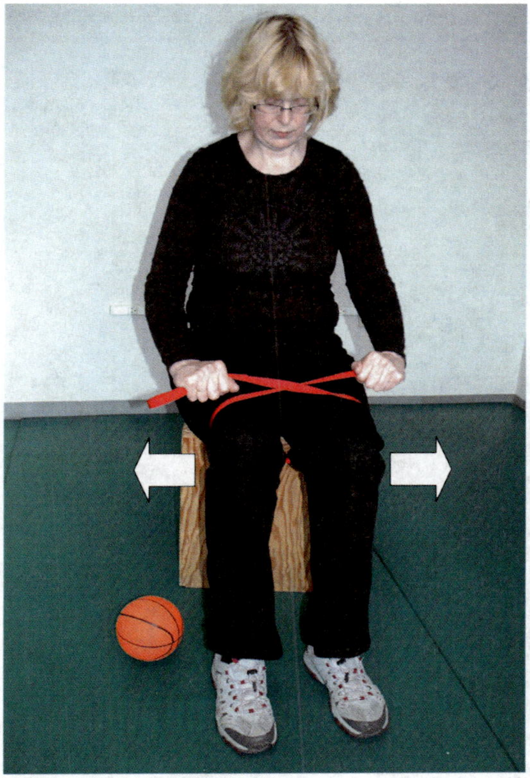

Fig. 8.86 Unleash the legs. While holding the leash firmly, push your legs apart

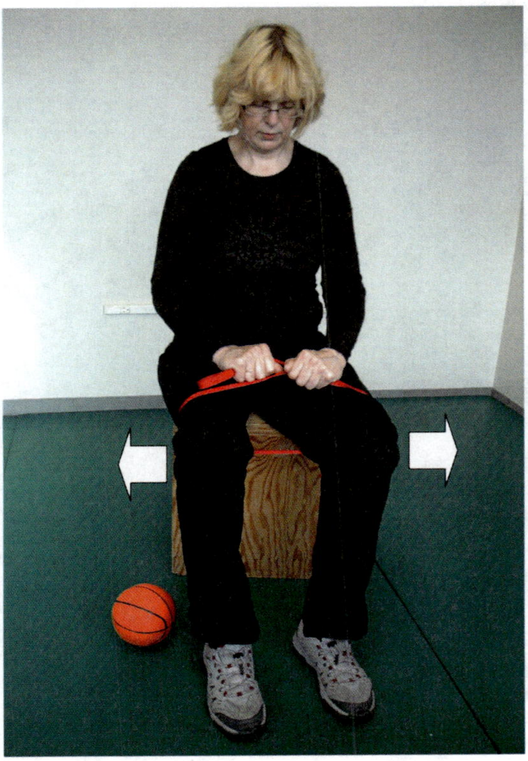

Fig. 8.87 Unleash the legs. Hold the leash tightly so your legs come apart slowly

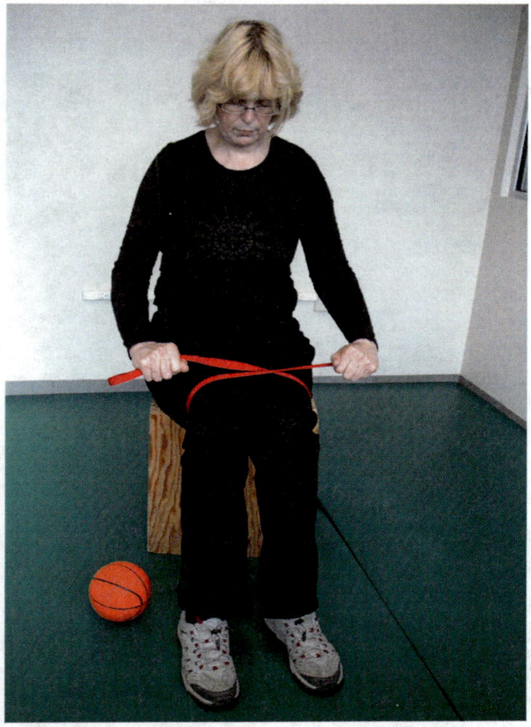

Fig. 8.88 Unleash the legs. Return to the start position

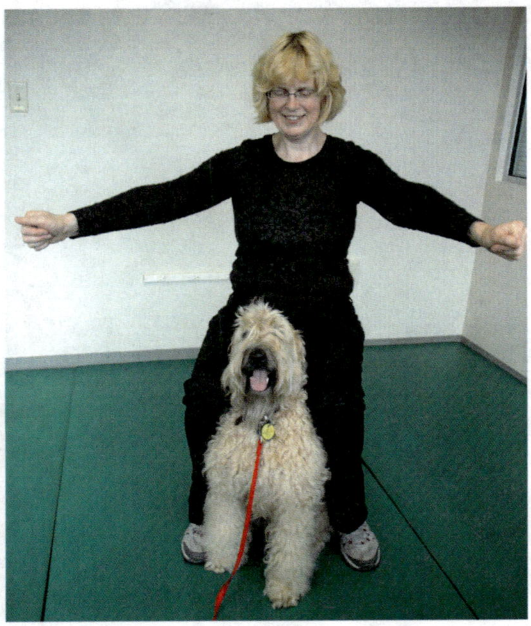

Fig. 8.89 Pet the dog. Start position. Sit down and place your dog in front of you

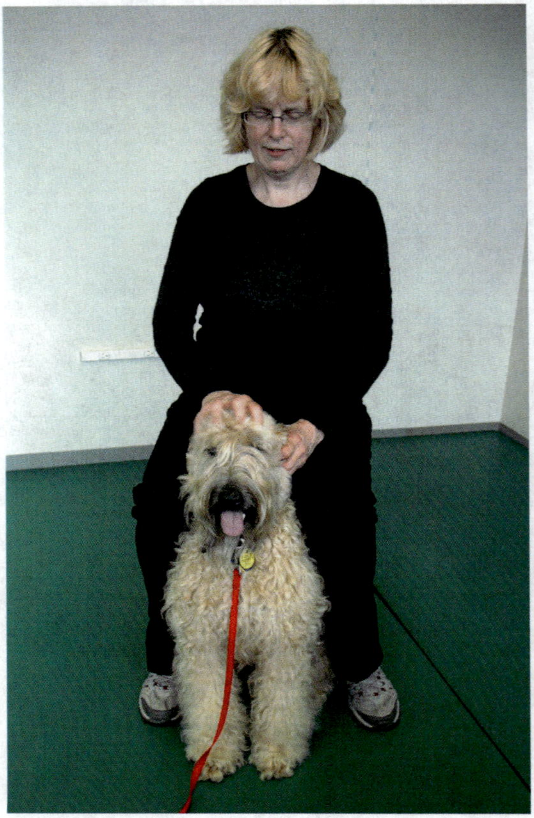

Fig. 8.90 Pet the dog. Massage your dog and stroke his fur

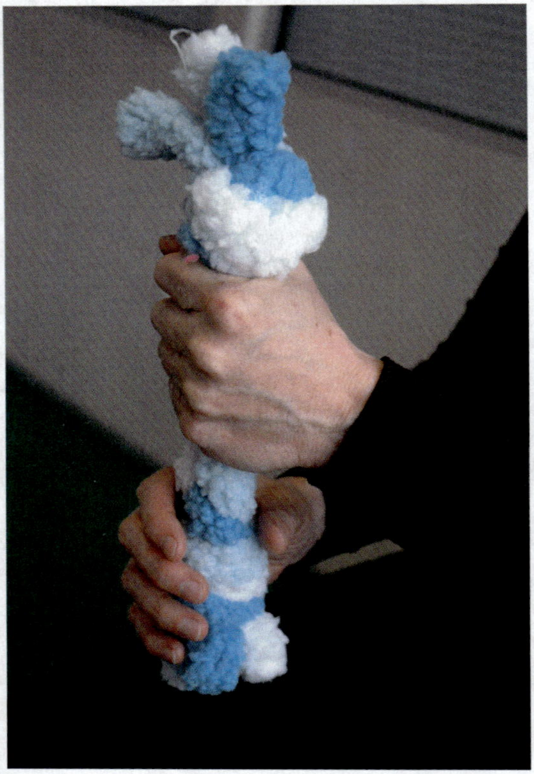

Fig. 8.91 Grip a clean dog toy. Start position

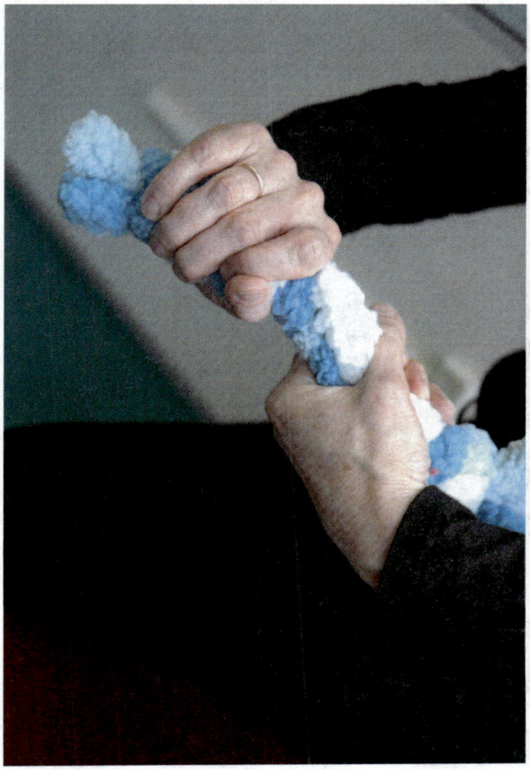

Fig. 8.92 Grip a clean dog toy. Squeeze and twist the toy

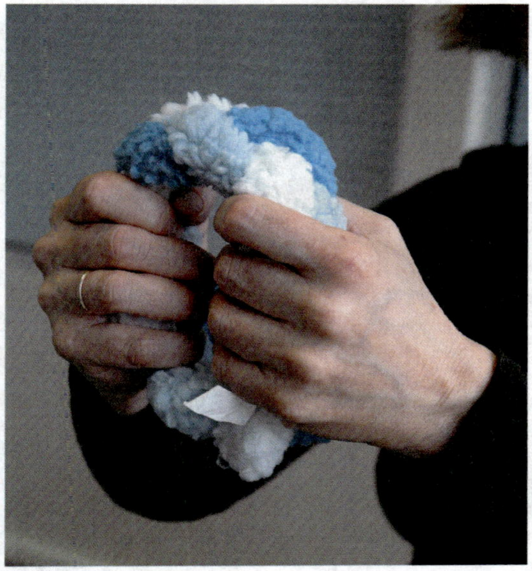

Fig. 8.93 Grip a clean dog toy. Bend the toy

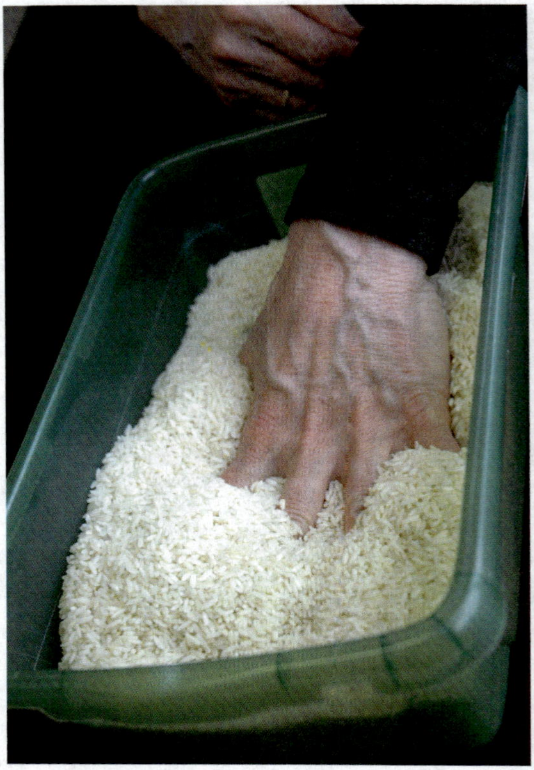

Fig. 8.94 Rice squeeze. Start position. Put your hand in a container filled with uncooked rice

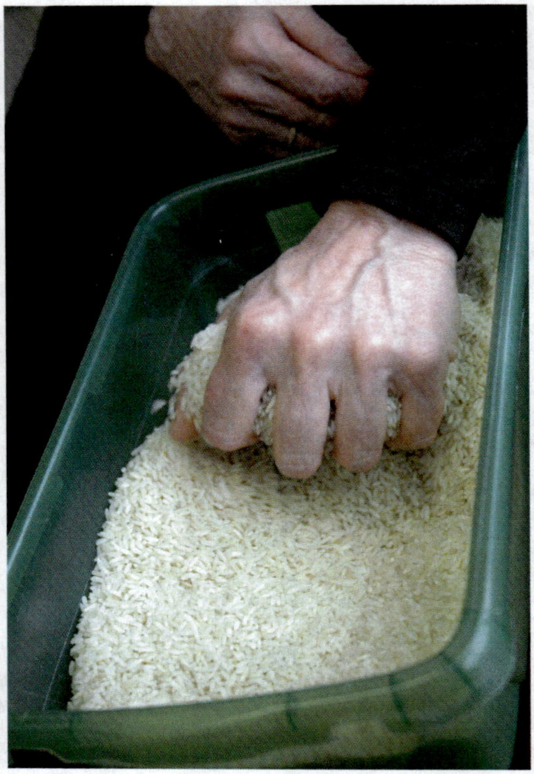

Fig. 8.95 Rice squeeze. Grab a fistful of rice

(Box 4). Walking has also been linked to health benefits for cancer patients (Chap. 7). Walking is considered to be moderate intensity when individuals can still carry on a conversation while walking but cannot sing. Patients should not feel out of breath or "winded" while walking or exercising.

Using a walking log can be a helpful motivational tool that tracks progress and ensures patients are progressing exercise at an appropriate pace. A sample exercise log is provided (Boxes 5 and 6).

Box 4 *Patient Instruction Sheet*: Tips for Starting a Walking Program

- Your walking goal should be to walk every day.
- Begin your walking program by walking on a level surface without hills.
- Walk a short distance that is comfortable for you and pay attention to your walking pattern.
- Your starting walking distance should be the distance you can walk comfortably before you feel fatigue or pain or notice that you are changing your walking pattern.
- Plan to walk every day. Initially, you will walk the distance you determined was comfortable for you.
- After 3 or 4 days, you may try making a small increase in your walking distance if you are not too sore. If you were comfortably walking 1 block as your starting walk, try adding an extra ¼ block so you will be walking 1 and ¼ blocks each day.
- Stay at your new distance for at least 3 or 4 days before increasing by another small amount. Wait until you are comfortable at the new distance before adding more. If the new distance makes you fatigued, gives you pain, or results in you changing your walking pattern, go back to the walking distance that was previously comfortable. Stay at that distance for 3–4 days before trying to increase again. This time, increase by a smaller amount.
- On treatment days or days when you are feeling more fatigued, still walk but go a shorter distance. You might also try dividing your walk into smaller segments, perhaps doing half of your usual walk in the morning and the other half in the afternoon.
- If you do miss walking days, you may have to start at a shorter distance on your next walking day. Do not try to walk extra to "catch up" for days you might have missed.

Box 5 *Patient Instruction Sheet*: Weekly Exercise Diary

- Starting distance should be a distance you can walk comfortably without increasing symptoms.
  - When you are regularly walking at this distance for three or four days, you may increase your walking distance by no more than ¼ of the previous comfortable distance. Do not make any additional increases for at least three days.
- When first starting stretching and strengthening exercises, plan to do about 5 min daily. Increase gradually by several minutes every 3–4 days.
- Try to divide your exercise throughout the day. You may break up walking and stretching/strengthening sessions into shorter segments done more than once daily.
- You will probably want to reduce exercise intensity on treatment days or days when symptoms are more problematic.
- If you are uncomfortable with your exercise more than two days in a row, reduce the intensity level (for example, decrease the distance walked and reduce the number of exercise repetitions). Find a comfortable level and stay at that level for three to four days before increasing.

(continued)

Box 5 (continued)

Day	Distance walked	Minutes spent doing stretches and/or strengthening exercises	Days with decreased exercise: Treatment day	Days with decreased exercise: High symptom day	Comfort with exercise: Comfortable	Comfort with exercise: Uncomfortable
Sun						
Mon						
Tues						
Wed						
Thurs						
Fri						
Sat						

Box 6 Sample of a Completed Diary

- At the end of week 1, the patient appropriately reduced exercise on a chemotherapy day; however, she then tried to "make up" for decreased exercise by advancing her program too quickly on the days following chemotherapy.
- She appropriately reduced her walking to a previously comfortable level during week 2 and was better able to tolerate and benefit from her exercise program.

Week 1

Day	Distance walked	Minutes spent doing stretches and/or strengthening exercises	Days with decreased exercise: Treatment day	Days with decreased exercise: High symptom day	Comfort with exercise: Comfortable	Comfort with exercise: Uncomfortable
Sun	1 Block	5 min			X	
Mon	1 Block	5 min			X	
Tues	1 Block	5 min			X	
Wed	1¼ Blocks	5 min			X	
Thurs	1¼ Blocks	7 min			X	
Fri	½ Block	4 min	Chemo	Fatigue	X	
Sat	1¼ Block	7 min		Fatigue		X

Week 2

Day	Distance walked	Minutes spent doing stretches and/or strengthening exercises	Days with decreased exercise: Treatment day	Days with decreased exercise: High symptom day	Comfort with exercise: Comfortable	Comfort with exercise: Uncomfortable
Sun	2 Blocks	7 min		Fatigue		X
Mon	2 Blocks	7 min		Fatigue and pain		X
Tues	1¼ Blocks	7 min			X	
Wed	1¼ Blocks	7 min			X	
Thurs	½ Blocks	7 min	Chemo	Fatigue	X	
Fri	1 Block	7 min		Fatigue	X	
Sat	1 Block	9 min			X	

Summary

- Stretching and strengthening exercises incorporating a dog theme can make exercising more enjoyable and improve exercise compliance.
- Patients with metastatic disease or treatments likely to result in osteoporosis (e.g., hormonal therapies for breast cancer) will generally need to reduce exercise intensity and avoid high-impact exercise (e.g., running or jumping).
- Daily exercise should incorporate some stretching and strengthening exercises.
- Walking can be an ideal exercise for cancer patients because it is an effective aerobic exercise, works large muscle groups, is convenient for most patients, and can be adjusted to suit individual abilities.

References

1. Pekmezi DW, Demark-Wahnefried W. Updated evidence in support of diet and exercise interventions in cancer survivors. Acta Oncol. 2011;50:167–78.
2. Doyle C, Kushi LH, Byers T, et al. Nutrition and physical activity during and after cancer treatment: an American Cancer Society guide for informed choices. CA Cancer J Clin. 2006;56:323–53.
3. Schmitz KH, Courneya KS, Matthews C, et al. American College of Sports Medicine roundtable on exercise guidelines for cancer survivors. Med Sci Sports Exerc. 2010;42:1409–26.
4. Lentino C, Visek AJ, McDonnell K, Dipietro L. Dog walking is associated with a favorable risk profile independent of moderate to high volume of physical activity. J Phys Act Health. 2012;9:414–20.
5. Nies MA, Motyka CL. Factors contributing to women's ability to maintain a walking program. J Holistic Nursing. 2006;24:7–14.
6. Temple V, Rhodes R, Wharf Higgins J. Unleashing physical activity: an observational study of park use, dog walking, and physical activity. J Phys Act Health. 2011;8:766–74.
7. Peel E, Douglas M, Parry O, Lawton J. Type 2 diabetes and dog walking: patients' longitudinal perspectives about implementing and sustaining physical activity. Br J Gen Pract. 2010;60:570–7.
8. Foundation for Cancer Research & Wellness. The exercise prescription. http://www.cancerrecovery.org/site/News2?page=NewsArticle&id=7227&news_iv_ctrl=0. Accessed May 2011.
9. Rajarajeswaran P, Vishnupriya R. Exercise in cancer. Indian J Med Paediatr Oncol. 2009;30:61–70.
10. Marcus DA. Fit As Fido: Follow Your Dog to Better Health. Bloomington, IN: iUniverse; 2008.
11. Shamley D, Srinaganathan R, Oskrochi R, Lascurain-Aquirrebeña I, Sugden E. Three-dimensional scapulothoracic motion following treatment for breast cancer. Breast Cancer Res Treat. 2009;118:315–22.

9 Incorporating Companion Dogs into Cancer Rehab: Practical Tips for Adding a Dog into the Home During Cancer Treatment and Recovery

Key Chapter Points

- The responsibility of caring for a companion dog owned by a cancer patient often must be shared by other family members during treatment.
- Adult, medium–large, easy-to-train breeds are often better choices for individuals with health problems.
- Cancer patients who are not able to have a companion dog may benefit from scheduled therapy dog visits.

Keywords
Breed • Fall risk • Puppy • Selection

Mayo Clinic oncologist Edward Creagan, MD, said, "I prescribe pets to a third of my cancer patients to help them cope with the rigors of their terrible disease" [1]. While adding a dog to a household can be very beneficial for many patients, this addition should only occur after careful consideration of the needs of the cancer patient and other members in the household to ensure that the needs of both humans and the dog can be consistently met. In addition, contingency plans for dog care need to be available when the demands for the ill patient may increase.

Considerations Before Adding a Companion Dog

Adding a dog to the family requires substantial ongoing work to ensure the dog will be properly trained and cared for. In some cases where a household member has an ongoing medical condition, the addition of a dog can add undue burden to an already overtaxed caregiver for the patient. Interest and availability of individuals to train and provide ongoing dog care, an appropriate environment, and available financial resources need to be considered in advance of bringing a companion dog into a home (Table 9.1). A dog should not be added to a home unless those adults who will likely need to care for the dog are enthusiastic and motivated about adding this responsibility.

A survey of cancer patients with pets undergoing chemotherapy highlighted that, while dog ownership may be beneficial for cancer patients, the responsibility of caring for a dog during illness often needs to be shared [2]. In this survey, 4 in 5 participants had received help caring for their pet from family members since receiving their diagnosis (Fig. 9.1). Two patients noted they did not acquire another pet because of their cancer, and one reported surrendering a pet. In addition, a

D.A. Marcus, *Therapy Dogs in Cancer Care: A Valuable Complementary Treatment*,
DOI 10.1007/978-1-4614-3378-1_9, © Springer Science+Business Media New York 2012

Table 9.1 Requirements for adding a companion dog to a home with someone with a medical illness

Dog needs	Required for adding a companion dog	Companion dog should probably not be added
Adult caregiver for dog	Person primarily responsible for dog care must be interested in adding a dog to the home If the person who will be primarily responsible for the dog is a patient with active health problems, a second interested adult should be present who can assume dog care when necessary (e.g., increased symptoms and treatment days) Person responsible for the dog should be motivated for basic dog training and daily dog exercise	Primary patient caregiver is already overburdened
Environment	Fenced yard, tie out, or runner available	Dog's caregiver is unable to commit to daily walks, maintain yard free of dog excrement, or clean unwanted accidents in the home
Other household members	No unstable psychiatric illness in any household member	Any household member is violent, abusive, or has anger control issues Individual who would be the primary caregiver for the dog has dementia
Finances	Surplus funds are available to cover costs for dog food, grooming, boarding, veterinary care, and other typical dog expenses	Insufficient funds

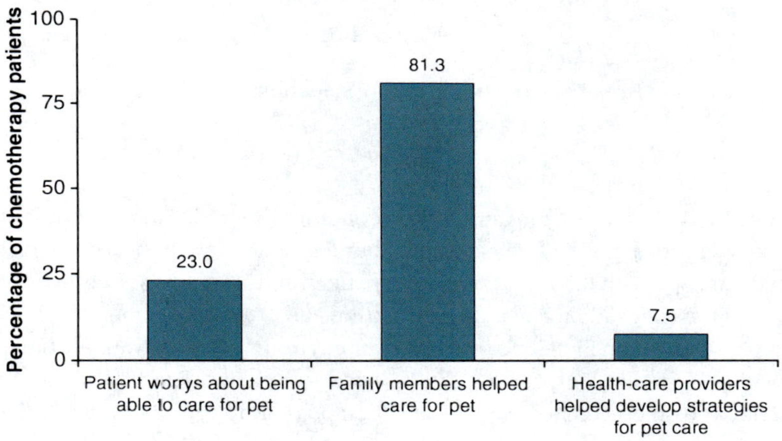

Fig. 9.1 Companion pet issues for patients undergoing chemotherapy (Based on [2])

minority of chemotherapy patients worked with their health-care provider to identify strategies for dog care.

Choosing an Appropriate Dog

Characteristics to be considered when selecting a dog include age, size, and breed characteristics (Table 9.2). Resources to identify appropriate breeds include dog breeders, individuals who show particular breeds, and breed-specific rescue workers. These individuals can be valuable resources for information on typical breed attributes and the difficulties associated with certain breeds.

Smaller or more active dogs may be more inclined to get underfoot and precipitate falls. A survey of emergency departments evaluated falls caused by pets [3]. Falls occurred from

Table 9.2 Characteristics to consider when adding a companion dog to a home with medical illness

Dog feature	Desirable characteristics	Undesirable traits
Age	Older dogs often have established personalities and behavior patterns, are less active and require less training, and are less likely to inadvertently bump, push, pull, or jump on a person who might become injured	Puppies require substantially more care and training than older dogs. In addition, dog personality will be more apparent in an older dog who will be easier to assess for appropriateness as an addition to a particular home
Size	Medium to larger dogs often move more slowly and are less likely to cause falls	Small dogs can easily get underfoot and cause unexpected falls, especially in older individuals or those with balance problems
Breed	Breeds that are less active and easier to train are often more desirable when a household has a member with an ongoing health problem	Highly protective, territorial, high-energy, and stubborn breeds can be difficult and time-consuming to train and manage. These dogs require a greater time commitment that can be overburdensome in a household where someone has an active medical condition

Box 1 Breed options for family with someone with a medical illness

More desirable breeds are easy going, obedient, and lower activity dogs	High-energy, territorial, protective, and stubborn breeds are not ideal choices
• Bichon Frise	• Akita
• Cavalier King Charles Spaniel	• Border Collie
• Cocker Spaniel	• Chihuahua
• Adult English Setter	• Chow Chow
• Golden Retriever	• German Shepherd
• Greyhound (when fenced yard is available)	• Husky
• Irish Wolfhound	• Terrier breeds
• Adult Labrador Retriever	
• Pomeranian	
• Pug	

chasing pets, falling or tripping over pets, or being pulled or pushed by pets. These data support attending to obedience training to minimize dog behaviors linked with increased fall risk.

Taking Advantage of Dog-Related Benefits When Adding a Companion Dog Is Not Appropriate

Dog-related health benefits can be provided by therapy dogs to individuals when the full-time responsibility of dog ownership is too much of a burden for a patient or the patient's family members. Therapy dog visits can often be arranged through therapy dog organizations (see Chap. 10), local hospital volunteer offices, or hospice facilities. Individuals might also contact local dog shelters and dog clubs that train dogs for therapy dog work to see how patients might receive visits from certified therapy dogs. The advantage of visits from a therapy dog is that the dog is trained and experienced in providing comforting attention to individuals with illnesses and the needs of the dog are addressed by the therapy dog's handler.

Expectations for Therapeutic Benefits

Therapy dogs have been trained to be calm and provide comfort and cheer, with patients often finding a therapeutic impact with the initial visit with a therapy dog. Benefits may be somewhat delayed with a companion dog that will require some period of adjustment into a new home, during which time it will likely be less attentive to the humans within the home. While spending time with a dog is therapeutic, there will be an adjustment period for a new dog added to a home. Puppies tend to be self-absorbed and may be less interested in providing cuddle time than exploring their environment, eating, and sleeping. Older dogs often require a period of adjustment when added to a new home, as they discover and become comfortable both with the environment and the individuals within their new home. (Chapter 10 lists resources that offer proven advice from expert dog trainers on successfully adding either a puppy or older dog into a home, as well as training guides. These should be read in advance of adding a dog to the home.)

It is also important to recognize that dogs have their own needs and will need time to be alone, time to play, and time to rest. A dog should not be expected to be continuously available for a human's needs. Individuals who require more consistent interaction from a dog may be more appropriate candidates for service dogs (Chap. 2).

Summary

- Adding a companion dog to a home requires careful consideration of the needs of both the individuals within the home and the new dog.
- Selecting a potential companion dog requires researching breed characteristics, determining household members' ability to care for a puppy versus an older dog who may already be housebroken and less energetic, and carefully evaluating personality characteristics of an individual dog.
- In most cases, family members will be required to provide at least some dog care for a cancer patient with a companion pet during the course of cancer treatment.
- Cancer patients unable to have a companion pet may benefit from scheduled therapy dog visits.

References

1. Creagan E. A scientific look at the human-animal bond. PAWSitive Interaction 2002 White Paper. Available at www.pawsitiveinteraction.com/pdf/a_scientific_look.pdf. Accessed September 2011.
2. Larson BR, Looker S, Herrera DM, et al. Cancer patients and their companion animals: results from a 309-patient survey on pet-related concerns and anxieties during chemotherapy. J Canc Educ. 2010;25:396–400.
3. Stevens JA, Teh SL, Haileyesus T. Dogs and cats as environmental fall hazards. J Safety Res. 2010;41:69–73.

Resources 10

Internet Resources

Therapy Dog Organizations

- United States and international therapy dog certification programs:
  - Delta Society
    - http://www.deltasociety.org
  - Therapy Dogs, Inc.
    - http://www.therapydogs.com
  - Therapy Dogs International
    - http://www.tdi-dog.org
- Regional therapy dog organizations:
  - Angel Paws in central Ohio
    - http://www.angelpawstherapy.org
  - Animal Friends in western Pennsylvania
    - http://www.thinkingoutsidethecage.org
  - Gabriel's Angels in southern Arizona
    - http://www.gabrielsangels.org/
  - Pacific Animal Therapy Society in British Columbia, Canada
    - http://patspets.ca/wordpress/
  - St. John Ambulance across Canada
    - http://www.sja.ca

American Kennel Club Therapy Dog Certification

- American Kennel Club's Canine Good Citizen Program
  - http://www.akc.org/events/cgc/
- Information on the American Kennel Club's therapy dog title award
  - http://www.akc.org/akctherapydog/about.cfm

Service Dog Organizations

- Assistance Dogs International
  - http://www.assistancedogsinternational.org/
- Canine Companions for Independence
  - http://www.cci.org
- Canine Support Teams in southern California
  - http://www.caninesupportteams.org/
- Guide Dogs of America
  - http://www.guidedogsofamerica.org/1/
- Medical Detection Dogs
  - http://medicaldetectiondogs.org.uk/
- The Seeing Eye (the oldest guide dog school)
  - http://www.seeingeye.org
- Shore Service Dogs in Maryland
  - http://www.shoreservicedogs.com

Exercise Instructions for Cancer Patients

- The Cancer Council of Western Australia has produced a comprehensive and detailed exercise instruction manual, "Guidelines for Implementing Exercise Programs for Cancer Patients." Available at http://www.cancerwa.asn.au/patients/staying-well/#exercise. Accessed December 2011.

D.A. Marcus, *Therapy Dogs in Cancer Care: A Valuable Complementary Treatment*,
DOI 10.1007/978-1-4614-3378-1_10, © Springer Science+Business Media New York 2012

- Schmitz KH, Courneya KS, Matthews C, et al. American college of sports medicine roundtable on exercise guidelines for cancer survivors. Med Sci Sports Exerc 2010;42: 1409–26.
- van Weert E, Hoekstra-Weebers JE, May AM, et al. The development of an evidence-based physical self-management rehabilitation programme for cancer survivors. Patient Educ Couns 2008;71:169–90.

Books

Complementary Medicine During Cancer Care

- Markman M, Cohen L. Integrative oncology: incorporating complementary medicine into conventional cancer care (current clinical oncology). Totowa: Humana Press; 2010.
- American Cancer Society. American cancer society complete guide to complementary & alternative cancer therapies. Atlanta: American Cancer Society; 2009.
- Block K. Life over cancer: the block center program for integrative cancer treatment, New York: Bantam Books; 2009.
- Servan-Schreiber D. Anticancer. A New Way of Life, new edition. New York: Viking Penguin; 2009.

Therapy Dog Books

- Marcus DA. The power of wagging tails: a doctor's guide to dog therapy and healing. New York: Demos Health Publishing; 2011.
- Altschiller D. Animal-assisted therapy. Westport: Greenwood; 2011.
- Hammond C. On Toby's terms. Gardena: Bettie Youngs Books Publishing; 2010.
- Joseph M. Moments with Baxter: comfort and love from the world's best therapy dog. San Diego: Sage Press; 2009.
- Pichot T. Transformation of the heart: tales of the profound impact therapy dogs have on their humans. Bloomington: iUniverse; 2009.
- Butler K. Therapy dogs today: their gifts, our obligation. Norman: Funpuddle; 2004.

Therapy Dog Training Books

- American Kennel Club. Citizen Canine. Irvine: Kennel Club Books; 2010.
- Fine A. Handbook on animal-assisted therapy, 3rd ed. San Diego: Academic; 2010.
- Lind N. Animal assisted therapy activities to motivate and inspire. Lombard: PYOW sports marketing; 2009.
- Davis KD. Therapy dogs. Training your dog to reach others. 2nd ed. Wenatchee: Dogwise Publishing; 2002.

Therapy Dog Books for Children

- Hammond C. Toby, the pet therapy dog, and his hospital friends. Gardena: Bettie Youngs Books Publishing; 2011.
- Raus H. Ben: the very best furry friend. Saxonburg: Pylon Publishing; 2011.
- Fedorovich D. The adventures of Sheila the therapy dog. Parker: Outskirts Press; 2007.
- London S. Rocky's trip to the hospital. Burlington: Kristar Publishing; 2003.
- Calmenson S. Rosie: a visiting dog's story. New York: Clarion Books; 1994.

Healing Power of Companion Pets

- Miller J. Healing companions: ordinary dogs and their extraordinary power to transform lives. Franklin Lakes: Career Press; 2010.
- Sakson S. Paws & effect: the healing power of dogs. New York: Spiegel & Grau; 2007.
- Becker M. The healing power of pets: harnessing the amazing ability of pets to make and keep people happy and healthy. New York: Hyperion; 2002.

Books for Adding a Companion Dog into the Home

- Benjamin CL. Mother knows best: the natural way to train your dog. New York: Hungry Minds; 1985.
- McConnell P, Scidmore B. The puppy primer. 2nd ed. Black Earth: McConnell Publishing; 2010.

- McConnell P. Love has no age limit: welcoming an adopted dog into your home. Black Earth: McConnell Publishing; 2011.
- Miller P. Do over dogs. Give your dog a second chance for a first class life. Wenatchee: Dogwise Publishing; 2010.

Exercising With Your Dog

- Marcus DA. The power of wagging tails: a doctor's guide to dog therapy and healing. New York: Demos Health Publishing; 2011.
- Cole-MacMurray K, Nishimoto S. See spot run: 100 ways to work out with your dog. Beverly: Quarry Books; 2010.
- Marcus DA. Fit as fido: follow your dog to better health, Bloomington: iUniverse; 2008.
- Becker M, Kushner R. Fitness unleashed! a dog and owner's guide to losing weight and gaining health together. New York: Three Rivers Press; 2006.

Index

D.A. Marcus, *Therapy Dogs in Cancer Care: A Valuable Complementary Treatment*,
DOI 10.1007/978-1-4614-3378-1, © Springer Science+Business Media New York 2012

Received
JAN -3 13
Mission College Library

Printed by Publishers' Graphics LLC
SO20120824